Advances in MDCT

Guest Editors

DUSHYANT V. SAHANI, MD
VAHID YAGHMAI, MD

RADIOLOGIC CLINICS OF NORTH AMERICA

www.radiologic.theclinics.com

January 2009 • Volume 47 • Number 1

SAUNDERS an imprint of ELSEVIER, Inc.

W.B. SAUNDERS COMPANY
A Division of Elsevier Inc.

1600 John F. Kennedy Boulevard • Suite 1800 • Philadelphia, Pennsylvania 19103-2899

http://www.theclinics.com

RADIOLOGIC CLINICS OF NORTH AMERICA Volume 47, Number 1
January 2009 ISSN 0033-8389, ISBN 13: 978-1-4160-6349-0, ISBN 10: 1-4160-6349-8

Editor: Barton Dudlick
Developmental Editor: Theresa Collier

Radiologic Clinics of North America (ISSN 0033-8389) is published bimonthly in January, March, May, July, September, and November by Elsevier Inc., 360 Park Avenue South, New York, NY 10010-1710. Business and Editorial Offices: 1600 John F. Kennedy Boulevard., Suite 1800, Philadelphia, PA 19103-2899. Customer Service Office: 11830 Westline Industrial Drive, St. Louis, MO 63146. Periodicals postage paid at New York, NY and additional mailing offices. Subscription prices are USD 328 per year for US individuals, USD 487 per year for US institutions, USD 160 per year for US students and residents, USD 383 per year for Canadian individuals, USD 611 per year for Canadian institutions, USD 473 per year for international individuals, USD 611 per year for international institutions, and USD 230 per year for Canadian and foreign students/residents. To receive student and resident rate, orders must be accompanied by name of affiliated institution, date of term and the signature of program/residency coordinatior on institution letterhead. Orders will be billed at individual rate until proof of status is received. Foreign air speed delivery is included in all *Clinics* subscription prices. All prices are subject to change without notice. **POSTMASTER:** Send address changes to *Radiologic Clinics of North America*, Elsevier Journals Customer Service, 11830 Westline Industrial Drive, St. Louis, MO 63146. **Customer Service: 1-800-654-2452 (US and Canada). From outside of the United States and Canada, call 1-314-453-7041. Fax: 1-314-453-5170. E-mail: JournalsCustomerService-usa@elsevier.com (for print support) and JournalsOnlineSupport-usa@elsevier. com (for online support).**

Reprints. For copies of 100 or more of articles in this publication, please contact the Commercial Reprints Department, Elsevier Inc., 360 Park Avenue South, New York, New York 10010-1710. Tel.: (+1) 212-633-3812; Fax: (+1) 212-462-1935; E-mail: reprints@elsevier.com.

Radiologic Clinics of North America also published in Greek Paschalidis Medical Publications, Athens, Greece.

Radiologic Clinics of North America is covered in *MEDLINE/PubMed (Index Medicus), EMBASE/Excerpta Medica, Current Contents/Life Sciences, Current Contents/Clinical Medicine, RSNA Index to Imaging Literature, BIOSIS, Science Citation Index,* and *ISI/BIOMED.*

Printed in the United States of America.

Contributors

GUEST EDITORS

DUSHYANT V. SAHANI, MD
Associate Professor of Radiology, Harvard
Medical School; and Director of Computed
Tomography, Department of Radiology,
Massachusetts General Hospital, Boston,
Massachusetts

VAHID YAGHMAI, MD
Associate Professor and Medical Director
of CT, Department of Radiology, Northwestern
University-Feinberg School of Medicine, Chicago,
Illinois

AUTHORS

GORKA BASTARRIKA, MD, PhD
Department of Radiology and Radiological
Science, Medical University of South Carolina,
Charleston, South Carolina; and Department
of Radiology, Clinica Universitaria, Universidad
de Navarra, Pamplona, Spain

NATALIE BRAUN, BS
Research Assistant, Department of Radiology,
Mayo Clinic, Rochester, Minnesota

JODIE CHRISTNER, PhD
Research Fellow, Department of Radiology,
Mayo Clinic, Rochester, Minnesota

DOMINIK FLEISCHMANN, MD
Associate Professor; and Director, Computed
Tomography, Department of Radiology Stanford
University Medical Center Stanford, California

JOEL G. FLETCHER, MD
Department of Radiology, Mayo Clinic, Rochester,
Minnesota

LUIS GUIMARAES, MD
Department of Radiology, Mayo Clinic, Rochester,
Minnesota

ROBERT HARTMAN, MD
Department of Radiology, Mayo Clinic, Rochester,
Minnesota

PATRICK A. HEIN, MD
Department of Radiology, Campus Charité Mitte,
Charité–Universitaetsmedizin Berlin, Berlin,
Germany

YOSHIDA HIROYUKI, PhD
Research Director, Three-Dimensional Imaging,
Department of Three-Dimensional Imaging,
Massachusetts General Hospital, Harvard Medical
School, Boston, Massachusetts

DAVID M. HOUGH, MD
Department of Radiology, Mayo Clinic, Rochester,
Minnesota

JAMES E. HUPRICH, MD
Department of Radiology, Mayo Clinic, Rochester,
Minnesota

AYA KAMAYA, MD
Assistant Professor, Department of Radiology,
Stanford University Medical Center, Stanford,
California

AVINASH R. KAMBADAKONE, MD, FRCR
Research Scholar, Division of Abdominal Imaging and Intervention, Department of Radiology, Massachusetts General Hospital, Boston, Massachusetts

CHRISTIAN KLOETERS, MD
Department of Radiology, Campus Charité Mitte, Charité–Universitaetsmedizin Berlin, Berlin, Germany

JAMES KOFLER, PhD
Assistant Professor of Radiologic Physics, Department of Radiology, Mayo Clinic, Rochester, Minnesota

CARLOS J. LEDEZMA, MD
Morristown Memorial Hospital, Department of Radiology, Morristown, New Jersey

YEONG SHYAN LEE, MD
Department of Radiology and Radiological Science, Medical University of South Carolina, Charleston, South Carolina; and Department of Diagnostic Radiology, Tan Tock Seng Hospital, Singapore

CYNTHIA H. McCOLLOUGH, PhD
Professor of Radiologic Physics, Department of Radiology, Mayo Clinic, Rochester, Minnesota

ERIK MITTRA, MD, PhD
Fellow, Division of Nuclear Medicine, Stanford Hospital and Clinics, Stanford, California

HANSEL J. OTERO, MD
Research Fellow, Applied Imaging Science Laboratory, Department of Radiology, Brigham and Women's Hospital and Harvard Medical School, Boston, Massachusetts

ANDREW N. PRIMAK, PhD
Research Associate, Department of Radiology, Mayo Clinic, Rochester, Minnesota

ANDREW QUON, MD
Assistant Professor, Division of Nuclear Medicine, Stanford Hospital and Clinics, Stanford, California

PATRIK ROGALLA, MD
Professor of Radiology, Department of Radiology, Campus Charité Mitte, Charité–Universitaetsmedizin Berlin, Berlin, Germany

BALAZS RUZSICS, MD, PhD
Department of Radiology and Radiological Science, Medical University of South Carolina, Charleston, South Carolina

FRANK J. RYBICKI, MD, PhD
Director, Applied Imaging Science Laboratory; Director of Cardiac CT and Vascular CT/MRI, Noninvasive Cardiovascular Imaging and Department of Radiology, Brigham and Women's Hospital; and Associate Professor of Radiology, Harvard Medical School, Boston, Massachusetts

DUSHYANT V. SAHANI, MD
Associate Professor of Radiology, Harvard Medical School; and Director of Computed Tomography, Department of Radiology, Massachusetts General Hospital, Boston, Massachusetts

U. JOSEPH SCHOEPF, MD, FAHA
Department of Radiology and Radiological Science, Medical University of South Carolina, Charleston, South Carolina; and Division of Cardiology, Department of Medicine, Medical University of South Carolina, Charleston, South Carolina

ANAND K. SINGH, MD
Research Fellow, Department of Three-Dimensional Imaging, Massachusetts General Hospital, Harvard Medical School, Boston, Massachusetts

MICHAEL L. STEIGNER, MD
Staff, Applied Imaging Science Laboratory; Attending Physician, Noninvasive Cardiovascular Imaging and Department of Radiology, Brigham and Women's Hospital; and Instructor in Radiology, Harvard Medical School, Boston, Massachusetts

NAOKI TAKAHASHI, MD
Department of Radiology, Mayo Clinic, Rochester, Minnesota

SANDRA TOCHETTO, MD
Department of Radiology, Northwestern University-Feinberg School of Medicine, Chicago, Illinois

MAX WINTERMARK, MD
University of California, Department of Radiology, Neuroradiology Section, San Francisco, California

VAHID YAGHMAI, MD
Associate Professor and Medical Director of CT, Department of Radiology, Northwestern University-Feinberg School of Medicine, Chicago, Illinois

JUDY YEE, MD
Professor and Vice Chair of Radiology and Biomedical Imaging, University of California, San Francisco; and Chief of Radiology, VA Medical Center, San Francisco, California

LIFENG YU, PhD
Assistant Professor of Radiologic Physics, Department of Radiology, Mayo Clinic, Rochester, Minnesota

Contents

Sixty-four–slice CT typified the dramatic race in technical development in radiology. Featuring high spatial resolution with 0.5-mm thin slices and 0.3-second gantry revolution times, it has become state-of-the-art technology in CT imaging shortly after its clinical introduction. Three-dimensional tube modulation together with adaptive x-ray shutters led to significant dose reduction to the patients while improving image quality because of implementation of optimized reconstruction algorithms. The latest innovations—new detector materials, dual-layer detector, dual-source and dynamic volume CT—represent the pinnacles in CT imaging, pursuing different directions to further clinical applications of CT.

A fundamental understanding of early arterial and parenchymal contrast medium (CM) dynamics is the basis for the design of CT scanning and injection protocols for state-of-the-art cardiovascular and body CT applications. Although normal parenchymal enhancement is primarily controlled by the total iodine dose injected per body weight, arterial enhancement is controlled by the iodine flux, the injection duration, and cardiac output. The technical capabilities of modern CT equipment allow and require precise scan timing to synchronize data acquisition with the desired phase of vascular enhancement (for CTA) and parenchymal enhancement (for liver and pancreatic CT). Automated tube current modulation and weight-based injection protocols allow individual optimization of radiation exposure and reduce interindividual variability of CM enhancement.

In recent years, the media has focused on the potential danger of radiation exposure from CT, even though the potential benefit of a medically indicated CT far outweighs the potential risks. This attention has reminded the radiology community that doses must be as low as reasonably achievable (ALARA) while maintaining diagnostic image quality. To satisfy the ALARA principle, the dose reduction strategies described in this article must be well understood and properly used. The use of CT must also be justified for the specific diagnostic task.

> Dual-energy CT refers to the use of CT data representing two different energy spectra and allows for the possibility of differentiating and classifying tissue to obtain material-specific images. Dual-energy CT data can be acquired using various CT hardware platforms, with numerous approaches also existing for display of anatomic and material-specific dual-energy information. Dual-source CT refers to the use of two x-ray sources and two x-ray detectors mounted on a single CT gantry and can be used in either a dual-energy or single-energy mode. This article summarizes and reviews current and potential applications for dual-energy and dual-source CT in the abdomen and pelvis.

> Advances in multidetector CT (MDCT) scanners have increased the pace of development of advanced postprocessing applications, such as virtual endoscopy (VE), segmentation and volumetry, and computer-aided postprocessing methods. Availability of thin-section MDCT data sets of isotropic voxel resolution ensures accuracy in structure segmentation, which is an important initial prerequisite on which the results of such advanced postprocessing applications are based. This article explains the technique of VE, segmentations and volumetry and various computer-aided post processing methods, with emphasis on their importance in the present clinical scenario.

> Multidetector CT now provides noninvasive coronary imaging, and patients with a low or intermediate probability of coronary artery disease can be imaged with radiation levels comparable to catheterization. Cardiac imaging drives rapid progress in CT hardware. To best apply evolving technology, imagers and referring clinicians need a solid understanding of spatial resolution, temporal resolution, volume coverage, and radiation dose. This article defines and discusses interactions between these parameters for state-of-the-art CT.

> With the widespread use of coronary CT angiography, new potential clinical indications are constantly being explored. Currently, 64-slice multidetector-row CT and dual-source CT are the benchmark for noninvasive coronary CT angiography; however, new technologies are already on the horizon. While significant obstacles still remain to be overcome, coronary CT angiography is closer than ever to fulfilling its promise of replacing invasive techniques in appropriate patient populations.

> A multimodal CT protocol provides a comprehensive noninvasive survey of acute stroke patients with accurate demonstration of the site of arterial occlusion and its hemodynamic tissue status. It combines widespread availability with the ability to

provide functional characterization of cerebral ischemia, and could potentially allow more accurate selection of candidates for acute stroke reperfusion therapy. This article discusses the individual components of multimodal CT and addresses the potential role of a combined multimodal CT stroke protocol in acute stroke therapy.

CT enterography is a new imaging modality that has distinct advantages over conventional CT, wireless capsule endoscopy, and barium examination. CT enterography is noninvasive and allows rapid mapping of disease activity before endoscopy and in cases where the endoscope cannot reach the diseased segment. CT enterography is readily available, is operator independent, and allows evaluation of extraenteric complications of small bowel disease. This article describes the latest techniques and applications of CT enterography.

CT colonography (CTC), also termed virtual colonoscopy, is increasingly accepted at sites throughout the world as a new effective tool for the diagnosis and screening of colorectal carcinoma. This article presents information of related issues of bowel cleansing, stool and fluid tagging, bowel distention and multidetector CT scanning parameters. The author presents discussion of interpretation of CTC, appropriate applications of CTC and potential complications.

Positron emission tomography (PET) and combined PET/CT provide powerful metabolic and anatomical information together in a single exam. This article reviews the fundamentals of PET physics, the state of the art and future directions in PET technology, and the current clinical applications of PET. The latter is quite diverse and includes oncology, cardiology, neurology, and infection and inflammation imaging, all with FDG as the tracer. Additionally, novel radiopharmeuticals are under development, many of which are target cellular processes that are more specific than glucose metabolism.

Perfusion CT has made tremendous progress since its inception and is gradually broadening its applications from the research realm into routine clinical care. This has been particularly noteworthy in the oncological setting, where perfusion CT is emerging as a valuable tool in tissue characterization, risk stratification and monitoring treatment effects especially assessing early response to novel targeted therapies. Recent technological advancements in CT have paved ways to overcome the initial limitations of restricted tissue coverage and radiation dose concerns. In this article, the authors review the basic principles and technique of perfusion CT and discuss its various oncologic and non-oncological clinical applications in body imaging.

Radiologic Clinics of North America

THE CLINICS ARE NOW AVAILABLE ONLINE!

Access your subscription at:
www.theclinics.com

GOAL STATEMENT

The goal of the *Radiologic Clinics of North America* is to keep practicing radiologists and radiology residents up to date with current clinical practice in radiology by providing timely articles reviewing the state of the art in patient care.

ACCREDITATION

The *Radiologic Clinics of North America* is planned and implemented in accordance with the Essential Areas and Policies of the Accreditation Council for Continuing Medical Education (ACCME) through the joint sponsorship of the University of Virginia School of Medicine and Elsevier. The University of Virginia School of Medicine is accredited by the ACCME to provide continuing medical education for physicians.

The University of Virginia School of Medicine designates this educational activity for a maximum of 15 *AMA PRA Category 1 Credits*™. Physicians should only claim credit commensurate with the extent of their participation in the activity.

The American Medical Association has determined that physicians not licensed in the US who participate in this CME activity are eligible for 15 *AMA PRA Category 1 Credits*™.

Credit can be earned by reading the text material, taking the CME examination online at http://www.theclinics.com/home/cme, and completing the evaluation. After taking the test, you will be required to review any and all incorrect answers. Following completion of the test and evaluation, your credit will be awarded and you may print your certificate.

FACULTY DISCLOSURE/CONFLICT OF INTEREST

The University of Virginia School of Medicine, as an ACCME accredited provider, endorses and strives to comply with the Accreditation Council for Continuing Medical Education (ACCME) Standards of Commercial Support, Commonwealth of Virginia statutes, University of Virginia policies and procedures, and associated federal and private regulations and guidelines on the need for disclosure and monitoring of proprietary and financial interests that may affect the scientific integrity and balance of content delivered in continuing medical education activities under our auspices.

The University of Virginia School of Medicine requires that all CME activities accredited through this institution be developed independently and be scientifically rigorous, balanced and objective in the presentation/discussion of its content, theories and practices.

All authors/editors participating in an accredited CME activity are expected to disclose to the readers relevant financial relationships with commercial entities occurring within the past 12 months (such as grants or research support, employee, consultant, stock holder, member of speakers bureau, etc.). The University of Virginia School of Medicine will employ appropriate mechanisms to resolve potential conflicts of interest to maintain the standards of fair and balanced education to the reader. Questions about specific strategies can be directed to the Office of Continuing Medical Education, University of Virginia School of Medicine, Charlottesville, Virginia.

The faculty and staff of the University of Virginia Office of Continuing Medical Education have no financial affiliations to disclose.

The authors/editors listed below have identified no financial or professional relationships for themselves or their spouse/partner:

Gorka Bastarrika, MD, PhD; Natalie Braun, BS; Barton Dudlick (Acquisitions Editor); Dominik Fleischmann, MD; Luis Guimaraes, MD; Patrick A. Hein, MD; David M. Hough, MD; James E. Huprich, MD; Avinash R. Kambadakone, MD, FRCR; Theodore E. Keats, MD (Test Author); Christian Kloeters, MD; James Kofler, Jr., PhD; Carlos J. Ledezma, MD; Yeong Shyan Lee, MD; Erik Mittra, MD, PhD; Hansel J. Otero, MD; Balazs Ruzsics, MD, PhD; Anand K. Singh, MD; Michael L. Steigner, MD; Naoki Takahashi, MD; Sandra Tochetto, MD; and Vahid Yaghmai, MD (Guest Editor).

The authors/editors listed below have identified the following financial or professional relationships for themselves or their spouse/partner:

Jodie Christner, PhD is an industry funded research/investigator for Siemens Heathcare.

Joel G. Fletcher, MD is an industry funded research/investigator for GE Healthcare and Siemens Medical Solutions.

Robert Hartman, MD is a consultant for Siemens and serves on the Advisory Board for American Medical Systems.

Yoshida Hiroyuki, PhD owns a patent with Hologic/R2 and MEDIAN Technology.

Aya Kamaya, MD is an industry funded research/investigator for Canon Inc.

Cynthia H. McCollough, PhD is an industry funded research/investigator for Bayer Healthcare and Siemens Medical Solutions.

Andrew N. Primak, PhD is an industry funded research/investigator for Siemens Heathcare.

Andrew Quon, MD is an industry funded research/investigator for Genentech.

Patrik Rogalla, MD has received occasional honoraria from Siemens Medical Solutions, Philips Medical Systems, and Toshiba Medical Systems.

Frank J. Rybicki, MD, PhD serves on the Advisory Boards and Speakers Bureaus and has received research grants from Toshiba Medical, Siemens Medical, and Bracco Diagnostics.

Dushyant V. Sahani, MD (Guest Editor) has received a grant from GE Healthcare.

U. Joseph Schoepf, MD, FAHA is an industry funded research/investigator for Bayer-Schering, Bracco, GE, Medrad, and Siemens, and is a consultant for Bayer-Schering, Bracco, GE, Medrad, Siemen, and Terarecon.

Max Wintermark, MD is an industry funded research/investigator for GE Healthcare and Philips Healthcare.

Judy Yee, MD is an industry funded research/investigator for GE Healthcare.

Lifeng Yu, PhD is an industry funded research/investigator for Xoran Technologies.

Disclosure of Discussion of Non-FDA Approved Uses for Pharmaceutical Products and/or Medical Devices.

The University of Virginia School of Medicine, as an ACCME provider, requires that all faculty presenters identify and disclose any off-label uses for pharmaceutical and medical device products. The University of Virginia School of Medicine recommends that each physician fully review all the available data on new products or procedures prior to clinical use.

TO ENROLL

To enroll in the Radiologic Clinics of North America Continuing Medical Education program, call customer service at 1-800-654-2452 or sign up online at http://www.theclinics.com/home/cme. The CME program is available to subscribers for an additional annual fee USD 205.

Preface

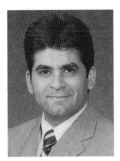 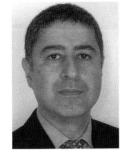

Dushyant V. Sahani, MD   Vahid Yaghmai, MD

Guest Editors

Since its introduction in 1972, computed tomography (CT) has made tremendous contributions in the realm of patient care and with the advent of multidetector CT (MDCT) technology, the landscape of medicine has been changed forever. There is hardly any speciality in medicine that has not benefited from the availability of CT, and MDCT technology has not only facilitated faster and more accurate diagnosis but also empowered CT to serve as an effective non-invasive alternative for screening and planning treatments in anatomically challenging areas. The inherent benefits of MDCT and its increasing demand have also stimulated advances in the data processing and image visualization technology. The workstations available commercially for image processing now have higher computational power and are loaded with sophisticated image visualization tools that have enhanced the image processing speed and enabled virtual navigation and image quantitation. Moreover, computer-aided detection is gaining tremendous interest with an intent to improve MDCT efficiency and accuracy. Coronary artery imaging and colon cancer screening with CT colonography are two glaring examples of transformation of patient care with an appropriate use of advances in CT and image processing technology. Evaluation of patients with stroke and cancer has been also revolutionized by employing various adaptations of CT such as tissue perfusion imaging and integrated PET/CT scanning.

Despite the availability of MDCT scanners for a decade, the technology remains in flux. In the recent past, 64-MDCT scanners were considered the top of the line equipments; however, several new innovations in CT are now available or emerging to embrace the patient care by using more detector rows (128-320 detector rows), new detector materials for higher sensitivity and ultrafast energy switching (Gemstone technology), two X-ray sources (dual-source CT), detectors with 2 layers to permit spectral analysis of the X-ray beam, and systems with flat-panel detectors (dynamic volume CT).

These exciting new opportunities available with MDCT would not have been feasible without focus and dedication of countless passionate physicians, scientists and engineers. We have a distinct privilege to introduce this issue of *Radiologic Clinics of North America* that focuses on these new or emerging technologies in MDCT. We are honoured that our panel of distinguished MDCT scientists have contributed articles to this issue in their respective area of expertise. We thank the *Radiologic Clinics of North America* for giving us this opportunity to present this interesting issue and also acknowledge the contribution of Barton Dudlick from Elsevier for his tremendous support on this project. We feel confident that this issue will enhance the reader's knowledge of newer

Radiol Clin N Am 47 (2009) xiii–xiv
doi:10.1016/j.rcl.2009.01.003

and emerging technology in MDCT and appropriate protocols for their use in the clinical practice while minimizing patient-related radiation risks.

Dushyant V. Sahani, MD
Department of Abdominal Imaging
Massachusetts General Hospital
55 Fruit Street, White-2-270
Boston, MA 02114

Vahid Yaghmai, MD
Department of Radiology
Northwestern University-Feinberg School of Medicine
676 N. Saint Clair, Suite 800
Chicago, IL 60611

E-mail addresses:
dsahani@partners.org (D.V. Sahani)
v-yaghmai@northwestern.edu (V. Yaghmai)

CT Technology Overview: 64-Slice and Beyond

Patrik Rogalla, MD*, Christian Kloeters, MD, Patrick A. Hein, MD

KEYWORDS

- CT • CT technology • Reconstruction techniques
- Radiation dose • Dual source CT • Dynamic volume CT

Since its introduction into clinical routine in 1972, computed tomography (CT) has made dramatic advances, most notably in recent years. All vendors today have 64-slice spiral CT scanners among their top-line offerings but the story by no means ends here: scanners with new detector materials for higher sensitivity and ultrafast energy switching, two x-ray tubes (dual-source CT), dual-layer detectors for spectral analysis of the x-ray beam, and systems with flat-panel detectors (dynamic volume CT) are further milestones of CT development in a modern clinical setting.

In 1917 Austrian mathematician Johann Radon presented an algorithm for creating an image from a set of measured data.[1] After further theoretic work by Cormack between 1950 and 1970, the British engineer Hounsfield built the first CT scanner in 1972. Hounsfield and Cormack were awarded the 1979 Nobel Prize in Medicine for their work. Hounsfield's prototype had a rotation time of about 300 seconds with a maximum image matrix of 80 × 80 pixels.[2,3] For comparison, today's 64-slice scanners have rotation times of 0.33 seconds with an image matrix of 512 × 512 pixels. Slice thickness is between 0.5 and 1 mm, and up to 64 slices can be acquired simultaneously. This comparison of performance nicely illustrates the rapid technical development CT technology has undergone over the last 30 years. Nevertheless, many fundamental principles, such as back projection and acquisition of 180° data, have not changed much since the first CT scanner was presented by Hounsfield.

Two other important developments were CT scanners of the fourth generation and electron beam CT (EBCT). Fourth-generation scanners have a stationary detector ring that does not rotate around the patient. The x-ray tube moves inside the detector ring. These scanners had the technical potential to achieve higher spatial resolution and faster rotation because less material is moved around the patient. The other technique, EBCT, was characterized by the complete absence of rotating components and the use of a centrally generated electron beam that was reflected by targets.[4,5] The absence of rotating mechanical parts enabled exposure times of 50 milliseconds; however, the limited overall x-ray energy generated by the electron beam precluded widespread use of the technology.

The conventional technique comprising a rotating gantry with a tube and detector opposing each other (third-generation CT scanners) has become the standard and is still used in state-of-the-art 64-slice CT scanners.

SIXTY-FOUR–SLICE TECHNOLOGY
Technical Evolution of 64-Slice CT

Following the presentation of the first 4-slice CT scanner in 1998, all other manufacturers also offered scanners enabling acquisition of four simultaneous slices per rotation. The next step was the development of 16-slice CT scanners parallel to slimmed-down versions for the simultaneous acquisition of 6, 8, or 10 slices. Another quantum leap in CT technology occurred in 2004 with the advent of scanners for the simultaneous acquisition of 64 slices per rotation. **Table 1** gives an overview of the current technology of 64-slice

Department of Radiology, Campus Charité Mitte, Charité – Universitätsmedizin Berlin, Charitéplatz 1, 10117 Berlin, Germany
* Corresponding author.
E-mail address: rogalla@charite.de (P. Rogalla).

Radiol Clin N Am 47 (2009) 1–11
doi:10.1016/j.rcl.2008.10.004
0033-8389/08/$ – see front matter © 2009 Elsevier Inc. All rights reserved.

Table 1
Summary of the current 64-slice CT scanners

Manufacturer	Scanner	No. of Slices	Slice Thickness	Detector Width	Rotation Time(s)
GE	LightSpeed VCT	64	0.625	40.0 mm	0.35
Philips	Brilliance	64	0.625	40.0 mm	0.40
Siemens	Sensation 64	2 × 32 (FFS)	0.6	28.8 mm	0.33
	Definition AS	64	0.6	38.4 mm	0.30
Toshiba	Aquilion 64	64	0.5	32.0 mm	0.35

Abbreviations: FFS, flying focal spot; s, seconds.

scanners from four manufacturers in respect to number of slices, slice thickness, total detector coverage, and gantry rotation time. Diagrams of the different multislice detector configurations used in the first multislice scanners are represented in **Fig. 1**. Advent of the 4-slice CT technology sparked an intense debate about the most promising and efficient detector configuration. **Fig. 2** presents diagrams of today's detector configurations, showing that all vendors now use the matrix configuration (symmetric arrangement of detectors of identical size).

Spatial and Contrast Resolution

The spatial resolution that can be achieved depends on many factors. In the XY-direction (axial plane), the high-contrast spatial resolution is determined by the number of projections (sampling frequency) and the number of detectors. With scanners from all vendors, high-resolution scans should not be acquired with the fastest gantry rotation, because the sampling rate stays usually constant and more projections are available when longer gantry rotation times are selected. The spatial resolution currently achieved on scanners from all manufacturers varies from 0.33 to 0.47 mm (high-contrast mode, ie, for bones). In this respect, the flying focal spot (FFS) technique (in marketing erroneously used for doubling the

nominal slice numbers) is beneficial because the moving focus on the tube anode doubles the number of projections.[6,7] This technique improves nominal high-contrast spatial resolution but fewer photons reach the detector per exposure because the photons are divided between two spots.

Resolution for low-contrast objects is determined by numerous other factors, including the reconstruction algorithm used, detector efficiency, and above all by filtering of the x-ray beam (**Fig. 3**). Less filtering makes the beam softer and yields a higher-contrast image but is also associated with higher radiation exposure because soft radiation is more readily absorbed by biologic tissue. Conversely, more filtering yields lower contrast images while reducing the radiation exposure. The effect may be neglected on unenhanced CT scans but becomes clearly apparent on scans obtained after administration of an iodine-based contrast agent mainly because of the differences in absorption of radiation of different energy by iodine. This effect (voltage dependence of CT attenuation) is one of the principles underlying the clinical use of dual-energy CT.[8]

Reconstruction Techniques

A major problem to be solved with the advent of 64-slice CT was that the cone beam geometry no longer allowed direct reconstruction of axial

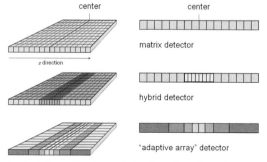

Fig. 1. Schematic view of the first four-slice detector configurations.

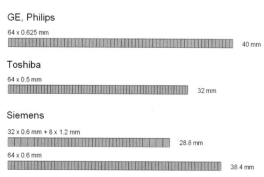

Fig. 2. Currently available 64-slice detector configurations.

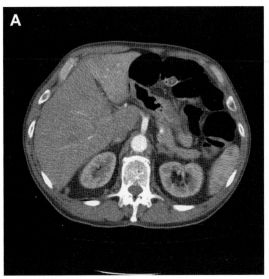 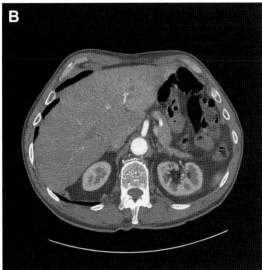

Fig. 3. Comparison of two different 64-slice CT scanners: the patient was first imaged on a CT scanner with thicker primary x-ray beam filtering. Three months later, the patient was imaged on a different CT unit with a thinner primary beam filter. The type, concentration, injection speed, and total amount of contrast agent and the scanning delay were identical. Note the attenuation difference in the aorta (228 HU in *A*, 279 HU in *B*).

images. Two basic approaches are currently used to generate CT images:

Rebinning algorithms. Advanced single-slice rebinning (ASSR) and its extension and generalization are algorithms optimized for small cone angles as they occur in 64-slice CT.[9] The algorithm reduces three-dimensional (3D) cone beam data to tilted two-dimensional slices by minimizing the deviation of the reconstruction plane from the spiral for each reconstruction position, and currently runs on both 16-slice and 64-slice CT scanners. In a second step, the data are sorted into angulated pseudoaxial slices using 2D filtered back projection. In a third step, the oblique slices are interpolated to parallel transaxial slices. The ASSR algorithm operates efficiently and requires fairly little computing power to reconstruct images of clinically acceptable image quality.[10] Representative examples for rebinning algorithms are the adaptive multiplanar reconstruction algorithm (AMPR) and the conjugate ray reconstruction (weighted hyperplane reconstruction).[11]

The second reconstruction principle used in 64-slice CT is based on sorting of raw data and represents an extension of the Feldkamp 3D convolution back-projection technique to multisection spiral scanning.[12] The Feldkamp algorithm was originally introduced for sequential scanning. In the raw data space, which is typically four times as large as the image data space, the signals from the individual detector rows are computed in such a way that axial images in parallel orientation are directly obtained from the raw data. Sorting of the raw data requires considerable processor power and more powerful computers. Direct 3D filtered back projection of raw data is superior to rebinning algorithms in homogeneous distribution of image noise and uniform slice thickness in particular for scanners with larger cone angles. Examples of the Feldkamp modifications are the Cobra algorithm and the TCOT algorithm.

Iterative reconstruction techniques, based on back and forward projection promising significant noise reduction, have been proposed since the early times of CT technology. The rapid advances in scanning performance exceeded the advances in computing power, however, so that today's 64-slice CT units all use filtered back-projection algorithms for image reconstruction as described previously. One may project that in the near future with broader availability of parallel processor technology, iterative image reconstruction algorithms will mature and reach the stage of clinical usefulness.

In single-slice spiral CT, the pitch factor (table feed relative to the collimation) did not affect image noise but higher pitch factors resulted in thicker slices and increasingly blurred anatomy. Typical pitch factors used in spiral CT ranged between 1 and 2. In multislice spiral CT, in particular 64-slice CT, the pitch factor does not affect the slice sensitivity profile of the reconstructed section but faster table feed (higher pitch value) increases image noise because fewer photons are available for image reconstruction. This effect is compensated for on all scanners by automatically increasing the tube current (mA value) when a higher pitch factor is selected. It is thus no longer possible to reduce the radiation dose by simply choosing a higher pitch factor (which was possible on spiral CT scanners). The image quality achieved with all currently available implementations of reconstruction algorithms may vary with the pitch factor. In terms of image quality, it is therefore not recommended to freely select the pitch factor, although this is technically feasible. On most 64-slice scanners, optimal image quality is obtained when using pitch values slightly less than 1 because computation of supplementary projections obtained by overlapping scanning generally results in higher image quality.

Means for Radiation Dose Reduction

While maintaining image quality, 64-slice CT scanners reduce the radiation exposure compared with earlier generations of scanners. This effect is mainly due to a reduction of the overbeaming effect (**Fig. 4**), but improved reconstruction techniques, more sensitive detector material, and more efficient DAS units (amplifying units behind the detectors) also contribute to the reduction of radiation exposure. An important innovation of 64-slice CT is the anatomic masking of the x-ray beam.[13] All reconstruction algorithms require 180° projection data for reconstructing the first and the last image in the spiral acquisition. At least

half an extra rotation is therefore required at each end of the scan run to ensure reconstruction of the required target anatomy range; this is known as overranging/overscanning and substantially contributes to the overall radiation exposure. Its relative contribution is especially high when a small volume is scanned using a high pitch factor and wide detectors (**Fig. 5**). For instance, the additional exposure due to overranging may be up to 100% when examining the inner ear using 64-slice CT with a width of the scan volume of 4 cm. Overranging can be completely eliminated by implementing x-ray shutters that move synchronously with the table feed at either end of the spiral. This option is meanwhile available on the scanners from three vendors.

Adapting the tube load to the patient's size and shape with the aim to keep image noise constant throughout the entire study has proved to lower the radiation dose to the minimum required. Both in-plane (XY-axis) and longitudinal (Z-axis) dose modulation is embedded in 64-slice CTs from all vendors.

An important advantage of 64-slice CT over 16-slice scanners is that it enables more reliable cardiac imaging. The number of nondiagnostic cardiac CT examinations has been reduced, primarily because the images can be reconstructed from fewer cardiac cycles. Nevertheless, the increase in sensitivity and specificity for detecting relevant coronary artery stenosis is small.[14] A substantial increase in patient dose results from helical acquisition in cardiac CT. Regardless of the number of x-ray tubes, the table feed must be sufficiently slow that projection data of 180° gantry rotation are available for image reconstruction at all points in time and space even in patients who have variable heart rate. Overlapping scanning with very low pitch factors is required with 64-slice CT to enable image reconstruction throughout the scan area and for all time points of the cardiac cycle. Clinical pitch values range from 0.15 to

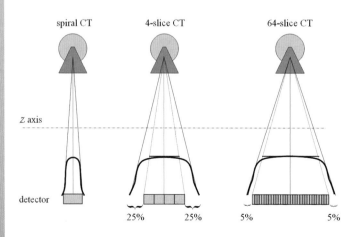

spiral CT   4-slice CT   64-slice CT

z axis

detector

25%   25%   5%   5%

Fig. 4. To ensure uniform exposure of the multislice detector, the x-ray beam shutter opening is wider than the width of the detector. This technique is referred to as overbeaming and can markedly increase radiation exposure in multislice CT when scanning a small body area. On 64-slice scanners, the overbeaming effect has become less influential compared with 4-slice scanners because of improved shutter techniques and the geometrically wider detectors. It accounts for only 5% to 10% of the overall radiation exposure in current 64-slice scanners.

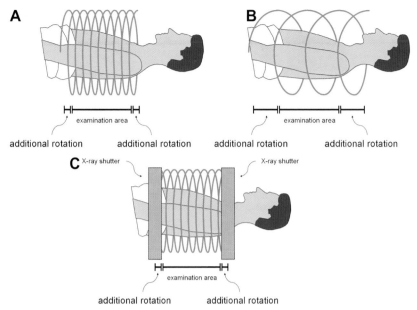

Fig. 5. The effect of overranging/overscanning increases with the detector width and the pitch used (*A*, *B*). The smaller the scan field, the larger the extra radiation exposure due to the overscanning effect. The additional radiation dose may increase up to 100% when scanning small children or the inner ear, for example. X-ray shutters synchronized to the table movement block the unnecessary radiation that occurs on either end of the spiral acquisition (*C*).

0.25, resulting in a marked increase in radiation exposure compared with a non-gated normal CT scan of the same anatomic area. Incremental, prospectively gated scanning protocols (so-called "step-and-shoot" technique) reduce radiation exposure because of the lack of overlapping data acquisition but preclude dynamic evaluation with calculation of ejection fraction and analysis of cardiac motion.[15]

Options for reducing the radiation exposure of cardiac 64-slice CT are available from all vendors and include:

Optimized pitch factor, adapted to the heart rate
Reduced-voltage scan protocols
Use of bow-tie filters or a smaller scan field of view
Tube current modulation and use of a smaller safety window (padding) for variable heart rates
Denoising filter technology in image postprocessing

Effective exposure time of 64-slice CT can be easily determined from the gantry rotation time. Because 180° projection data are necessary, the effective exposure time in single-tube systems is half the rotation time in milliseconds. The fastest gantry rotation currently achieved is 300

milliseconds, corresponding to a resolution of 150 milliseconds. The effective exposure time can be further reduced using multisegment reconstruction (**Fig. 6**), but this reconstruction technique requires a smaller pitch and therefore increases radiation exposure.[16]

Overlapping Reconstruction

With spiral CT, image quality of 3D reconstructions and multiplanar reformations can be improved by using up to 50% overlapping image reconstruction, mainly because of the bell-shaped configuration of the sensitivity profile in spiral CT. In 64-slice CT, on the other hand, the individual slices have a nearly rectangular sensitivity profile, which is why overlapping reconstruction of 50% of the nominal slice thickness appears superfluous; 20% overlap has proved to be perfectly adequate to improve the image quality of 3D views. Greater overlap merely increases the number of slices, slows down the workstation, and requires more storage capacity without an appreciable improvement in image quality (**Fig. 7**).

ADVANCES BEYOND 64-SLICE TECHNOLOGY
Dual-Source CT

A milestone in the development of CT technology was the advent of so-called dual-source CT, which

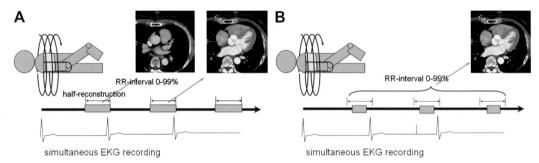

A half-reconstruction · RR-interval 0-99% · simultaneous EKG recording

B RR-interval 0-99% · simultaneous EKG recording

Fig. 6. Diagrams of the two reconstruction techniques used in 64-slice cardiac CT. In half-scan reconstruction (*A*), each image is reconstructed from a single cardiac cycle. The temporal resolution (reconstruction window) therefore corresponds to half the gantry rotation time. When the image is reconstructed over several cardiac cycles (*B*), the calculated exposure time is shortened accordingly. This technique is more susceptible to variations in cardiac motion between two beats.

has been described in many articles since its introduction in 2005.[17] The following short overview should only serve as a summary.

The dual-source CT is equipped with two x-ray tubes and two corresponding detectors. The two acquisition systems are mounted onto the rotating gantry with an angular offset of 90°. The first detector array covers the maximum field of view (FOV) of the scan (50 cm), whereas the second detector array is limited to a smaller FOV (26 cm) because of space limitations on the gantry (**Fig. 8**). Each detector array consists of a total of 40 detectors; 32 rows with 0.6-mm effective thickness are centrally located, framed by four rows with 1.2-mm effective thickness on both sides (see **Table 1**). By using the FFS technique, two overlapping sets of 32 slices are merged for reconstruction of 64 slices per gantry rotation with an overlap of 0.3 mm. The axial image reconstruction is handled using the modified AMPR. With the shortest gantry rotation

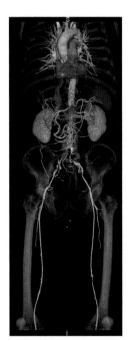

Fig. 7. Thin-slice CT angiography with volume rendering. The axial source images were 0.5 mm thick, reconstructed with 0.4-mm increment. Higher degree of overlap would only increase the number of slices and slow down the workstation speed but not result in a relevant improvement of image quality.

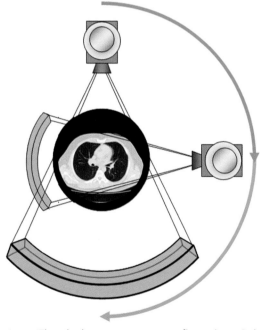

Fig. 8. The dual-source gantry configuration. Only a 90° gantry rotation is necessary to collect 180° of projection data, resulting in a temporal window of 83 milliseconds for ECG-gated cardiac imaging. Because both tubes can be loaded with different voltages, simultaneous data acquisition at two kV settings is possible allowing for analysis of tissue composition.

time of 0.33 seconds, this technique led to two major technical improvements:

Improved temporal resolution of cardiac CT scans resulting from the simultaneous use of both x-ray tubes for reconstruction. In this way, the nominal temporal resolution is reduced by half, enabling reconstruction with markedly fewer motion artifacts (**Fig. 9**). The comparatively higher temporal resolution has been shown to reduce motion artifacts and thus leads to a broader clinical application, for instance, in patients who have medical contraindications to β-blockers and higher heart rates, or in patients in an emergency situation diagnosed for chest pain triage.[18]

Dual-energy acquisition. The two tubes are operated with different voltages. This technique for the first time enables simultaneous acquisition of two scans (ie, without a delay) with different voltage. The principle of dual-energy scanning is not new and has been used in clinical CT for 30 years. What is new is the option of acquiring both scans simultaneously and applying tissue decomposition for tissue analysis.[8] Dual-energy acquisition techniques open up many new diagnostic options, such as the characterization of gallstones or kidney stones,[19] the computation of virtual noncontrast images, and the generation of pure iodine images (see **Fig. 9**).

Alternatively, both tubes can be used to increase the radiation dose, which may offer a diagnostic benefit in severely obese patients. Because the tubes are arranged with 90° offset in the gantry system, however, scattered radiation from one tube originating in the patient's body may reach the detector system belonging to the second tube. Because scattered radiation does not contain diagnostic information but results in a detector signal, the image quality may be slightly reduced, visible as pronounced artifacts mainly in the periphery of the object and as reduced accuracy of HU values that may drop up to 36 units.[20] It has been shown that correction algorithms may compensate for the "capping" artifacts and restore homogeneity in the reconstructed image but result in increased image noise of up to 14% in the center and up to 19% in the image periphery.

New Detector Materials

Another milestone in CT technology lies in the development of new detector materials that exhibit

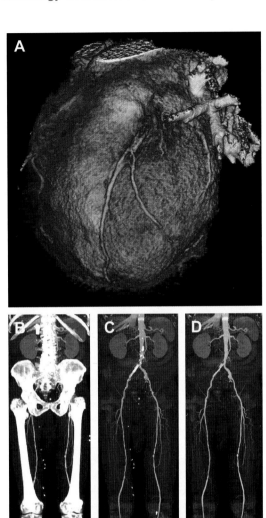

Fig. 9. (A) Dual-source CT of the heart. Despite the heart rate of 120 beats per minute, the coronary arteries exhibit only small motion artifacts. The second tube was used to shorten the temporal window to 83 milliseconds. CT angiography (B) using dual-energy technique in a patient who had multiple stents. The bone subtraction is facilitated by automatic bone detection. Because of the different absorption characteristics of calcium and iodine at 140 and 80 kV, calcified plaques (C) can be separated from the vascular lumen in dual-energy CT and subtracted from the maximum-intensity projection (D).

higher sensitivity to radiation and allow faster sampling rates. There is a new scintillator that features a negligible afterglow in conjunction with a 100-fold faster reaction time, allowing for recording of 7000 views per second. Implementation of the new scintillator may be one of the prerequisites for single-source ultra-fast dual energy switching, promising almost simultaneous spatial and temporal registration and material decomposition without the limitation of a reduced FOV due to the second smaller detector in dual-source CT. Approximately 50% fewer beam-hardening artifacts, metal artifact reduction, and further improvements in contrast-to-noise ratio are some of the benefits resulting from the new scintillator.

Double-Layer Detectors

Dual energy may be principally achieved either by radiating the object with two different energy spectra from a single source through fast voltage switching or from multiple sources operating at different voltages, or by analyzing the energy spectrum on the detector side. The latter would be best realized by using an energy-sensitive detector, which is physically possible but is several years from being able to be implemented in a clinical environment. A simple but effective solution lies in a double-layer detector design. The upper layer predominantly receives photons with lower energy and the lower layer receives photons with higher energy. Summing the signal from both detector layers returns the full signal as in a single-layer detector, but separate readouts from both layers allow for simple spectral analysis of the x-ray beam. This technology is currently under clinical evaluation.

Dynamic Volume CT

Two scanners have recently been introduced pioneering the future direction in CT development: expanding the detector coverage with potential elimination of spiral scanning for specific applications. The 128-slice scanner carries a fluid metal cooled x-ray tube and a tiled detector with 128 rows at 0.625-mm thickness (projected in the rotation axis of the gantry) and a novel two-dimensional anti-scatter grid. The detector covers 8 cm and exhibits increased dose efficiency. Further technical highlights are the ultrafast gantry rotation of 270 milliseconds leading to a centrifugal force of 40 times the gravitational acceleration, FFS in cardiac imaging, and arrhythmia rejection. The following scanning modes are featured:

Spiral scanning with 8-cm detector coverage (**Fig. 10**). To avoid significant overranging effects, the x-ray shutter is moved synchronous to the table feed as explained earlier (sliding collimation).

Joggle mode. The table moves back and forth between two table positions to expand the effective coverage for dynamic imaging.

Step-and-shoot mode. This mode, designed for low-dose cardiac scanning, overcomes the lack of full anatomic coverage of the entire heart. The heart is scanned within the minimum of three beats (one beat is

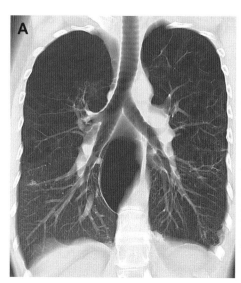
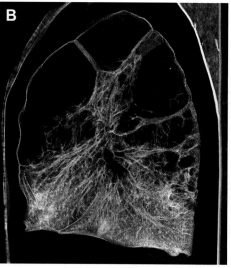

Fig. 10. Severe emphysema reconstructed as thick-slice slab (*A*) and using volume rendering technique (*B*). Axial scans were obtained with the 128-slice CT scanner in spiral mode (128 × 0.625 mm, sliding collimation). Total scanning duration: 2 seconds.

necessary for table movement to the next position). Because of the cone beam geometry necessitating some overlap between two consecutive scans, the effective coverage depends on the scan field-of-view and typically varies between 12 and 14 cm.

The climax in detector coverage is represented currently by the 320-slice dynamic volume CT scanner, comprising a conventional gantry with an aperture of 70 cm and a 70-kW x-ray tube with an opposing solid-state detector. The detector is 16 cm in width along the rotational axis of the gantry and consists of 320 rows of 0.5-mm thick elements, the current pinnacle in the nominal number of slices that can be scanned per gantry rotation. Each detector row consists of 896 elements, which are read out 900 to 3600 times per rotation, depending on the gantry revolution time. Revolution times can be varied between 350 milliseconds to 3 seconds for 360° data acquisition. A maximum of 640 slices with 50% spatial overlap can be reconstructed from each gantry rotation.

The cone beam angle of 15.2° is a function of the detector width and the tube focus-to-detector distance as compared with an angle of 3.05° for 64–detector row CT scanners of the same series. The source data are reconstructed using an exact cone beam algorithm, which nearly completely eliminates all artifacts typically degrading cone beam CT.[21] The geometric configuration of the scan area resulting from the geometry of the x-ray beam when scanning with a stationary table results in images with masked data as seen in the coronal

plan. The missing image data (truncation) could theoretically be reconstructed from the raw data[22] but the computation power necessary to do so exceeds the capacity of current-generation computers.

Three new scanning modes are available:

Stitching mode. Wide volume coverage is achieved by sequentially moving the table and stitching together the acquired scans. The time required for shifting the table between scans ranges between to 1.2 and 1.5 seconds. The overlap necessary between two consecutive scans typically amounts to 17% and depends on the scan field, which in most cases is determined by the diameter of the patient. Patient movement during the scan may cause visible stair-step artifacts or contour disruptions at the stitched positions. In helical scanning, the same patient movement would present as a widespread motion blur.

ECG-gated non-spiral single beat cardiac scan.[23] Because of the detector coverage of 16 cm, the entire heart can be imaged without table motion. Multiple applications, such as single-rotation imaging with arrhythmia rejection or dynamic imaging over an entire cardiac beat, are possible and clinically used.

Dynamic volume scanning provides volumetric imaging over time, offering functional analysis of entire organs (Fig. 11). Because there is no table movement during scanning, each individual volume demonstrates

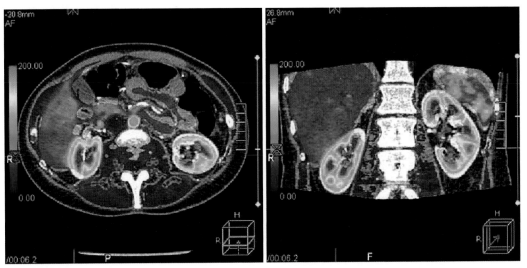

Fig. 11. Example of perfusion imaging of the kidneys, calculated with the maximum-slope technique. Note the truncated rhomboid shape of the coronally reformatted image caused by the cone geometry of the x-ray beam in dynamic volume CT.

just one instance in time. Dynamic scanning can be performed as a continuous acquisition with uninterrupted radiation exposure or as an intermittent series with variable intervals ranging from 0.5 to 30 seconds between acquisitions. Additionally, because a low-dose technique is preferable, several rotations can be combined to generate one time-averaged acquisition to reduce noise and improve image quality.

One of the reasons CT is so popular for perfusion studies is that there is a linear relationship between the concentration of contrast medium in a tissue and the resulting CT attenuation, which enables use of simple perfusion models. The detector widths that were available before the advent of 128- and 320–detector row CT presented a major obstacle to whole-organ coverage. An important issue in perfusion imaging, however, is to obtain diagnostic information with a reasonable radiation exposure, which increases with the number of scans acquired. Only strict use of low-dose techniques (eg, 80 kV with dramatically reduced tube current) will restrict radiation exposure to the scope of a conventional diagnostic CT examination. What remains to be determined is how the display of function and the calculation of organ and tumor perfusion with powerful computers will actually translate into clinical benefits for the patient.

SUMMARY

Following the introduction of spiral CT technology into clinical practice in 1988, the advantages of being able to scan larger areas of anatomy in a single breath-hold quickly became apparent. Because of the limited detector width available in conventional helical CT scanners, however, a slice thickness of 5 to 10 mm had to be used, resulting in multiplanar reconstructed images with much poorer resolution compared with axial images. Multidetector configurations consisting of several rows along the patient's longitudinal axis dramatically improved spatial imaging with the additional benefit of shorter scan times. Now 64–detector row CT scanners are available from all vendors with detectors varying in width from 2.8 to 4 cm allowing acquisition of slices ranging from 0.5 to 0.625 mm in thickness, which provides reconstruction with isotropic resolution in all reformatting planes. The clinically achievable spatial resolution in 64-slice CT lies in the range of 0.33 to 0.47 mm for high-contrast objects.

All vendors offering 64-slice CTs use reconstruction techniques that more or less compensate for the cone shape of the x-ray fan beam.

Direct reconstruction from raw data is computationally more expensive but superior to algorithms with approximation techniques. Tube modulation techniques are standard in 64-slice CTs, whereas adaptive x-ray shutters for elimination of unnecessary x-ray exposure on either end of the spiral acquisition represent a novel approach and have only recently been introduced.

The most recent milestones in CT development are the dual-source CT technology, ultra-fast voltage switching with new scintillator material and double-layer detector configuration inaugurating novel clinical applications, including tissue decomposition and dynamic volume CT on the one hand, and on the other hand rendering true perfusion imaging possible. One might expect that in light of recent advances in CT technology, CT will continue to play a pace-maker role for improvements in medical imaging on the whole.

ACKNOWLEDGMENTS

The authors express their special thanks to Dr. Thomas Werncke and Professor Mathias Prokop for contributing the clinical images used in **Figs. 9** and **10**.

REFERENCES

1. Cormack AM. 75 years of radon transform. J Comput Assist Tomogr 1992;16:673.
2. Hounsfield GN. The E.M.I. scanner. Proc R Soc Lond B Biol Sci 1977;195:281–9.
3. Hounsfield GN. Computerized transverse axial scanning (tomography): part I. Description of system 1973. Br J Radiol 1995;68:H166–72.
4. Rumberger JA, Lipton MJ. Ultrafast cardiac CT scanning. Cardiol Clin 1989;7:713–34.
5. Kloeters C, Dushe S, Dohmen PM, et al. Evaluation of left and right ventricular diastolic function by electron-beam computed tomography in patients with passive epicardial constraint. J Comput Assist Tomogr 2008;32:78–85.
6. Mori I. Antialiasing backprojection for helical MDCT. Med Phys 2008;35:1065–77.
7. Kyriakou Y, Kachelriess M, Knaup M, et al. Impact of the z-flying focal spot on resolution and artifact behavior for a 64-slice spiral CT scanner. Eur Radiol 2006;16:1206–15.
8. Hawkes DJ, Jackson DF, Parker RP. Tissue analysis by dual-energy computed tomography. Br J Radiol 1986;59:537–42.
9. Kachelriess M, Fuchs T, Schaller S, et al. Advanced single-slice rebinning for tilted spiral cone-beam CT. Med Phys 2001;28:1033–41.

10. Kachelriess M, Schaller S, Kalender WA. Advanced single-slice rebinning in cone-beam spiral CT. Med Phys 2000;27:754–72.

11. Hsieh J, Toth TL, Simoni P, et al. A generalized helical reconstruction algorithm for multidetector row CT. Radiology 2001;221(P):217 [abstract].

12. Taguchi K, Aradate H. Algorithm for image reconstruction in multi-slice helical CT. Med Phys 1998;25:550–61.

13. Flohr T, Stierstorfer K, Wolf H, et al. Principle and performance of a dynamic collimation technique for spiral CT. Radiology Society of North America 2007;SSA16–04.

14. Lembcke A, Hein PA, Enzweiler CN, et al. Acute myocardial ischemia after aortic valve replacement: a comprehensive diagnostic evaluation using dynamic multislice spiral computed tomography. Eur J Radiol 2006;57:351–5.

15. Hsieh J, Londt J, Vass M, et al. Step-and-shoot data acquisition and reconstruction for cardiac x-ray computed tomography. Med Phys 2006;33:4236–48.

16. Blobel J, Baartman H, Rogalla P, et al. Spatial and temporal resolution with 16-slice computed tomography for cardiac imaging. RöFo 2003;175:1264–71.

17. Flohr TG, McCollough CH, Bruder H, et al. First performance evaluation of a dual-source CT (DSCT) system. Eur Radiol 2006;16:256–68.

18. Rist C, Johnson TR, Becker CR, et al. New applications for noninvasive cardiac imaging: dual-source computed tomography. Eur Radiol 2007;17(Suppl 6):F16–25.

19. Scheffel H, Stolzmann P, Frauenfelder T, et al. Dual-energy contrast-enhanced computed tomography for the detection of urinary stone disease. Invest Radiol 2007;42:823–9.

20. Kyriakou Y, Kalender WA. Intensity distribution and impact of scatter for dual-source CT. Phys Med Biol 2007;52:6969–89.

21. Mori S, Endo M, Komatsu S, et al. A combination-weighted Feldkamp-based reconstruction algorithm for cone-beam CT. Phys Med Biol 2006;51:3953–65.

22. Leng S, Zhuang T, Nett BE, et al. Exact fan-beam image reconstruction algorithm for truncated projection data acquired from an asymmetric half-size detector. Phys Med Biol 2005;50:1805–20.

23. Rybicki FJ, Otero HJ, Steigner ML, et al. Initial evaluation of coronary images from 320-detector row computed tomography. Int J Cardiovasc Imaging 2008;24:535–46.

Optimal Vascular and Parenchymal Contrast Enhancement: The Current State of the Art

Dominik Fleischmann, MD*, Aya Kamaya, MD

KEYWORDS

- Computed tomography
- Contrast medium enhancement • CT angiography
- Cardiac CT • CT liver • CT pancreas

Multislice or multidetector-row CT (MDCT) is a rapidly evolving technology. The development of more powerful and sophisticated x-ray tubes, advances in detector design with increasing numbers of detector rows mounted on ever-faster rotating gantry systems, and sophisticated reconstruction algorithms have led to substantial gains in spatial and temporal resolution, volume coverage, and acquisition speed. Although these developments offer new opportunities in cardiovascular and body CT imaging, protocol design and contrast medium (CM) delivery become more difficult and less forgiving at the same time.

Several traditional concepts of CM injection conceived in the single–detector row CT era still apply today. For example, the relationship between the total volume of CM injected and the degree of opacification of the normal liver parenchyma will not change in the foreseeable future, because this relationship is controlled by pharmacokinetics—the respective volumes of distribution of a radiographic contrast agent in the extracellular space. Scan timing is also not critical for imaging of the liver in a portal venous phase, even with the fastest scanner.

Substantially more sophistication is needed, however, when modern CT technology is used to take advantage of rapid changes of CM opacification because of differences in organ perfusion, for example in imaging of hypervascular liver lesions, the pancreas, or perfusion itself, and for imaging of the cardiovascular system. Understanding the early CM dynamics is a prerequisite for the design of scanning and injection protocols in all these instances, and correct scan timing is critical.

This article first explains the fundamentals of arterial and parenchymal CM enhancement, followed by a discussion about how user-selectable parameters (injection flow rate, injection volume, and injection duration) affect the respective time attenuation responses. Although practical examples of injection strategies are demonstrated, these reflect implementations for current, rapidly evolving scanner technology. The pharmacokinetic principles, however, apply more generally, and also allow the reader to design his or her own future strategy of data acquisition and CM delivery, independent of the scanner used.

CONTRAST MEDIA FOR COMPUTED TOMOGRAPHY

All currently used angiographic x-ray CM are water-soluble derivates of symmetrically iodinated benzene (triiodobenzene). The diagnostic use of x-ray CM is exclusively based on the physical ability of iodine to absorb x-rays. The increase in CT numbers observed in a given vessel or tissue after

Department of Radiology, Stanford University Medical Center, 300 Pasteur Drive, Room S-072, Stanford, CA 94305-5105, USA
* Corresponding author.
E-mail address: d.fleischmann@stanford.edu (D. Fleischmann).

Radiol Clin N Am 47 (2009) 13–26
doi:10.1016/j.rcl.2008.10.009

CM administration is directly proportional to the local iodine concentration.[1]

The selection of intravenous CM for CT is primarily governed by safety considerations and the rate of expected adverse reactions. Nonionic CM are generally safer than ionic CM[2–5] and thus preferable in the setting of CT.[6] The contraindications and precautions for the use of intravenous radiographic CM also apply to its use in CT. Guidelines for patient screening, premedication, and recognition and management of acute adverse reactions have been published elsewhere.[7–9]

Currently there is no consensus if or to what extent iso-osmolar contrast agents[10] reduce the risk for CM-induced nephropathy (CIN) in patients who have impaired renal function compared with low-osmolar agents, notably in the setting of intravenous injections for CTA.[11,12] If patients at risk for CIN undergo a CT study, it is important, however, to ensure that serum creatinine levels are being followed up adequately.

PHARMACOKINETICS AND PHYSIOLOGY OF ARTERIAL AND PARENCHYMAL ENHANCEMENT

All angiographic x-ray CM are extracellular fluid markers. After intravenous administration they are rapidly distributed between the intravascular and extravascular interstitial spaces.[13] Traditional pharmacokinetic studies on CM have concentrated on the phase of elimination rather than on the early phase of CM distribution. For the time frame relevant to modern CT, however, it is this particularly complex phase of early CM distribution and redistribution that determines vascular enhancement and enhancement of well-perfused organs.

Vascular enhancement and parenchymal organ enhancement are dominated by different kinetics. For nonvascular CT (eg, imaging of the liver during a parenchymal phase) the degree of organ opacification correlates closely with the volume of CM (iodine) administered and is inversely related to a patient's body weight (a surrogate parameter for extracellular space).

Arterial enhancement, on the other hand, is not immediately related to CM volume. Arterial enhancement is controlled by two key factors, or key rules, as summarized in **Box 1**:[14] (a) the amount of iodinated CM delivered per unit of time, which, for a given iodine concentration, is the injection flow rate (mL/s), and (b) the injection duration, in seconds. The injection flow rate multiplied by the injection duration equals the CM volume, so CM volume does indirectly play a role, notably because most power injectors require that a CM injection is keyed into the injector interface as CM volume and flow rate. It is substantially

---

Box 1
Key rules of early arterial contrast medium dynamics and their consequences

Key rules of arterial enhancement

Rule 1: Arterial enhancement is proportional to the iodine administration rate

Arterial opacification can be increased by

- increasing the injection flow rate and/or by
- increasing the iodine concentration of the contrast medium

Rule 2: Arterial enhancement increases cumulatively with the injection duration

- longer CM injections increase arterial enhancement
- a minimum injection duration of approximately 10s is always needed to achieve adequate arterial enhancement

Rule 3: Individual enhancement is controlled by cardiac output

- cardiac output is inversely proportional to arterial opacification
- increasing or decreasing both the injection rate and the injection volumes to body weight reduces the interindividual variability of arterial enhancement

---

more useful to consider injection protocols for cardiovascular CT as injection flow rate times injection duration. For example, an intravenous CM injection described as 100 mL at 5 mL/s should be understood as 5 mL/s for 20 seconds, because the latter can be more intuitively translated into the expected strength and length of a desired vascular enhancement phase. The importance of thinking about injection protocols as injection flow rate times the injection duration cannot be overemphasized. It is the most important step to an intuitive understanding of cardiovascular injection protocols, and also reflected in the first two key rules listed in **Box 1**.

Early Arterial Contrast Medium Dynamics

Time attenuation responses to intravenously injected CM vary between vascular territories and even more so between different individuals, but they all share the same basic principles.[14] **Fig. 1** illustrates the early arterial CM dynamics as observed in the aorta: When a 16-mL test bolus of CM is injected intravenously, it causes an arterial enhancement response in the aorta after a certain time interval. The time interval needed for the CM to arrive in the arterial territory of interest is referred to as the contrast medium transit time (t_{CMT}), an important landmark for scan timing. The arterial time attenuation response itself consists of two phases. The first peak of the time attenuation response is referred to as the "first pass" effect. This peak is followed by the "recirculation" phase; a characteristic of this phase is that the tail of the time attenuation curve does not return to zero after the first pass, but undulates or rebounds above the baseline. This tail is only in part caused by true recirculation of opacified blood from highly perfused organs, such as the brain and the kidney, and for the most part it is

a consequence of bolus broadening. It is important, however, to acknowledge its existence, because it explains the somewhat unintuitive effect of the injection duration on vascular enhancement.

Effect of injection flow rate on arterial enhancement (Rule 1)

For a given patient and vascular territory, the degree of arterial enhancement is directly proportional to the iodine administration rate. **Fig. 1** shows that when the injection rate is doubled from 4 mL/s to 8 mL/s, or more precisely, if the iodine administration rate is increased from 1.2 g to

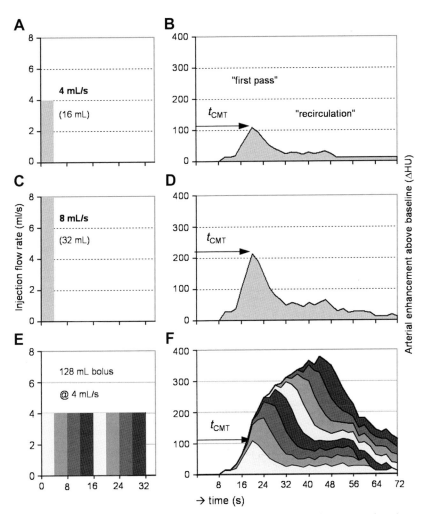

Fig. 1. Simple additive model illustrating the effects of injection flow rate and injection duration on arterial enhancement. Intravenous CM injection (*A*) causes an arterial enhancement response (*B*), which consists of an early first-pass peak and a lower recirculation effect. Doubling the injection flow rate (doubling the iodine administration rate) (*C*) results in approximately twice the arterial enhancement (*D*). The effect of the injection duration (*E*) can be regarded as the sum (time integral) of several enhancement responses (*F*). Note that because of the asymmetric shape of the test-enhancement curve and recirculation effects, arterial enhancement following an injection of 128 mL (the time integral of eight consecutive 16 mL) increases continuously over time. (*Adapted from* Fleischmann D. Contrast-medium administration. In: Catalano C, Passariello R, editors. Multidetector-row CT angiography. Berlin, Heidelberg, New York: Springer; 2005. p. 41; with permission.)

2.4 g of iodine per second (if 300 mg I/mL CM is used) the corresponding enhancement response is twice as strong. Note that changing the iodine concentration of the contrast agent has the same proportional effect on arterial enhancement as changing the injection flow rate.

There are physiologic and practical limitations to increasing the injection flow rates, however. Injection flow rates of 8 mL/s or greater have been shown to not directly translate into stronger enhancement,[15] possibly because of pooling in the central venous system with reflux into the inferior vena cava, a phenomenon that can be observed with even moderate or low flow rates in patients who have significantly decreased cardiac output. High injection flow rates are also limited by the size of the intravenous cannula, most of which would not allow injection rates greater than 6 mL/s for an 18 G cannula, even if warmed (and thus less viscous) contrast agents are used.

Effect of injection duration on arterial enhancement (Rule 2)

The effect of increasing (or shortening) the injection duration is more difficult to understand than the direct relationship of the iodine administration rate, but it is equally important. One intuitive way to think about the effect of the injection duration is shown in **Fig. 1**. A longer injection duration of, for example, 32 seconds (128 mL total volume) can be considered as the sum of eight subsequent injections of small test boluses of 4 seconds' duration (16 mL each). Each of these eight test boluses has its own effect (first pass and recirculation) on arterial enhancement. Under the assumption of a time-invariant linear system,[16] the cumulative enhancement response to the entire 128-mL injection equals the sum (time integral) of each enhancement response to their respective eight test boluses.[14] Note that the recirculation effects of the earlier test boluses overlap (and thus sum up) with the first-pass effects of later test boluses, resulting in the typical continuous increase of arterial enhancement over time.

Physiologic parameters affecting vascular enhancement (Rule 3)

The degree of arterial enhancement following the same intravenous CM injection is highly variable between individuals. Even in patients considered to have normal cardiac output, mid aortic enhancement may range from 140 HU to 440 HU (a factor of three) between patients.[17] If body weight is taken into account, the average aortic enhancement ranges from 92 to 196 HU/mL/kg (a factor of two).[18] Adjusting the CM injection rates (and volumes) to body weight therefore reduces interindividual differences of arterial enhancement, but it does not completely eliminate them. Body-weight adjustment of injections is nevertheless recommended, at least for patients who have small (<60 kg) and large (>90 kg) body size. We adjust all our CT protocols (body and cardiovascular) for patient physique by grouping them in five body-weight groups (**Tables 1–4**). This approach is a practical compromise that allows individualization of CM delivery while avoiding the need for a calculator.

The fundamental physiologic parameter affecting arterial enhancement is cardiac output and,

---

Table 1
Integrated 64-channel CT acquisition and injection protocol for abdominal CT angiography

Acquisition	64 × 0.6 mm (Number of Channels × Channel Width); Automated Tube Current Modulation (250 Quality Reference mAs)		
Pitch	Variable (depends on volume coverage, usually <1.0)		
Scan time	Fixed to 10 s (in all patients)		
Injection duration	Fixed to 18 s (in all patients)		
Scanning delay	t_{CMT} + 8s (scan starts 8 seconds after CM arrives in the aorta, as established with automated bolus triggering)		
Contrast medium	High concentration (350–370 mg I/mL)		
Injection flow rates and volumes	Individualized to body weight		
	Body weight (kg)	CM flow rate (mL/s)	CM volume (mL)
	<55	4.0	72
	56–65	4.5	81
	66–85	5.0	90
	86–95	5.5	99
	>95	6.0	108

Table 2
Injection protocol for 64-channel coronary CT angiography

Scan Time; Injection Duration (Scan Time + 8 s)		≤6 s; 14 s (6 s + 8 s)	8 s; 16 s (8 s + 8 s)	10 s; 18 s (10 s + 8 s)	12 s; 20 s (12 s + 8 s)
Body Weight	CM Flow Rate (mL/s)		CM Volume (mL)		
<55 kg	4.0	55	64	72	80
56–65 kg	4.5	65	72	81	90
66–85 kg	5.0	70	80	90	100
86–95 kg	5.5	75	88	99	110
>95 kg	6.0	85	96	108	120

CM 370 mg I/mL concentration. Scanning delay is t_{CMT} + 8s.

to a lesser extent, central blood volume. Cardiac output is inversely related to the degree of arterial enhancement, particularly in first-pass dynamics.[19] This relationship can be understood intuitively when thinking about a CM injection as flow of iodine (iodine molecules per second), injected into a larger flow of blood (mL of blood per second). The relative amount of flow of iodine into the flow of blood determines the iodine concentration in the blood, and thus its CT attenuation. Arterial enhancement is therefore lower in patients who have high cardiac output, but it is stronger in patients who have low cardiac output (despite the delayed t_{CMT} in the latter).

Enhancement of Normal Liver Parenchyma

Parenchymal enhancement results less from the opacification of blood vessels and more from CM distribution into the extravascular interstitial space of an organ or tissue.[13] The dynamics of hepatic CM enhancement are also influenced by the dual blood supply of the liver, with most hepatic blood flow (approximately 80%) derived from the portal venous system, where any CM bolus is substantially broadened (and delayed) within the splanchnic vasculature.

The enhancement of normal liver parenchyma is much lower than vascular enhancement, and also occurs much later than arterial enhancement (approximately 40 or 50 seconds after aortic enhancement). Scan timing for parenchymal (hepatic venous phase) liver imaging can also be chosen empirically, approximately 70 seconds or later after start of an injection. The hepatic venous enhancement phase (also referred to as the portal venous phase) is also comparably long, and the contrast to low-attenuation liver

Table 3
Integrated 64-channel CT acquisition and injection protocol for lower extremity CTA

Acquisition	64 × 0.6 mm (Number of Channels × Channel Width); Automated Tube Current Modulation (250 Quality Eeference mAs)
Pitch	Variable (depends on volume coverage, usually <1.0)
Scan time	Fixed to 40 s (in all patients)
Injection duration	Fixed to 35 s (in all patients)
Scanning delay	t_{CMT} + 3s (minimum delay)
Contrast medium	High concentration (350–370 mg I/mL)
Injection flow rates and volumes (biphasic)	Maximum flow rate for first 5 s of injection, continued with 80% of this flow rate for 30 s, followed by 30 mL saline flush.
	Body weight (kg) — CM volumes and biphasic flow rates
	<55 — 20 mL (4.0 mL/s) + 96 mL (3.2 mL/s)
	56–65 — 23 mL (4.5 mL/s) + 108 mL (3.6 mL/s)
	66–85 — 25 mL (5.0 mL/s) + 120 mL (4.0 mL/s)
	86–95 — 28 mL (5.5 mL/s) + 132 mL (4.4 mL/s)
	>95 — 30 mL (6.0 mL/s) + 144 mL (4.8 mL/s)

Table 4
Liver and pancreas CT 64-channel injection protocol

High Concentration CM (370 mg I/mL) Injection (∼1.6 mL/kg Body Weight) in 30 s	
Body Weight	Injection Volume @ Flow Rate
<121 lb (<55 kg)	90 mL @ 3.0 mL/s
121–143 lb (<65 kg)	100 mL @ 3.5 mL/s
143–187 lb (75 kg default)	120 mL @ 4.0 mL/s
187–209 lb (>85 kg)	135 mL @ 4.5 mL/s
>209 lb (>95 kg)	150 mL @ 5.0 mL/s

lesions remains adequate for as long as CM has not diffused into the interstitial spaces of low-attenuation solid liver lesions, making them potentially isodense to surrounding normal liver parenchyma. Certain liver lesions, notably well-differentiated hepatocellular carcinomas, remain or become hypoattenuating even later, in the so-called "delayed" or equilibrium/post-equilibrium phase, which occurs approximately 3 to 5 minutes after contrast delivery. Delayed-phase imaging may improve the sensitivity of hepatocellular carcinoma (HCC) in cirrhotic livers.[20,21] Even later imaging (10–15 minutes or more) depicts CM retention in fibrous components of neoplasms, such as tumor capsules and cholangiocellular carcinomas.[22–24]

Enhancement of normal liver parenchyma—and thus the contrast to low-attenuation liver lesions—is independent of the injection flow rate, but is directly proportional to the total amount of CM (iodine) delivered. The main physiologic parameter affecting the strength of CM enhancement of normal liver parenchyma is body weight. Although body weight may not be the best surrogate marker for extracellular fluid space, notably in obese patients, it is more readily available than lean body weight.[25] As a ballpark rule, 500 to 600 mg of iodine per kilogram of bodyweight achieves adequate hepatic parenchymal enhancement. Adjustment of CM volume to body size is again recommended, as described previously (see **Table 4**).

Enhancement of Hypervascular Liver Lesions

The enhancement dynamics of so-called "hypervascular" liver lesions is fundamentally different when compared with normal liver parenchyma (**Fig. 2**). Such lesions are characterized by their systemic arterial rather than portal venous blood supply, and therefore demonstrate an earlier enhancement than surrounding normal liver parenchyma, somewhat comparable to the enhancement of the spleen. Scan timing is critical to maximize the contrast (attenuation difference) between

hypervascular lesions and normal liver parenchyma. Because hypervascular liver lesion opacification increases slightly later than opacification of the supplying artery, it is best to image such lesions as late as possible, yet before the surrounding liver parenchyma has a chance to increase the background attenuation from portal venous CM. This particular phase of enhancement is commonly referred to as the late arterial phase and occurs approximately 10 to 15 seconds after CM arrival in the aorta.[26] Note that at that time the portal vein branches (but not the parenchyma or hepatic veins) will be slightly opacified, hence the alternative term "portal venous inflow phase" (see **Fig. 2**).

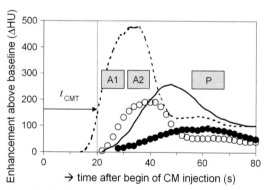

Fig. 2. Early CM dynamics of the liver. Hepatic vascular and parenchymal time attenuation curves modeled for an injection duration of 20 seconds. Normal hepatic parenchymal enhancement (*solid circle*) is comparably low and delayed relative to enhancement of the portal vein (*solid line*). The enhancement of a hypervascular liver lesion (*open circle*) follows arterial enhancement (*dashed line*), and thus slightly precedes portal venous and hepatic parenchymal enhancement. The early arterial phase (A1) begins immediately after the contrast medium transit time (t_{CMT}). The late arterial phase (A2) begins 10 to 15 seconds after the t_{CMT} and provides the best contrast between hypervascular liver lesion and normal liver parenchyma. The parenchymal phase (hepatic venous phase) occurs approximately 40 seconds after the t_{CMT}.

Because of their intimate relationship to arterial contrast dynamics, the enhancement of hypervascular liver lesions can be controlled by the same parameters that affect arterial enhancement: Fast injection flow rates and high-concentration CM (overall greater iodine flux) result in stronger enhancement of hypervascular lesions and thus increased lesion-to-background contrast.[27,28] Scan timing is critical, obviously, and should be chosen relative to the arrival of CM (t_{CMT}) in the abdominal aorta.

Enhancement of the Pancreas

The enhancement kinetics of other solid organs, such as the normal pancreas, also follow arterial dynamics. There is a longer delay necessary to increase the opacification of the interstitial spaces of the organ of interest, and hence to increase the contrast to the ductal system and the lesion-to-background contrast for hypovascular pancreatic lesions, such as most adenocarcinomas. Pancreatic imaging thus also benefits from high iodine flux and accurate scan timing relative to the t_{CMT},[29] but also improves with larger CM volumes. Scan timing is critical, and best lesion-to-background contrast is achieved approximately 20 to 25 seconds after CM arrival in the aorta[29,30] (for injection durations of 30 seconds, and scan times of approximately 5 seconds). Enhancement of the celiac and superior mesenteric arteries and the splenic vein remains strong in this phase also. The superior mesenteric vein is often not well opacified in this phase. The degree of pancreatic enhancement is also affected by a patient's body weight, and adjusting the iodine dose and the injection flow rate (to maintain constant injection durations) to body weight decreases the variability of pancreatic enhancement between individuals.[31]

If hypervascular pancreatic lesions are suspected or known and followed (eg, neuroendocrine tumors) the delay can be chosen shorter, before normal pancreatic tissue has enhanced strongly. A delay of approximately 10 to 15 seconds after aortic opacification is adequate. Again, high iodine administration rates are beneficial.

SYNCHRONIZING CONTRAST MEDIUM ENHANCEMENT WITH CT DATA ACQUISITION

A fixed, empiric scanning delay remains adequate for many routine CT applications. For example, for routine CM-enhanced thoracic CT, small to moderate amounts of CM suffice to delineate the hilar vessels. A fixed scanning delay of approximately 40 to 50 seconds also allows opacification of tumors or pleural enhancement. With fast scanners, the thorax can be scanned within a few seconds (3–6 seconds), and the data acquisition should be initiated approximately 10 seconds after the entire bolus has been injected to avoid artifacts from unopacified contrast in the great thoracic veins. As an example, we inject 1 mL/kg body weight within 30 seconds, and use a fixed delay of 40 seconds in this instance. For routine chest-abdomen-pelvis CT we inject 1.6 mL/kg body weight in 40 seconds, and scan after a fixed delay of 70 seconds.

Fixed, empiric scanning delays cannot be recommended for cardiac or vascular CT, (and also dedicated phase-sensitive scans for liver and pancreas imaging) because the arterial t_{CMT} is prohibitively variable between individual patients, ranging from as short as 8 to as long as 40 seconds in patients who have cardiovascular diseases. The scanning delay (the time interval between the beginning of a CM injection and the initiation of CT data acquisition) needs to be timed relative to the t_{CMT} of the vascular territory of interest. With fast MDCT acquisitions the t_{CMT} itself does not necessarily serve as the scanning delay, as was the case with slower single-detector CT systems, but the t_{CMT} rather serves as a landmark relative to which the scanning delay can be individualized. Depending on the vessels of interest an additional delay relative to the t_{CMT} can be selected. In CTA, this additional delay may be as short as 2 seconds (t_{CMT} + 2s), but often slightly longer delays of 5 or 8 seconds are used (t_{CMT} + 8s). The notation "t_{CMT} + 8s" means that the scan is initiated 8 seconds after the CM has arrived in the target vasculature. Even longer relative delays are used for early-arterial or late-arterial phases of the liver and for pancreatic imaging, as described previously. Transit times can be easily determined using either a test-bolus injection or an automatic bolus triggering technique.

Test Bolus

The injection of a small test bolus (15–20 mL) while acquiring a low-dose dynamic (non-incremental) CT acquisition is a reliable means to determine the t_{CMT} from the intravenous injection site to the arterial territory of interest.[32] The t_{CMT} equals the time-to-peak enhancement interval measured in a region of interest (ROI) placed within a reference vessel (see **Fig. 1**). The advantage of using a test bolus is its reliability and accuracy in predicting the t_{CMT}, notably for cardiac and coronary CTA. Theoretically, the information contained in the time-attenuation response to a test bolus can also be exploited to predict and individually tailor the subsequent injection to achieve a desired enhancement plateau.[16,33]

Automated Bolus Triggering

For automated bolus triggering, a circular ROI is placed into the target vessel on a nonenhanced image.[34] While CM is injected, a series of low-dose non-incremental scans are obtained and the attenuation within the ROI is monitored. The t_{CMT} equals the time when a predefined enhancement threshold (trigger level) is reached (eg, 100 ΔHU). For technical reasons, however, the CT acquisition cannot begin immediately and automated bolus triggering causes a slight delay relative to the t_{CMT}. This inherent delay depends on the scanner model and on the longitudinal distance between the monitoring series and the starting position of the scan. Also, if a prerecorded breath-holding command is programmed into the CT acquisition, this increases the minimal delay before a scan can be initiated. The minimal trigger delay after CM arrival when using automated bolus triggering is usually 2 seconds, which can be ignored when designing an injection protocol. If a longer trigger delay is necessary or intentionally chosen (eg, 8 seconds, t_{CMT} + 8s), the injection duration needs to be increased accordingly to guarantee a long enough enhancement phase within the vascular territory of interest. Bolus triggering is a robust and practical technique for routine use and has the advantage of not requiring an additional test bolus injection, thus decreasing the total contrast used. It also eliminates unwanted organ enhancement (eg, renal collecting system) in the subsequent full bolus study.

SCANNING AND INJECTION PROTOCOL DESIGN

The design of CT protocols aims at standardizing the sequence of events for a wide array of CT studies, which are routinely applied on a daily basis. CT protocols are tailored to the organ of interest and optimized for a given scanner. The sequence of acquisitions (digital radiograph for selecting the scanning range, precontrast, postcontrast, and delayed acquisitions, and so forth) with their respective technical acquisition and reconstruction parameters (kVp, mAs, detector configuration, pitch, rotation time, slice thickness/interval, reconstruction kernel, and so forth) are preprogrammed into the scanner menu. Injection parameters are kept as a separate paper or electronic file; however, this may change in the future and injection protocols may be stored in the memory of a power injector or on the scanner console.

A detailed discussion of the trade-offs of CT image acquisition and reconstruction parameters is beyond the scope of this article, but two recent developments deserve special attention in the context of scanning and injection protocol design: automated tube current modulation and acquisition speed.

Automated Tube Current Modulation

Modern CT scanners are equipped with powerful x-ray tubes and the complex relationship between tube power, gantry rotation time, pitch, and image noise make manual selection of exposure parameters unintuitive and may result in unnecessarily high radiation exposure (notably in slim individuals) or suboptimal image quality with excessive noise (typically in very obese patients). Automated tube current modulation is available on all modern CT scanners and should be used in all protocols, with a few exceptions (head, and ECG gated scans). The various techniques of automated tube current modulation substantially decrease the wide range of noise observed between different patient studies (**Fig. 3**) but also result in more uniform noise within a given CT study by delivering more dose where it is needed (eg, lateral projections through the shoulders, pelvis), and reducing the tube output for projections through tissue with less x-ray absorption.[35,36] The practical implementations of automated tube current modulation—notably the user input—differ significantly between scanner manufacturers, but the principle is that the user selects a desired/acceptable image quality (quality reference mAs) or image noise (noise index) rather than selecting a particular tube current.

Advantages and Disadvantages of Fast CT Acquisitions

All modern CT scanners (notably 64-channel systems and beyond) allow fast data acquisition with short scan times, which has several obvious advantages. Shorter scan times allow for easier breath-holding and are the prerequisite for imaging during dedicated phases of organ enhancement. Fast gantry rotations are also fundamental for cardiac imaging because the gantry rotation time directly translates into temporal resolution. In the setting of cardiovascular CT applications, shorter scan times also allow for the use of less total CM volumes and larger anatomic coverage. Fast scan times also come with potential disadvantages. First, short scan times usually need faster CM injections, and the traditional strategy of selecting the injection duration equal to the scan time is no longer adequate. Second, fast data acquisitions may in fact be too fast in situations in which vascular opacification is delayed because of pathologic conditions. For example, opacification of large aneurysms may take several seconds

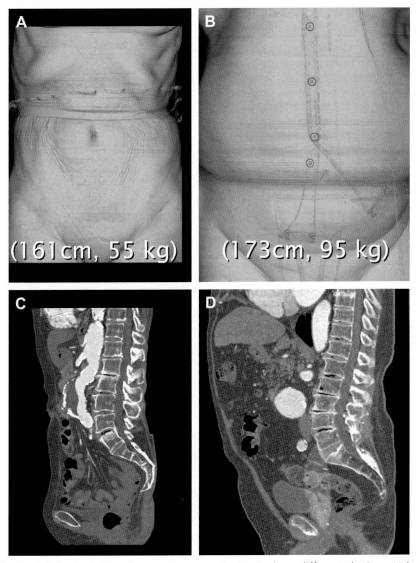

Fig. 3. Individualized abdominal CT angiograms in two patients who have different physique. Volume-rendered images of an 81-year-old slim (55 kg) woman (A) and an 83-year-old obese (95 kg) man (B) illustrate different body habitus of two patients who underwent abdominal CT angiograms using automated tube current modulation and body weight–adjusted CM injections. Corresponding sagittal reformations (C, D) demonstrate comparable image quality (image noise, arterial opacification) despite markedly different patient physique. Identical selection of 250 quality reference mA with automated tube current modulation resulted in 136 effective mA in the slim patient (A), but in 270 effective mA in the obese patient (B).

because of slow mixing of opacified blood with non-opacified blood, and filling of arteries distal to significantly diseased vessels may also substantially delay the propagation of an intravenously injected bolus downstream. This delay is most commonly encountered in lower extremity CTA for peripheral arterial disease.[37]

In the single-detector CT era one would aim at selecting the fastest possible table speed; this is not necessarily the best choice with modern CT equipment. Deliberately scanning at a moderate table speed, or allowing the bolus a head start, is a more appropriate and reliable strategy. Another benefit of not using the fastest possible acquisition speed is that slower scans (with submaximal gantry rotation speed and submaximal pitch) provide a considerable cushion of tube power, which may be needed in large and obese patients to maintain acceptable image noise.

Contrast Medium Injection Strategies for Cardiovascular CT

The traditional paradigm of injection protocol design for CTA aims at choosing an injection flow rate and injection duration that match the scan time. Scan times for CTA vary widely, however, and may range from more than 30 seconds for a thoracoabdominal CTA using a 4-channel MDCT to as short as 4 seconds for an abdominal CTA using a 64-channel MDCT. Even shorter scan times will become possible in the near future. No universal strategy of CM injection for cardiovascular CT can therefore be applied to all scanners.

Basic strategy: injection time equals scan time

The traditional injection strategy for CTA, derived in the era of single-slice CT, was to inject CM for a duration that is equal to the scan time. For a 40-second abdominal CTA acquisition, the injection duration would also be 40 seconds, resulting in a fairly large CM dose of 160 mL if a typical injection flow rate of 4 mL/s was used. Scan timing was determined either by using a test bolus or by bolus tracking.

This basic strategy is still useful for many CTA applications and for cardiac CT, whenever scan times are in the range of 10 to 20 seconds. Over the years of CT evolution with increasingly shorter scan times, the injection flow rates have increased from 4 mL/s to 5 mL/s and even 6 mL/s. At the same time, the iodine concentration of the CM used has also increased from the traditional 300 mg I/mL to 350, 370, or 400 mg I/mL at most institutions. This increase is not at all surprising, because the lower opacification from shorter injections (a consequence of Rule 2) has to be compensated for by increasing the iodine flux (see Rule 1) (**Fig. 4**). By increasing the injection flow rate from 4 to 5 mL/s and using a contrast agent with, for example, 350 rather than 300 mg I/mL concentration, the iodine flux and thus arterial enhancement is increased by 45%.

Basic strategy with additionally increased scanning delay

With even faster scanners it became readily apparent that the basic strategy (injection duration equals scan time) alone is not applicable for scan times well below 10 seconds. The obvious solution is simply to increase the injection duration and to increase the scanning delay accordingly; in other words, make use of Rule 2. Note that with this approach the injection duration is no longer equal to but is longer than the scan time, and the scanning delay is not equal to but is longer than the tCMT (see **Fig. 4**).

Strategies for 64-channel CT and beyond: the paradigm shift

As opposed to the previous strategies, wherein the injection duration was chosen to match the scan time (plus increased delay), the technical capabilities of modern 64-channel scanners allow a reversal of the traditional paradigm: we no longer select the injection duration based on the scan time, but we select the scan time based on a injection protocol that allows good opacification with reasonable injection flow rates for a wide range of patients. The average injection flow rate is a moderate 5 mL/s, which allows down-regulating (≤4 mL/s) and up-regulating (≥6 mL/s) the flow rates according to patients' physiology.

Our current integrated scanning and CM injection strategy for 64-channel CTA is, therefore, to deliberately slow down the CT acquisition and, importantly, use the same scan time for a given vascular territory for every patient (the pitch thus varies between patients and tube output is controlled by automated tube current modulation). When the same scan time is used for all patients, one can always use the same injection duration also, which simplifies individualizing the flow rates (and volumes) for different patient physiology. For example, we use a fixed scan time of 10 seconds for abdominal CTA, with an injection duration of 18 seconds, and a scanning delay of tCMT + 8 seconds, as determined by bolus triggering (see **Table 1**). This strategy allows breath-holding for virtually all patients. It results in reliably strong arterial enhancement because of high iodine flux and increased scanning delay relative to the tCMT, while avoiding excessive injection flow rates. Image noise is constant within and across individuals by using automated tube current modulation.

A similar approach is used for other vascular territories. Slight modifications are needed for cardiac CT and for lower extremity CTA. In cardiac CT, the scan time cannot be predetermined, because gantry rotation time and pitch have to be adapted to the heart rate. Scan times are reasonably similar across patients to allow individualizing the injection flow rates and volumes (see **Table 2**). Instead of flushing the veins with saline alone, it is advantageous to flush the veins with diluted contrast (70%–80% saline, 20%–30% CM) to maintain right ventricular opacification.

Lower extremity CTA benefits from deliberately slowing down the acquisition even more. Because of the potentially slow propagation of a CM bolus within a diseased lower extremity arterial tree, we always use a scan time of 40 seconds.[37–39] The injection duration is always 35 seconds; this is possible because the data acquisition follows the bolus

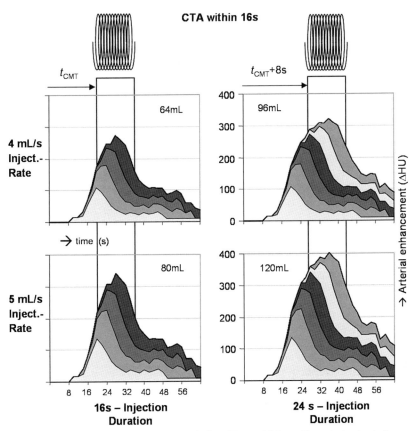

CTA within 16s

t_{CMT} $t_{CMT}+8s$

64mL   96mL

4 mL/s
Inject.-
Rate

→ time (s)

→ Arterial enhancement (ΔHU)

80mL   120mL

5 mL/s
Inject.-
Rate

8 16 24 32 40 48 56   8 16 24 32 40 48 56

16s – Injection Duration   **24 s – Injection Duration**

Fig. 4. Strategies to improve arterial enhancement with fast CT acquisitions. Two strategies to increase arterial enhancement compared with what can be achieved from a 16-second injection at 4 mL/s (*upper left panel*) can be used alone or in combination. Increasing the injection rate from 4 to 5 mL/s increases the enhancement approximately 20% (*lower left panel*). Alternatively, one can also increase the injection duration and the scanning delay, taking advantage of the increase of enhancement with longer injection durations (*right upper panel*). Maximum enhancement can be achieved when both the injection rate (or the iodine concentration) and the injection duration are increased (*right lower panel*) simultaneously. (*From* Fleischmann D. Present and future trends in multiple detector-row CT applications: CT angiography. Eur Radiol 2002;12:S11; with permission.)

down the arterial tree and the injection duration can therefore be shorter than the scan time (see **Table 3**).

Contrast Medium Injection Strategies for 64-Channel Multidetector-Row CT of the Liver and Pancreas

For CT studies of the liver, the scanning and injection protocols are adapted to the clinical indication. Routine abdomen or chest-abdomen-pelvis CT scans aim at imaging of the liver during a hepatic venous phase only. The acquisition parameters are chosen to cover the entire anatomic area of interest. We adjust the CM volume to patient weight (~ 1.6 mL/kg body weight of 350 mg I/mL CM, injected within 40 seconds) and use a simple fixed scanning delay of 70 seconds in this instance.

Dedicated liver studies are acquired at predefined phases of enhancement. Each acquisition is short, approximately 3 to 5 seconds. The selection of image acquisition windows is timed relative to the CM arrival in the aorta (t_{CMT}). Early arterial phase images are generally used for pure arterial imaging and anatomic mapping, such as in preoperative evaluation for living related liver donor evaluation. Our routine triphasic liver CT includes a late arterial phase (for optimal visualization of suspected hypervascular lesions), a hepatic venous phase, and a 3-minute delayed phase. Recent studies have found the 3-minute delayed phase images highly useful in detecting well-differentiated hepatocellular carcinomas that wash out relative to the adjacent liver, which otherwise may have been missed on arterial or portal venous phase images.[20] Occasionally a post-equilibrium 10- to 15-minute delayed phase is used instead of, or in addition to, the 3-minute delayed-phase scan in cases such as suspected or known cholangiocarcinoma.

Table 5
Enhancement phases and scanning delays for 64-channel CT of the liver

	Enhancement Phase	Timing	Indication/Role
0	Noncontrast	NA	Recurrent pyogenic cholangitis, postembolization
(A)	Early arterial phase	t_{CMT} + 8s	CTA, arterial mapping
B[a]	Late arterial phase	t_{CMT} + 16s	Assessment of hypervascular liver lesions
C[a]	Portal venous phase (hepatic venous phase)	t_{CMT} + 50s (or 35 s after B)	Assessment of hypoattenuating liver lesions, relationship of portal and hepatic veins to lesion
D[a]	Delayed—equilibrium phase	~3 min	Detection of well-differentiated HCCs with early washout, retention of contrast in hemangiomas
(E)	Delayed—post-equilibrium phase	~10–15 min	Assess for delayed retention of contrast in cholangiocarcinoma

[a] Phases B + C represent a biphasic liver protocol; B + C + D represent a triphasic liver protocol.

Nonenhanced scans are not routinely included in our triphasic liver protocols, but may be helpful in the setting of recurrent pyogenic cholangitis wherein intrahepatic biliary stones are best seen on noncontrast images. Noncontrast images may also be useful in the setting of post–chemo infusion to differentiate retained chemo-infused material from contrast enhancement. Even if noncontrast images are not obtained, chemo-infused material should also be easily detected and identifiable on the 3- to 5-minute delayed images. For phase-selective liver CT, the injection volumes and flow rates are again adjusted to body weight groups (see **Table 4**). The specific timing parameters are given in **Table 5**. Automated tube-current modulation is always used.

Our dedicated pancreatic CT protocol includes a nonenhanced scan, a contrast-enhanced scan optimized for pancreatic parenchymal enhancement (pancreatic phase), and a hepatic venous phase, which also includes the liver. We use the same CM volumes and flow rates, adjusted to

Table 6
Enhancement phases and scanning delays for 64-channel CT of the pancreas

	Enhancement Phase	Timing	Indication/Role
0	Noncontrast	NA	Routinely obtained to localize pancreas and assess for pancreatic calcifications
(A)	Arterial phase	t_{CMT} + 8s	Optional, alternative for B, for suspected/known hypervascular lesions (eg, neuroendocrine tumors)
B	Pancreatic phase	t_{CMT} + 25s	Assessment of hypovascular (and often also hypervascular) pancreatic lesions, relation to pancreatic duct, degree of encasement of arteries by pancreatic tumor
C	Portal venous phase (hepatic venous phase)	25 s after B (40 s after A)	Assessment of perivenous tumor extension and evaluation of hypoattenuating liver lesions

body weight, as for the dedicated liver studies, and scan timing is accomplished with automated bolus triggering relative to aortic enhancement **(Table 6)**, which differs from the liver protocol.

SUMMARY

CM delivery remains an integral part of state-of-the arte body and cardiovascular CT. Although CT technology continues to evolve, the physiologic and pharmacokinetic principles of arterial and parenchymal enhancement will remain unchanged in the foreseeable future. A basic understanding of early CM dynamics thus provides the foundation for the design of current and future CT scanning and injection protocols. With these tools at hand, CM use can be optimized for a wide variety of clinical CT applications and optimized for each patient while exploiting the full capabilities of this powerful imaging technology.

REFERENCES

1. Dawson P, Blomley MJ. Contrast media as extracellular fluid space markers: adaptation of the central volume theorem. British Journal of Radiology 1996;69: 717–22.
2. Hill JA, Winniford M, Cohen MB, et al. Multicenter trial of ionic versus nonionic contrast media for cardiac angiography. The iohexol cooperative study. Am J Cardiol 1993;72:770.
3. Katayama H, Yamaguchi K, Kozuka T, et al. Adverse reactions to ionic and nonionic contrast media. A report from the Japanese committee on the safety of contrast media. Radiology 1990;175:621.
4. Palmer FJ. The RACR survey of intravenous contrast media reactions. Final report. Australas Radiol 1988; 32:426.
5. Wolf GL, Arenson RL, Cross AP. A prospective trial of ionic vs nonionic contrast agents in routine clinical practice: comparison of adverse effects. AJR Am J Roentgenol 1989;152:939.
6. Hopper KD. With helical CT, is nonionic contrast a better choice than ionic contrast for rapid and large IV bolus injections? AJR Am J Roentgenol 1996;166:715.
7. Manual on contrast media, version 6. Reston (VA): American College of Radiology; 2008.
8. Thomsen HS, editor. Contrast media: safety issues and user guidelines, 1st edition. (Medical radiology - diagnostic imaging and radiation oncology), New York: Springer; 2005.
9. Thomsen HS, Morcos SK. Management of acute adverse reactions to contrast media. Eur Radiol 2004;14:476.
10. Aspelin P, Aubry P, Fransson SG, et al. Nephrotoxic effects in high-risk patients undergoing angiography. N Engl J Med 2003;348:491.
11. Barrett BJ, Katzberg RW, Thomsen HS, et al. Contrast-induced nephropathy in patients with chronic kidney disease undergoing computed tomography: a double-blind comparison of iodixanol and iopamidol. Invest Radiol 2006;41:815.
12. Katzberg RW, Barrett BJ. Risk of iodinated contrast material–induced nephropathy with intravenous administration. Radiology 2007;243:622.
13. Dawson P, Blomley MJ. Contrast agent pharmacokinetics revisited: I. Reformulation. Acad Radiol 1996; 3(Suppl 2):S261.
14. Fleischmann D. Present and future trends in multiple detector-row CT applications: CT angiography. Europ Radiol 2002;12:S11.
15. Claussen CD, Banzer D, Pfretzschner C, et al. Bolus geometry and dynamics after intravenous contrast-medium injection. Radiology 1984;153:365.
16. Fleischmann D, Hittmair K. Mathematical analysis of arterial enhancement and optimization of bolus geometry for CT angiography using the discrete Fourier transform. J Comput Assist Tomogr 1999;23:474.
17. Sheiman RG, Raptopoulos V, Caruso P, et al. Comparison of tailored and empiric scan delays for CT angiography of the abdomen. AJR Am J Roentgenol 1996;167:725.
18. Hittmair K, Fleischmann D. Accuracy of predicting and controlling time-dependent aortic enhancement from a test bolus injection. J Comput Assist Tomogr 2001;25:287.
19. Bae KT, Heiken JP, Brink JA. Aortic and hepatic contrast medium enhancement at CT. Part II. Effect of reduced cardiac output in a porcine model. Radiology 1998;207:657.
20. Iannaccone R, Laghi A, Catalano C, et al. Hepatocellular carcinoma: role of unenhanced and delayed phase multi-detector row helical CT in patients with cirrhosis. Radiology 2005;234:460.
21. Lim JH, Choi D, Kim SH, et al. Detection of hepatocellular carcinoma: value of adding delayed phase imaging to dual-phase helical CT. Am J Roentgenol 2002;179:67.
22. Asayama Y, Yoshimitsu K, Irie H, et al. Delayed-phase dynamic CT enhancement as a prognostic factor for mass-forming intrahepatic cholangiocarcinoma. Radiology 2005;238:150.
23. Keogan MT, Seabourn JT, Paulson EK, et al. Contrast-enhanced CT of intrahepatic and hilar cholangiocarcinoma: delay time for optimal imaging. AJR Am J Roentgenol 1997;169:1493.
24. Lacomis J, Baron R, Oliver J 3rd, et al. Cholangiocarcinoma: delayed CT contrast enhancement patterns. Radiology 1997;203:98.
25. Ho LM, Nelson RC, Delong DM. Determining contrast medium dose and rate on basis of lean

body weight: does this strategy improve patient-to-patient uniformity of hepatic enhancement during multi-detector row CT? Radiology 2007;243:431.

26. Foley WD, Mallisee TA, Hohenwalter MD, et al. Multiphase hepatic CT with a multirow detector CT scanner. AJR Am J Roentgenol 2000;175:679.

27. Awai K, Takada K, Onishi H, et al. Aortic and hepatic enhancement and tumor-to-liver contrast: analysis of the effect of different concentrations of contrast material at multi-detector row helical CT. Radiology 2002;224:757.

28. Schima W, Hammerstingl R, Catalano C, et al. Quadruple-phase MDCT of the liver in patients with suspected hepatocellular carcinoma: effect of contrast material flow rate. Am J Roentgenol 2006;186:1571.

29. Schueller G, Schima W, Schueller-Weidekamm C, et al. Multidetector ct of pancreas: effects of contrast material flow rate and individualized scan delay on enhancement of pancreas and tumor contrast. Radiology 2006;241:441.

30. Kondo H, Kanematsu M, Goshima S, et al. MDCT of the pancreas: optimizing scanning delay with a bolus-tracking technique for pancreatic, peripancreatic vascular, and hepatic contrast enhancement. Am J Roentgenol 2007;188:751.

31. Yanaga Y, Awai K, Nakayama Y, et al. Pancreas: patient body weight tailored contrast material injection protocol versus fixed dose protocol at dynamic CT. Radiology 2007;245:475.

32. Van Hoe L, Marchal G, Baert AL, et al. Determination of scan delay-time in spiral CT-angiography: utility of a test bolus injection. J Comput Assist Tomogr 1995;19:216.

33. Fleischmann D, Rubin GD, Bankier AA, et al. Improved uniformity of aortic enhancement with customized contrast medium injection protocols at CT angiography. Radiology 2000;214:363.

34. Birnbaum BA, Jacobs JE, Langlotz CP, et al. Assessment of a bolus-tracking technique in helical renal CT to optimize nephrographic phase imaging. Radiology 1999;211:87.

35. Mastora I, Remy-Jardin M, Delannoy V, et al. Multidetector row spiral CT angiography of the thoracic outlet: dose reduction with anatomically adapted online tube current modulation and preset dose savings. Radiology 2004;230:116.

36. Rizzo S, Kalra M, Schmidt B, et al. Comparison of angular and combined automatic tube current modulation techniques with constant tube current ct of the abdomen and pelvis. Am J Roentgenol 2006;186:673.

37. Fleischmann D, Rubin GD. Quantification of intravenously administered contrast medium transit through the peripheral arteries: implications for CT angiography. Radiology 2005;236:1076–82.

38. Fleischmann D, Hallett RL, Rubin GD. CT angiography of peripheral arterial disease. J Vasc Interv Radiol 2006;17:3.

39. Fleischmann D. Contrast-medium administration. In: Catalano C, Passariello R, editors. Multidetector-row CT angiography. Berlin, Heidelberg, New York: Springer; 2005. p. 41.

Strategies for Reducing Radiation Dose in CT

Cynthia H. McCollough, PhD*, Andrew N. Primak, PhD,
Natalie Braun, BS, James Kofler, PhD, Lifeng Yu, PhD,
Jodie Christner, PhD

KEYWORDS

- CT • Radiation dose • Cardiac CT • Dose reduction
- Automatic exposure control • Effective dose

BACKGROUND AND SIGNIFICANCE

High-end CT systems allow acquisition of isotropic volumetric data sets that permit high quality reformatted images and images with less than 1 mm slice thickness. These capabilities have greatly expanded the usefulness of CT, and CT usage has correspondingly increased, replacing more and more radiographic examinations. In 1990, approximately 13 million CT scans were performed in the United States.[1] In 2000, the number of CT scans more than tripled to approximately 46 million.[1] The estimated number of CT scans for 2006 is 62 million.[1] With high-quality CT imaging being performed more frequently, patients can benefit from a quicker and more accurate diagnosis and precise anatomic information for planning therapeutic procedures. Despite the tremendous contributions of CT to modern health care, however, some attention must also be given to the small health risk associated with the ionizing radiation received during a CT examination.

CT scanners create cross-sectional images by measuring x-ray attenuation properties of the body from many different directions. Currently, the radiation dose associated with a typical CT scan (1–14 mSv depending on the examination) is comparable to the annual dose received from natural sources of radiation, such as radon and cosmic radiation (1–10 mSv), depending on where a person lives.[2] The health risk to an individual from exposure to radiation from a typical CT scan is thus comparable to background levels of radiation. Considering the growing population of people undergoing CT scans, however, the implications of CT radiation dose on public health effects may be significant, although considerable debate exists regarding this assumption. One study suggested that as much as 0.4% of all current cancers in the United States may be attributable to the radiation from CT studies based on CT usage data from 1991 to 1996.[1] When organ-specific cancer risk was adjusted for current levels of CT usage, it was determined that 1.5% to 2% of cancers may eventually be caused by the ionizing radiation used in CT.[1] This study and a similar series of previous articles[3,4] received considerable attention from the public media. One positive effect of the media attention was that the CT community was obliged to review the amount of radiation prescribed for CT scans, especially for pediatric patients. This review ultimately resulted in an aggressive effort to minimize CT doses and optimize image quality. Concurrently, new technologies, such as automatic exposure control (AEC), were in development, and were eventually made commercially available for all current CT systems. The use of AEC greatly enhances and simplifies efforts to decrease patient dose.

The media reporting on the risk of CT radiation doses has had a negative effect on the public's perception of CT imaging and radiation, influenced by the sensationalist and alarmist tone of the news stories. Phrases such as "…dangerous radiation from 'super X-rays'…"[5] and comparisons to atomic bomb survivors[6] exploit the public's general apprehension of radiation. Although informing the public of potential health risks—even small

Department of Radiology, Mayo Clinic, 200 First Street SW, Rochester, MN 55905, USA
* Corresponding author.
E-mail address: mccollough.cynthia@mayo.edu (C.H. McCollough).

Radiol Clin N Am 47 (2009) 27–40
doi:10.1016/j.rcl.2008.10.006
0033-8389/08/$ – see front matter

risks—is not inappropriate, journalistic responsibility should ensure that the data are presented so as not to exaggerate or present the risk estimates in a manner that can be easily misinterpreted by a population that, in general, is not sufficiently knowledgeable in radiation or radiobiology to accurately assess the information. Such alarmist articles are a public disservice in that they cause unnecessary stress to patients, or in some cases may persuade a patient to decline a CT scan that could have a positive health impact. The latter case cannot be overstated because low-level radiation risk estimates, which are derived primarily from atomic bomb survivors and have considerable uncertainties at low doses (<100 mSv), give no consideration to the medical benefit of a CT scan. There is no question that the benefit of an appropriately indicated CT scan far exceeds the associated estimated risk or that CT providers need to prescribe the minimal amount of radiation required to obtain images adequate for evaluating the patient's condition. In general, the medical community needs to better educate the public to the risks and benefits associated with CT so that they can make informed decisions regarding their health care.

BRIEF TUTORIAL ON THE MEASUREMENT OF RADIATION OUTPUT FOR CT
Scanner Output

The computed tomography dose index (CTDI) is the primary metric used in CT to describe the radiation output from a scanner. It is a measure of the amount of radiation delivered from a series of contiguous irradiations to a pair of standardized acrylic phantoms. It is, however, measured from one axial CT scan (one rotation of the x-ray tube).[7-10] The CTDI was defined in the early days of CT, when dose assessments were made using thermoluminescent dosimeters and multiple axial scans, each one incremented from the previous scan by the nominal beam width. This procedure was not only time consuming and laborious, but also required many scans (exposures) for each beam width, phantom size, tube potential setting (kV), and position in the field of view (FOV, periphery or center). The resultant parameter was referred to as the multiple-scan average dose (MSAD), which was typically a factor of two to three times higher than the peak radiation dose from one axial scan. Shope and Gagne[9] demonstrated the mathematical equivalence between the scan intensive MSAD and the CTDI, which is able to be measured using only one scan (one gantry rotation), when certain criteria are met with

regard to the length of the ionization chamber and the length of the clinical scan being assessed.

The theoretically perfect equivalence of MSAD and CDTI is not achieved in many clinical scenarios, but because of the speed and ease of CTDI measurements, the use of MSAD declined. CTDI is now used internationally following a standardized measurement technique. Several variants of CTDI exist that describe specific steps in the measurement and calculation processes. These include the $CTDI_{100}$ and the weighted CTDI ($CTDI_w$). These parameters are described in multiple publications.[11-13]

Volume CT dose index
The CTDI variant that is currently of most relevance is the volume CTDI ($CTDI_{vol}$). This parameter accounts for gaps or overlaps between the x-ray beams from consecutive rotations of the x-ray source and variations in dose across the FOV. The $CTDI_{vol}$ provides a single parameter, based on a directly and easily measured quantity, which describes the radiation delivered to the scan volume for a standardized (CTDI) phantom.[13] The SI units are milligray (mGy). $CTDI_{vol}$ is a useful indicator of the radiation output for a specific examination protocol, because it takes into account protocol-specific information, such as pitch. $CTDI_{vol}$ is not a direct measurement of dose; it is a standardized measure of radiation output in the CT environment.[14]

Dose-length product
To better represent the overall energy delivered by a given scan protocol, the $CTDI_{vol}$ can be integrated along the scan length to compute the dose-length product (DLP),[7] where the DLP (in mGy-cm) is equal to $CTDI_{vol}$ (in mGy) times scan length (in cm). The DLP reflects the integrated radiation output (and thus the potential biologic effect) attributable to the complete scan acquisition. An abdomen-only CT examination might have the same $CTDI_{vol}$ as an abdomen/pelvis CT examination, but the latter examination would have a greater DLP, proportional to the greater z-extent of the scan volume.

Effective Dose

Effective dose, E, is not a measurement of dose, but rather a concept that reflects the stochastic risk (eg, cancer induction) from an exposure to ionizing radiation.[15,16] It is typically expressed in the units of millisieverts. Effective dose reflects radiation detriment averaged over gender and age and its use has several limitations when applied to medical populations.[15-18] In particular, it uses a mathematical model for a "standard" body in its calculation[19] and is hence not an appropriate risk indicator for any one individual. It does, however, facilitate the comparison of biologic effect between diagnostic examinations of different types or having different acquisition parameters.[15,16] By comparing patient effective dose to background radiation dose from natural sources, which in the United States averages 3 mSv per year with a range across the United States from 1 to 10 mSv,[2] patients and their families are better able to put the risk associated with medical doses into perspective.

The European Working Group for Guidelines on Quality Criteria in CT has proposed a generic estimation method for effective dose.[7] A set of coefficients k, where the values of k depend only on the region of the body being scanned (**Table 1**),[20–21] were determined in relation to the DLP. E (in mSv) can thus be estimated by multiplying the DLP value (in mGy-cm), which is reported on most CT systems, by the region-specific k coefficient (in mSv/(mGy-cm)).

The values of E predicted by DLP and the values of E estimated using more rigorous calculation methods are remarkably consistent, with a maximum deviation from the mean of approximately 10% to 15%.[22] Thus, the use of DLP to estimate E seems to be a reasonably robust method for estimating effective dose. However, effective dose alone does not give a complete picture of estimated radiation risk to specific radiation-sensitive organs or patients of a specific age or gender. For a complete picture, specific organ doses and age, gender, and organ-specific risk estimates are needed.

Recently the International Commission on Radiation Protection (ICRP) altered their recommendations regarding the relative radiation sensitivities of various organs and tissues. For the same exact scan performed on the same exact equipment and resulting in the same predicted organ doses, the value for effective dose differs depending on whether the recommendations from 1991 (ICRP 60) or 2007 (ICRP 103) are used.[15,18] The version of E (eg, ICRP 60 or ICRP 103) must be provided when a value of effective dose is given. The data presented in **Table 1** make use of the organ weighting factors from ICRP 60; the new values from ICRP103 have not yet been widely adopted.

JUSTIFICATION AND OPTIMIZATION
General Principles of "as Low as Reasonably Achievable"

The guiding principles for radiation protection in medicine are:

- Justification: The examination must be medically indicated.
- Optimization: The examination must be performed using doses that are as low as reasonably achievable (ALARA), consistent with the diagnostic task.
- Limitation: Although dose levels to occupationally exposed individuals (ie, the radiologist or technologist) are limited to levels recommended by consensus organizations, limits are not typical for medically necessary examinations or procedures.

As the growth in CT use increased, particularly in pediatric patients, and concern over the population dose from CT was expressed in the scientific literature and lay press,[3,4,23,24] it became clear that the responsible use of CT required adjustment of technique factors based on patient size (attenuation characteristics).[3,25,26] In response, the radiology community (radiologists, physicists, and

Table 1
Normalized effective dose per dose-length product for adults (standard physique) and pediatric patients of various ages over various body regions

Region of Body	k (mSv mGy^{-1} cm^{-1})				
	0-y-Old	1-y-Old	5-y-Old	10-y-Old	Adult
Head and neck	0.013	0.0085	0.0057	0.0042	0.0031
Head	0.011	0.0067	0.0040	0.0032	0.0021
Neck	0.017	0.012	0.011	0.0079	0.0059
Chest	0.039	0.026	0.018	0.013	0.014
Abdomen and pelvis	0.049	0.030	0.020	0.015	0.015
Trunk	0.044	0.028	0.019	0.014	0.015

Conversion factor for adult head and neck and pediatric patients assumes use of the head CT dose phantom (16 cm). All other conversion factors assume use of the 32-cm diameter CT body phantom.[20,21] These coefficients estimate effective dose as defined in ICRP report #60[15] and do not reflect the newly recommended tissue weighting values of ICRP #103.[18]

manufacturers) has worked to implement ALARA principles in CT imaging.[23,27–33] The guiding principle for dose management in CT is that the right dose for a CT examination takes into account the specific patient attenuation and the specific diagnostic task. For large patients, this means a dose increase is consistent with ALARA principles.

Additionally, each CT examination must be appropriate for the individual patient. Justification is a shared responsibility between requesting clinicians and radiologists. For medical exposures, the primary tasks of the imaging community are to work with ordering clinicians to direct patients to the most appropriate imaging modality for the required diagnostic task, and to ensure that all technical aspects of the examination are optimized, such that the required level of image quality can be obtained while keeping the doses as low as possible. The American College of Radiology Appropriateness Criteria provides evidence-based guidelines to help physicians in recommending an appropriate imaging test.[34] The European Commission guidelines and United Kingdom's Royal College of Radiologists document titled "Referral Guidelines for Imaging" also provide a detailed overview of clinical indications for imaging examinations, including CT.[35] A CT examination should thus be performed only when the radiation dose is deemed to be justified by the potential clinical benefit to the patient.

DOSE REDUCTION STRATEGIES
General Strategies

All dose-reduction strategies are predicated on the assumption that the CT scanner's radiation dose levels and image quality fall within manufacturer specifications and other general quality criteria. This goal can be accomplished through a quality control program that is designed and overseen by a qualified medical physicist.

Fixed tube current (technique charts)
Unlike traditional radiographic imaging, a CT image never looks "over-exposed" in the sense of being too dark or too light; the normalized nature of CT data (ie, CT numbers represent a fixed amount of attenuation relative to water) ensures that the image always appears properly exposed. As a consequence, CT users are not technically compelled to decrease the tube current-time product (mAs) for small patients, which may result in excess radiation dose for these patients. It is, however, a fundamental responsibility of the CT operator to take patient size into account when selecting the parameters that affect radiation dose, the most basic of which is the mAs.[27,30]

As with radiographic and fluoroscopic imaging, the operator should be provided with appropriate guidelines for mAs selection as a function of patient size. These are often referred to as technique charts. In CT, the tube current, exposure time and tube potential can all be altered to give the appropriate exposure to the patient. Users most commonly standardize the tube potential (kV) and gantry rotation time (s) for a given clinical application. The fastest rotation time should typically be used to minimize motion blurring and artifact, and the lowest kV consistent with the patient size should be selected to maximize image contrast.[36–41] Tube current is thus the primary parameter that is adapted to patient size.

Numerous investigators have shown that the manner in which mA should be adjusted as a function of patient size should be related to the overall attenuation, or thickness, of the anatomy of interest as opposed to patient weight, which is correlated to patient girth, but not a perfect surrogate for attenuation as a function of anatomic region.[25,26,42] The exception is for imaging of the head, wherein attenuation is relatively well defined by age because the primary attenuation comes from the skull and the process of bone formation in the skull is age dependent.

Clinical evaluations of mA-adjusted images have demonstrated that radiologists do not find the same noise level acceptable in small patients as in larger patients.[25] Because of the absence of adipose tissue between organs and tissue planes, and the smaller anatomic dimensions, radiologists tend to demand lower noise images in children and small adults relative to larger patients.[25,26,42,43] For CT imaging of the head, the mAs reduction from an adult to a newborn of approximately a factor of 2 to 2.5 is appropriate. For CT imaging of the body, typically a reduction in mAs of a factor of 4 to 5 from adult techniques is acceptable in infants,[42] whereas for obese patients, an increase of a factor of 2 is appropriate.[42] To achieve sufficient exposure levels for obese patients, either the rotation time or the tube potential may also need to be increased.

Tube current (mA) modulation
Extremely large variations in patient absorption occur with projection angle and anatomic region and are not considered when using a fixed tube current (**Fig. 1**). The projection with the most noise primarily determines the noise of the final image. Data acquired through body parts having less attenuation can thus be acquired with substantially less radiation without negatively affecting the final image noise.[38,44–47] In addition, it is also possible to reduce dose for projections of limited interest.

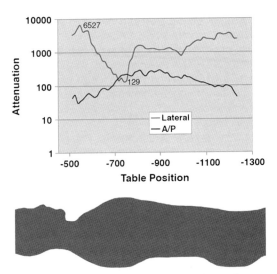

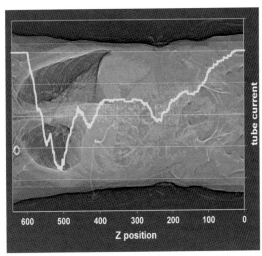

Fig. 1. Graph (top) of relative attenuation values as a function of table position and associated body region (bottom) shows almost three orders of magnitude of variation in attenuation, according to body region and projection angle. (From McCollough CH, Brue sewitz MR, Kofler JM Jr. CT dose reduction and dose management tools: overview of available options. Radiographics 2006;26(2):504; with permission.)

Fig. 2. Graph of relative tube current superimposed on a CT projection radiograph illustrates the concept of longitudinal dose modulation. The prescribed tube current curve is determined by using attenuation data from the CT projection radiograph and a manufacturer-specific algorithm (From McCollough CH, Bruesewitz MR, Kofler JM Jr. CT dose reduction and dose management tools: overview of available options. Radiographics 2006;26(2):506; with permission).

For example, in cardiac CT, decreasing mA during systole can significantly reduce dose to the patient. Tube current modulation may occur angularly about the patient, along the long axis of the patient, or incorporate both to adapt to attenuation differences within the patient.

Angular (x,y) mA modulation Angular (x,y) mA modulation addresses the variation in x-ray attenuation around the patient by varying the mA as the x-ray tube rotates about the patient (eg, in the anteroposterior [AP] versus lateral direction). The operator chooses the initial mA value, and the mA is modulated upward or downward from the initial value with a period of one gantry rotation. As the x-ray tube rotates between the AP and lateral positions, the mA can be varied according to the attenuation information from the CT radiograph (ie, scout image) or in near–real time according to the measured attenuation from the 180° previous projection.

Longitudinal (z) mA modulation Longitudinal (z) mA modulation addresses the varying attenuation of the patient among anatomic regions by varying the mA along the z axis of the patient (eg, shoulders versus the abdomen), as shown in **Fig. 2**. The operator must therefore provide as input to the algorithm the desired level of image quality, the paradigms for which are at present relatively manufacturer-specific.

Angular and longitudinal (x,y,z) mA modulation Angular and longitudinal (x,y,z) mA modulation combines the previous two methods to vary the mA during rotation and along the z axis of the patient. The operator must still indicate the desired level of image quality by one of the following methods. This results in the most comprehensive approach to CT dose reduction because the x-ray dose is adjusted according to the patient attenuation in all three dimensions.

Automatic exposure control
Overview It is technologically possible for CT systems to adjust the x-ray tube current in real time in response to variations in x-ray intensity at the detector,[36,47–49] much as fluoroscopic x-ray systems adjust exposure automatically. The modulation may be fully preprogrammed, occur in near–real time by using a feedback mechanism, or incorporate preprogramming and a feedback loop. These methods of adapting the tube current to patient attenuation, known generically as AEC, are analogous to photo timing in general radiography and have demonstrated reductions in dose of about 20% to 40% when image quality is appropriately specified. An exception to this trend occurs with obese patients. In large patients, the radiation dose is increased to ensure adequate image quality. Much of the additional x-ray dose is absorbed

by excess adipose tissue. Thus, doses to internal organs do not increase linearly with increases in tube current settings.[50,51] AEC is a broad term that encompasses not only tube current modulation (to adapt to changes in patient attenuation) but also determining and delivering the right dose for any patient (infant to obese) to achieve the diagnostic task.

Image quality selection paradigms for automatic exposure control systems Each manufacturer of CT systems uses a different method of defining the image quality in the user interface. GE uses a concept known as the Noise Index. The noise index is referenced to the standard deviation of pixel values in a specific size water phantom and is compared with patient attenuation measured from the CT radiograph (scout) to maintain image noise. Toshiba allows two ways to prescribe image quality in their Sure Exposure AEC algorithm: Standard Deviation and Image Quality Level. Like GE's Noise Index, Sure Exposure also compares the patient's CT radiograph (Scanogram) data to the standard deviation of a specific-attenuation water phantom. Philips uses a Reference Image from a satisfactory patient examination (Reference Case) stored in the system with which image quality for future examinations is to be matched. Siemens uses a Quality Reference mAs to define the effective mAs (= mAs/pitch) required to produce a specific image quality in an 80-kg patient (20 kg for pediatric cases) for a given protocol. For specific patients, the tube current is based on the CT radiograph (Topogram) and fine-tuned by an online feedback system.

Future dose-reduction strategies

Adjusting kV based on patient size There have been several physics and clinical studies on the use of lower tube potential (kV) in CT imaging to improve image quality or reduce radiation dose. The principle behind the benefit of lower kV in some clinical applications is this: The attenuation coefficient of iodine increases as photon energy decreases toward the k-edge energy of 33 kV. In many CT examinations involving the use of iodinated contrast media, the superior enhancement of iodine at lower tube potentials improves the conspicuity of hypervascular or hypovascular pathologies. The images obtained using lower tube potentials tend to be much noisier, however, mainly because of the higher absorption of low-energy photons by the patient. A tradeoff between image noise and contrast enhancement must therefore be made.

Fig. 3A shows the change of iodine CT number with tube potential for three different phantom sizes. The CT numbers of the iodine solution are larger at lower kVs than at higher kVs. With an increase in phantom size, CT numbers decrease because of beam hardening effects. Fig. 3B shows, for the same total radiation dose, image noise as the tube potential and phantom size change. For smaller phantom sizes, images acquired at different kVs have almost the same noise levels, with slightly higher noise for images acquired at 80 kV. With the increase of the phantom size, however, lower-kV scans yield images with higher noise levels compared with images attained at higher kVs. Fig. 3C combines the information from Fig. 3A and B to determine the change of contrast-to-noise ratio (CNR) as a function of tube potential and phantom size, where contrast is defined as the CT number of the iodine solution minus the CT number of background, which in this case was water (CT number ≈ 0 HU). The benefit of increased contrast enhancement at 80 kV is negated by increased noise for the large phantom size.

When the patient size is below some threshold, the use of a lower tube potential can generate better image quality than the higher tube potential, for the same radiation dose. Alternatively, dose can be reduced while maintaining the same image quality as a high tube potential image. Consequently, for a given patient size, an optimal tube potential exists that yields the best image quality (in, eg, CNR, lesion detectability) or the lowest radiation dose. This optimal tube potential is highly dependent on the patient size and the specific diagnostic task. For noncontrast CT examinations, the benefit of lower kV has not been established because soft tissue contrast is not highly dependent on the tube potential.

Iterative reconstruction Iterative reconstruction techniques have demonstrated the potential for improving image quality and reducing radiation dose in CT[52–56] relative to the currently used filtered back projection techniques. The most noticeable benefit of iterative reconstruction is that it is able to incorporate into the reconstruction process a physical model of the CT system that can accurately characterize the data acquisition process, including noise, beam hardening, scatter, and so forth. This ability allows for dramatic improvements in image quality, especially in the case of low-dose CT scans, in which the propagation of non-ideal data during the image reconstruction becomes more significant than in routine CT scanning. This benefit has long been used by nuclear medicine imaging, where the photon numbers are much smaller than in CT.

Iterative reconstruction is also superior to filtered back projection in handling insufficient data. Recent advances in iterative reconstruction

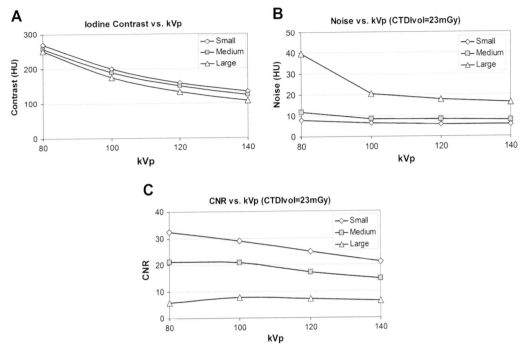

Fig. 3. (*A*) Graph of the CT number of a 2% iodine solution for small, medium, and large phantoms at various x-ray tube potentials. (*B*) Graph of noise (standard deviation of CT numbers within the water background) in images of small, medium, and large phantoms at different tube potentials. (*C*) Graph of the contrast-to-noise ratio (CT number of iodine solution divided by the background noise level) in small, medium, and large phantoms at different tube potentials.

allow a significant reduction in the number of required projection views, while still producing acceptable image quality. The use of iterative reconstruction techniques thus has the potential to substantially reduce the radiation dose in CT.[57–59] With computational power growing quickly, the clinical implementation of iterative reconstruction algorithms is within reach.[56]

Patient-Specific Dose Reduction Strategies

Pregnant patients

Imaging the pregnant patient presents a unique challenge to the radiologist because of the concern of radiation risk for the conceptus (embryo/fetus). Potential effects of radiation on the conceptus include prenatal death, intrauterine growth restriction, small head size, severe mental retardation, reduced intelligence quotient, organ malformation, and childhood cancer. The probability of any effects depends on the radiation dose to the conceptus (**Table 2**).[15,17,60–67]

Common indications for CT scanning in a pregnant patient include suspected appendicitis, pulmonary embolism, and urinary tract calculi. To minimize radiation exposure to the fetus, it is important to determine if the necessary diagnostic information can be obtained from an alternative non–radiation-based imaging modality. For nonacute symptoms, radiologists and physicians must also decide if immediate CT scanning is required or if CT scanning can be postponed until after the delivery.

For scanning body regions outside the abdomen and pelvis, such as chest CT for suspected pulmonary embolism, the dose to the fetus is extremely low (<0.1 mGy) because the scattered radiation levels fall off quickly away from the scan volume. For CT in a pregnant patient who has suspected appendicitis, the scan volume should be restricted to the necessary anatomy, and dual-pass (with and without contrast) studies should be avoided, if possible.[68,69] In CT for renal calculi in a pregnant patient, fetal dose can be reduced with use of low mAs, high pitch, and a limited scan range without substantially compromising the study quality.[70] For abdominal-pelvic CT, which directly irradiates the fetus, scan parameters (such as wider beam collimation, higher pitch, and lower mAs, kV, and scan range) can be selected to reduce the fetal dose to approximately 23 mGy per scan phase. Even for a routine dose level, biphase CT

Table 2
Probability of birthing healthy children who have no malformation or subsequent childhood cancer development for various radiation exposures during pregnancy

Dose to Conceptus (mGy)	Child has no Malformation (%)	Child will not Develop Cancer (%)	Child will not Develop Cancer or have a Malformation (%)
0	96	99.93	95.93
0.5	95.999	99.926	95.928
1.0	95.998	99.921	95.922
2.5	95.995	99.908	95.91
5.0	95.99	99.89	95.88
10.0	95.98	99.84	95.83
50.0	95.90	99.51	95.43
100.0	95.80	99.07	94.91

Data from Wagner LK, Lester RG, Saldana LR. Exposure of the pregnant patient to diagnostic radiations: a guide to medical management. Madison (WI): Medical Physics Publishing; 1997; with permission; and Wagner LK, Hayman LA. Pregnancy and women radiologists. Radiology 1982;145(2):559–62.

examination of the abdomen and pelvis, the probability of birthing a healthy baby decreases by only 0.5% (see **Table 2**).

Pediatric patients

The risk for cancer in children caused by radiation exposure is about two to three times higher than adults because pediatric patients have a longer life expectancy and their organs are more sensitive to radiation damage.[4,60–64] For newborns, the risk for cancer induction is essentially the same as in the second and third trimesters of pregnancy (see **Table 2**).

The best way to reduce the radiation dose to pediatric patients is to avoid unnecessary CT examinations and to look for alternative diagnostic imaging modalities with less or no exposure to ionizing radiation. Pediatric protocols with scanning parameters specifically designed for children must be used.[71,72] These protocols usually include tube current modulation,[39,47] a child-size bowtie filter and scanning field of view (FOV), or a weight- or size-based technique chart that can determine the appropriate kV or mAs for each patient.[73,74]

Automatic tube current modulation and manual technique charts are currently widely used. Additionally, lower kV values may be used, depending on patient size and clinical indication. For pediatric patients, because of less attenuation in the body, the noise level does not increase significantly with the decrease of kV for the same radiation dose. For iodine contrast-enhanced examinations, therefore, a lower kV can be used to improve the contrast enhancement without increasing the noise. Because of this, the benefit of image quality improvement or dose reduction is much more significant than in adult patients. Lower-kV

techniques have been actively investigated and are beginning to be widely used in pediatric CT.[26,41,73,74]

There are several factors that should be taken into account when lower-kV techniques are used in practice. First, because of the less efficient x-ray production of the tube at low kV values, the mAs has to be increased to avoid excessive noise levels. Second, for certain sized patients, a lower kV may not be appropriate. To address these issues, a weight or size-based kV/mAs technique chart should be used. Third, to avoid motion artifacts and decrease scan times in pediatric patients, a fast rotation time and a high helical pitch are desirable, which often limit the maximum mAs that can be used because of tube current limitations. In this situation, a higher kV may be necessary to avoid compromising the examination quality. Finally, although lower kV increases the contrast of iodine, it may not increase the contrast of tissues, lesions, and other pathologic structures without iodine uptake. The use of lower kV has to be carefully evaluated by radiologists and physicists for every particular type of pediatric examination.

Other specific dose-reduction strategies

Cardiac CT Dose in cardiac CT is a considerably more complex issue compared with noncardiac CT applications. There are two major reasons for this complexity. The first reason is that dose, noise, and pitch have different relationships in cardiac CT compared with noncardiac spiral CT.[75] The second reason is that dose in cardiac CT can depend on the patient's heart rate (HR).

In noncardiac multidetector CT (MDCT), noise depends on pitch. In cardiac spiral CT, however, noise is independent of pitch and depends only on the tube current-time product (mAs).[75] Additionally, because only a partial amount of the projection data from one gantry rotation is used for image reconstruction (to optimize the temporal resolution), relatively high mAs values are needed to provide an acceptable noise level for cardiac CT imaging, especially for cardiac CT angiography (CTA) examinations, which require the use of thin slices for better visualization of the coronary arteries.

A combination of relatively high mAs values with the low pitch values required in cardiac CT (dose is proportional to mAs/pitch) explains why cardiac CT examinations are associated with a higher radiation dose. Effective doses up to 21 mSv have been reported in the literature,[76] and the recent review by Achenbach and colleagues[77] claims that maximum organ dose values (based on Monte Carlo calculations) delivered during cardiac CT examinations can be as high as 50 to 100 mGv when no dose reduction measures are taken.

ECG-based tube current modulation is an important dose-reduction tool in cardiac CT.[38,78] The principle of ECG-based mA modulation is illustrated by **Fig. 4.** The percent dose reduction using ECG-based tube current modulation is higher for patients who have slow HRs compared with those who have high HRs, because the maximum mA time period is a smaller percentage of the time interval between successive R waves in the ECG (R-R interval) at low HR.

Additionally, the width of the maximum mA window must be carefully chosen to make sure that the data for the best cardiac phase (the one with the least motion artifact) is acquired with maximum tube current (hence, best image quality). Failure to properly set up the ECG-based tube current modulation parameters may compromise the

diagnostic quality of the cardiac examination. According to the dual-source coronary CTA study by Weustink and colleagues,[79] optimal windows for ECG-based tube current modulation for low (HR≤65 bpm), intermediate (65<HR<80 bpm), and high (HR≥80 bpm) HRs were at 60% to 76%, 30% to 77%, and 31% to 47% of the R-R interval, respectively.

Finally, for patients who have a very irregular HR, using ECG-based tube current modulation can compromise the diagnostic quality of the images if the optimal reconstruction window occurs during the reduced tube current interval. Some systems address this concern by automatically increasing the tube current to the maximum level when a statistical trend-analysis algorithm recognizes an R-R interval that is significantly different from the previous rhythm.[80]

One of the earliest studies of ECG-based tube current modulation reported dose savings of 30% to 50% for 4-slice CT.[78] A later study by Hausleiter and colleagues[81] reported effective dose estimates for coronary CTA using 64-slice CT of approximately 9.4 mSv with ECG-based tube current modulation and 14.8 mSv without tube current modulation.[81] One study of dual-source coronary CTA reported mean effective dose values of 7.8 to 8.8 mSv,[82] and another reported effective doses of 6.8, 13.4, and 4.2 mSv for low, intermediate, and high HR, respectively, when using the optimal windows for ECG-based tube current modulation.[79] The higher dose at intermediate HR is attributable to the need for a wider maximum tube current window.

ECG modulation cannot be combined with some other types of tube current modulation, such as angular modulation. Although it is possible to use z-modulation in cardiac CT, this is not widely available. The role of AEC in cardiac mode is typically limited to automatically adjusting the mAs values based on patient size.

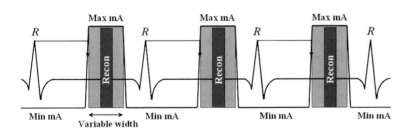

Fig. 4. ECG-based modulation of the tube current. The width of the temporal window having the maximum tube current (Max mA) can be selected by the user, whereas the temporal width of the image reconstruction window is fixed (Recon). For full quality images, the reconstruction window (darker gray time interval) should fall within the maximum mA window (lighter gray time interval). (*Courtesy of* Suhny Abbara, MD, Boston, MA).

Alternatively, technique charts may be used to manually choose the proper mAs settings based on patient size, the type of cardiac examination (eg, coronary calcium scoring versus coronary CTA), and the noise level accepted in the clinical practice. Appropriate use of lower kV values (80 or 100 kV) for coronary CTA examinations of smaller patients can further reduce radiation dose without compromising the image quality. A recent study by Leschka and colleagues[83] showed that dual-source coronary CTA with 100 kV is feasible in patients of normal weight and can produce a higher contrast-to-noise ratio at estimated effective doses as low as 4.4 mSv. In a study by Achenbach and colleagues,[77] a 74-year-old patient who had 63 kg body weight was scanned using 80-kV tube current and ECG-based tube current modulation, resulting in fully diagnostic image quality at an estimated effective dose of 3.0 mSv.

Additional dose reductions can be achieved using prospective ECG-triggering (ie, "step and shoot" acquisitions). The lack of overlapping beams at low spiral pitch values makes this mode dose efficient. This mode is not as reliable as the conventional spiral, retrospectively-gated mode, however, and requires a careful selection of patients having stable, low heart rates. Because there are no data collected outside the narrow acquisition window predicted to correspond to the best phase of the cardiac cycle, any sudden change in cardiac rhythm (eg, ectopic beat) can ruin image quality for the portion of the heart included in that axial scan. Nevertheless, a recent study by Scheffel and colleagues[84] concluded that prospectively triggered dual source CT coronary angiography allows for the accurate diagnosis of significant coronary stenoses at a low radiation dose in patients who have a regular HR. For 120 selected patients having an average heart rate of 59 ± 6 bpm (range 44–69 bpm), the reported mean effective dose was 2.5 ± 0.8 mSv (range 1.2–4.4 mSv).[84]

The susceptibility of prospectively triggered coronary CTA to artifacts caused by variations in cardiac cycle length or by the occurrence of ectopic beats can be reduced by using adaptively triggered sequential scans with dynamic temporal windows, where triggering for each cardiac cycle is adjusted according to the ECG trend and variability. In a study in which cardiac CT scans were simulated on the basis of 60 ECGs recorded during actual coronary CTA examinations, the adaptively triggered sequential scans provided 68% dose reduction relative to spiral cardiac CT with constant tube current, without compromising the reliability of image quality.[85] The standard sequential mode without adaptive triggering provided improved dose reductions (75%) but suffered from inconsistent availability of the optimal cardiac phase, missing it in 18% of the cases.

Selective in-plane shielding Selective shielding of radiation-sensitive tissues and organs during CT scanning has been proposed and products to implement this are commercially available. Their use is not generally recommended, however, because the dose reduction they provide can be readily achieved by decreasing x-ray tube current, which does not introduce noise or increase beam-hardening artifacts.

Shields made of thin sheets of flexible latex impregnated with bismuth and shaped to cover the eye lens, thyroid, or breasts can be used, respectively, during brain, cervical spine, or chest CT examinations. Dose savings to the superficially located target organ when using such shields have been reported to be 40% to 67% for adults[86–90] and 30% to 40% for children.[91,92] Most of these studies reported artifacts near the shields. Additionally, these studies overestimated organ dose reductions by assuming that organ doses are equivalent to the measured skin dose reductions.

A quantitative study by Geleijns and colleagues[93] assessed the tradeoff between absorbed dose and image quality for the use of selective shields. Using commercially available shields and an anthropomorphic phantom, image noise was experimentally quantified by the standard deviation of CT numbers in the target organ. Absorbed organ doses were also computed using a validated Monte Carlo method. With use of the shields, organ dose reductions of 26%, 27%, and 30% were found for the thyroid, eye lens, and breast, respectively, contrary to the larger savings reported elsewhere. For each organ, dose reduction was accompanied by increased noise and artifacts. This increase was most marked and most varied near the breast, where the noise increase ranged from a minimum of 50% (8 HU increased to 12 HU) near the shield center to a maximum of 100% (7.5 HU increased to 15 HU) near the shield edge. They additionally report that the same 30% dose reduction could be achieved by decreasing the x-ray tube current by 30%, yet with a smaller and more uniform noise increase of 20% to 30%; this is because while the dose shield attenuates the anterior x-ray beam and hence decreases anterior organ dose, it also attenuates x-rays coming from the posterior direction that have already contributed to organ dose and contain important image information.

SUMMARY

In recent years, the media has focused on the potential danger of radiation exposure from CT, even though the potential benefit of a medically indicated CT far outweighs the potential risks. This attention has reminded the radiology community that doses must be ALARA while maintaining diagnostic image quality. To satisfy the ALARA principle, the dose reduction strategies described in this article must be well understood and properly used. The use of CT must also be justified for the specific diagnostic task.

ACKNOWLEDGMENTS

The authors thank Kris Nunez and Megan Jacobsen for their help with the manuscript preparation and submission.

REFERENCES

1. Brenner DJ, Hall EJ. Computed tomography—an increasing source of radiation exposure. N Engl J Med 2007;357(22):2277–84.
2. National Council on Radiation Protection and Measurements. Ionizing radiation exposure of the population of the United States. Report no. 93. Bethesda (MD): National Council on Radiation Protection and Measurements; 1987. NCRP Report No. 93.
3. Donnelly LF, Emery KH, Brody AS, et al. Minimizing radiation dose for pediatric body applications of single-detector helical CT: strategies at a large children's hospital. AJR Am J Roentgenol 2001;176: 303–6.
4. Brenner DJ, Elliston CD, Hall EJ, et al. Estimated risks of radiation-induced fatal cancer from pediatric CT. AJR Am J Roentgenol 2001;176:289–96.
5. The Associated Press. Report links increased cancer risk to CT scans. The New York Times. November 29, 2007.
6. Khamsi R. CT scan radiation can equal nuclear bomb exposure. Available: NewScientist.com. News Service. Accessed May 11, 2007.
7. Jessen KA, Shrimpton PC, Geleijns J, et al. Dosimetry for optimisation of patient protection in computed tomography. Appl Radiat Isot 1999;50:165–72.
8. Nagel HD. Radiation exposure in computed tomography. 2nd edition. Frankfurt: COCIR; 2000.
9. Shope TB, Gagne RM, Johnson GC. A method for describing the doses delivered by transmission x-ray computed tomography. Med Phys 1981;8(4): 488–95.
10. American Association of Physicists in Medicine. Standardized methods for measuring diagnostic x-ray exposures. New York: AAPM; 1990. Report no. 31.
11. McNitt-Gray MF. AAPM/RSNA physics tutorial for residents: topics in CT. Radiation dose in CT. Radiographics 2002;22(6):1541–53.
12. American Association of Physicists in Medicine. The measurement, reporting and management of radiation dose in CT 2008. College Park (MD) Report No 96.
13. International Electrotechnical Commission. Medical electrical equipment. Part 2-44: particular requirements for the safety of x-ray equipment for computed tomography. IEC publication No. 60601-2-44. Ed. 2.1. Geneva, Switzerland: International Electrotechnical Commission (IEC) Central Office; 2002.
14. Boone JM. The trouble with $CTDI_{100}$. Med Phys 2007;34(4):1364–71.
15. International Commission on Radiological Protection. 1990 recommendations of the international commission on radiological protection (Report 60). Ann ICRP 1991;21(1–3).
16. McCollough CH, Schueler BA. Calculation of effective dose. Med Phys 2000;27(5):828–37.
17. International Commission on Radiological Protection. Recommendations of the international commission on radiological protection (ICRP #26). Oxford: The International Commission on Radiological Protection; 1977. ICRP Publication 26.
18. International Commission on Radiological Protection. 2007 recommendations of the international commission on radiological protection (ICRP Publication 103). Ann ICRP 2007;37:1–332.
19. Cristy M. Mathematical phantoms representing children of various ages for use in estimates of internal dose. Oak Ridge (TN): Oak Ridge National Laboratory; 1980. NUREG/CR-1159, ORNL/NUREG/TM-367.
20. Bongartz G, Golding S, Jurik A, et al. European guidelines for multislice computed tomography. Funded by the European Commission. Contract number FIGM-CT2000-20078-CT-TIP. March 2004.
21. Shrimpton PC, Hillier MC, Lewis MA, et al. National survey of doses from CT in the UK: 2003. Br J Radiol 2006;79(948):968–80.
22. McCollough CH. Patient dose in cardiac computed tomography. Herz 2003;28(1):1–6.
23. Haaga JR. Radiation dose management: weighing risk versus benefit. AJR Am J Roentgenol 2001; 177(2):289–91.
24. Nickoloff EL, Alderson PO. Radiation exposures to patients from CT: reality, public perception, and policy. AJR Am J Roentgenol 2001;177(2):285–7.
25. Wilting JE, Zwartkruis A, van Leeuwen MS, et al. A rational approach to dose reduction in CT: individualized scan protocols. Eur Radiol 2001; 11(12):2627–32.
26. Boone JM, Geraghty EM, Seibert JA, et al. Dose reduction in pediatric CT: a rational approach. Radiology 2003;228(2):352–60.
27. Linton OW, Mettler FA Jr. National conference on dose reduction in CT, with an emphasis on pediatric patients. Am J Roentgenol 2003;181(2):321–9.

28. Frush DP, Donnelly LF, Rosen NS. Computed tomography and radiation risks: what pediatric health care providers should know. Pediatrics 2003;112(4):951–7.

29. Golding SJ, Shrimpton PC. Commentary. Radiation dose in CT: are we meeting the challenge? Br J Radiol Jan 2002;75(889):1–4.

30. FDA. FDA public health notification: reducing radiation risk from computed tomography for pediatric and small adult patients. Pediatr Radiol 2002;32(4): 314–6.

31. Kalra MK, Maher MM, Toth TL, et al. Strategies for CT radiation dose optimization. Radiology 2004; 230(3):619–28.

32. Cody DD, Moxley DM, Krugh KT, et al. Strategies for formulating appropriate MDCT techniques when imaging the chest, abdomen, and pelvis in pediatric patients. AJR Am J Roentgenol 2004;182(4): 849–59.

33. International Commission on Radiological Protection. Managing patient dose in computed tomography, ICRP publication 87. Ann ICRP 2000;30(4):7–45.

34. The American College of Radiology appropriateness criteria. College Park (MD): American College of Radiology; 2008.

35. The Royal College of Radiologists. Making the best use of clinical radiology services: referral guidelines. 6th edition. 2007. London.

36. McCollough CH. Automatic exposure control in CT: are we done yet? Radiology 2005;237(3):755–6.

37. Funama Y, Awai K, Nakayama Y, et al. Radiation dose reduction without degradation of low-contrast detectability at abdominal multisection CT with a low-tube voltage technique: phantom study. Radiology 2005;237(3):905–10.

38. McCollough CH, Bruesewitz MR, Kofler JM Jr. CT dose reduction and dose management tools: overview of available options. Radiographics 2006; 26(2):503–12.

39. Nakayama Y, Awai K, Funama Y, et al. Abdominal CT with low tube voltage: preliminary observations about radiation dose, contrast enhancement, image quality, and noise. Radiology 2005;237(3):945–51.

40. Huda W, Ravenel JG, Scalzetti EM. How do radiographic techniques affect image quality and patient doses in CT? Semin Ultrasound CT MR 2002;23(5): 411–22.

41. Siegel MJ, Schmidt B, Bradley D, et al. Radiation dose and image quality in pediatric CT: effect of technical factors and phantom size and shape. Radiology 2004;233(2):515–22.

42. McCollough CH, Zink FE, Kofler J, et al. Dose optimization in CT: creation, implementation and clinical acceptance of size-based technique charts. Radiology 2002;225(P):591.

43. Kalra MK, Maher MM, Toth TL, et al. Techniques and applications of automatic tube current modulation for CT. Radiology 2004;233(3):649–57.

44. Graser A, Wintersperger BJ, Suess C, et al. Dose reduction and image quality in MDCT colonography using tube current modulation. AJR Am J Roentgenol 2006;187(3):695–701.

45. Greess H, Wolf H, Baum U, et al. Dose reduction in computed tomography by attenuation-based, online modulation of tube current: evaluation of six anatomical regions. Eur Radiol 2000;10(2):391–4.

46. Mulkens T, Bellinck P, Baeyaert M, et al. Use of an automatic exposure control mechanism for dose optimization in multi-detector row CT examinations: clinical evaluation. Radiology 2005;237(1): 213–23.

47. Haaga JR, Miraldi F, MacIntyre W, et al. The effect of mAs variation upon computed tomography image quality as evaluated by in vivo and in vitro studies. Radiology 1981;138(2):449–54.

48. Kalender WA, Wolf H, Suess C. Dose reduction in CT by anatomically adapted tube current modulation: phantom measurements. Med Phys 1999;26(11):2248–53.

49. Gies M, Kalender WA, Wolf H, et al. Dose reduction in CT by anatomically adapted tube current modulation: simulation studies. Med Phys 1999;26(11):2235–47.

50. Schmidt B. Dose calculations for computed tomography [dissertation]. Reports from the Insitute of Medical Physiks 2001;7 [in German].

51. Schmidt B, Kalender WA. A fast voxel-based Monte Carlo method for scanner- and patient-specific dose calculations in computed tomography. In: Guerra AD, editor, Physica Medica, vol 18. Erlangen, Germany: European Journal of Medical Physics; 2002. p. 43–53.

52. Nuyts J, De Man B, Dupont P, et al. Iterative reconstruction for helical CT: a simulation study. Phys Med Biol 1998;43(4):729–37.

53. Fessler JA, Ficaro EP, Clinthorne NH, et al. Grouped-coordinate ascent algorithms for penalized-likelihood transmission image reconstruction. IEEE Trans Med Imaging 1997;16(2):166–75.

54. Elbakri IA, Fessler JA. Statistical image reconstruction for polyenergetic X-ray computed tomography. IEEE Trans Med Imaging 2002;21(2):89–99.

55. Lasio GM, Whiting BR, Williamson JF. Statistical reconstruction for x-ray computed tomography using energy-integrating detectors. Phys Med Biol 2007; 52(8):2247–66.

56. Thibault JB, Sauer KD, Bouman CA, et al. A three-dimensional statistical approach to improved image quality for multislice helical CT. Med Phys 2007; 34(11):4526–44.

57. Candes EJ, Romberg J, Tao T. Robust uncertainty principles: exact signal reconstruction from highly incomplete frequency information. IEEE Trans Inf Theory 2006;52(2):489–509.

58. Sidky EY, Kao CM, Pan XH. Accurate image reconstruction from few-views and limited-angle data in divergent-beam CT. J Xray Sci Technol 2006;14(2):119–39.

59. Chen GH, Tang J, Leng S. Prior image constrained compressed sensing (PICCS): a method to accurately reconstruct dynamic CT images from highly undersampled projection data sets. Med Phys 2008;35(2):660–3.

60. Wagner LK, Lester RG, Saldana LR. Exposure of the pregnant patient to diagnostic radiations: a guide to medical management. Madison (WI): Medical Physics Publishing; 1997.

61. Wagner LK, Hayman LA. Pregnancy and women radiologists. Radiology 1982;145(2):559–62.

62. International Commission on Radiological Protection. Developmental effects of irradiation on the brain of the embryo and fetus. Ann ICRP 1986;16(4).

63. International Commission on Radiological Protection. Pregnancy and medical radiation. Ann ICRP 1999. Publication No 84.

64. National Council on Radiation Protection and Measurements. Medical radiation exposure of pregnant and potentially pregnant women. Bethesda (MD): National Council on Radiation Protection and Measurements; 1977. NCRP Report No. 54.

65. National Council on Radiation Protection and Measurements. Recommendations on limits for exposure to ionizing radiation. Bethesda (MD): National Council on Radiation Protection and Measurements; 1987. NCRP Report No. 90.

66. National Council on Radiation Protection and Measurements. Risk estimates for radiation protection. Bethesda (MD): NCRP; 1993. NCRP Report No. 115.

67. American Association of Physicists in Medicine. A primer on low-level ionizing radiation and its biological effects. New York: AAPM; 1986. Report no. 18.

68. Wagner LK, Huda W. When a pregnant woman with suspected appendicitis is referred for a CT scan, what should a radiologist do to minimize potential radiation risks? Pediatr Radiol 2004; 34(7):589–90.

69. Castro MA, Shipp TD, Castro EE, et al. The use of helical computed tomography in pregnancy for the diagnosis of acute appendicitis. Am J Obstet Gynecol 2001;184(5):954–7.

70. Forsted DH. CT of pregnant women for urinary tract calculi, pulmonary thromboembolism, and acute appendicitis. Am J Roentgenol 2002;178(5): 1285–6.

71. Huda W, Bushong SC. In x-ray computed tomography, technique factors should be selected appropriate to patient size. Med Phys 2001;28(8): 1543–5.

72. Frush DP, Donnelly LF. Helical CT in children: technical considerations and body applications. Radiology 1998;209(1):37–48.

73. Hollingsworth C, Frush DP, Cross M, et al. Helical CT of the body: a survey of techniques used for pediatric patients. AJR Am J Roentgenol 2003;180(2): 401–6.

74. Paterson A, Frush DP. Dose reduction in paediatric MDCT: general principles. Clin Radiol 2007;62(6): 507–17.

75. Primak AN, McCollough CH, Bruesewitz MR, et al. Relationship between noise, dose, and pitch in cardiac multi-detector row CT. Radiographics 2006; 26(6):1785–94.

76. Mollet NR, Cademartiri F, van Mieghem CA, et al. High-resolution spiral computed tomography coronary angiography in patients referred for diagnostic conventional coronary angiography. Circulation 2005;112(15):2318–23.

77. Achenbach S, Anders K, Kalender WA. Dual-source cardiac computed tomography: image quality and dose considerations. Eur Radiol 2008;18:1188–98.

78. Jakobs TF, Becker CR, Ohnesorge B, et al. Multislice helical CT of the heart with retrospective ECG gating: reduction of radiation exposure by ECG-controlled tube current modulation. Eur Radiol 2002;12(5):1081–6.

79. Weustink AC, Mollet NR, Pugliese F, et al. Optimal electrocardiographic pulsing windows and heart rate: effect on image quality and radiation exposure at dual-source coronary CT angiography. Radiology 2008;248(3):792–8.

80. McCollough CH, Primak AN, Saba O, et al. Dose performance of a 64-channel dual-source CT scanner. Radiology 2007;243(3):775–84.

81. Hausleiter J, Meyer T, Hadamitzky M, et al. Radiation dose estimates from cardiac multislice computed tomography in daily practice: impact of different scanning protocols on effective dose estimates. Circulation 2006;113(10):1305–10.

82. Stolzmann P, Scheffel H, Rentsch K, et al. Dual-energy computed tomography for the differentiation of uric acid stones: ex vivo performance evaluation. Urol Res 2008;36:133–8.

83. Leschka S, Stolzmann P, Schmid FT, et al. Low kilovoltage cardiac dual-source CT: attenuation, noise, and radiation dose. Eur Radiol 2008;18:1809–17.

84. Scheffel H, Alkadhi H, Leschka S, et al. Low-dose CT coronary angiography in the step-and-shoot mode: diagnostic performance. Heart 2008;94: 1132–7.

85. Raupach R, Bruder H, Primak AN, et al. Dose reduction strategies for CT cardiac imaging [abstract B-654]. ECR 2008 Book of Abstracts 18 (Suppl 1). Vienna: ECR; 2008. p.292.

86. Hein E, Rogalla P, Klingebiel R, et al. Low-dose CT of the paranasal sinuses with eye lens protection: effect on image quality and radiation dose. Eur Radiol 2002;12(7):1693–6.

87. Hopper KD, King SH, Lobell ME, et al. The breast: in-plane x-ray protection during diagnostic thoracic CT—shielding with bismuth radioprotective garments. Radiology 1997;205(3):853–8.

88. Hopper KD. Orbital, thyroid, and breast superficial radiation shielding for patients undergoing

diagnostic CT. Semin Ultrasound CT MR 2002; 23(5):423–7.

89. Hopper KD, Neuman JD, King SH, et al. Radioprotection to the eye during CT scanning. AJNR Am J Neuroradiol 2001;22(6):1194–8.

90. McLaughlin DJ, Mooney RB. Dose reduction to radiosensitive tissues in CT. Do commercially available shields meet the users' needs? Clin Radiol 2004; 59(5):446–50.

91. Fricke BL, Donnelly LF, Frush DP, et al. In-plane bismuth breast shields for pediatric CT: effects on radiation dose and image quality using experimental and clinical data. AJR Am J Roentgenol 2003; 180(2):407–11.

92. Perisinakis K, Raissaki M, Theocharopoulos N, et al. Reduction of eye lens radiation dose by orbital bismuth shielding in pediatric patients undergoing CT of the head: a Monte Carlo study. Med Phys 2005; 32(4):1024–30.

93. Geleijns J, Salvado Artells M, Veldkamp WJ, et al. Quantitative assessment of selective in-plane shielding of tissues in computed tomography through evaluation of absorbed dose and image quality. Eur Radiol 2006;16(10):2334–40.

Dual-Energy and Dual-Source CT: Is There a Role in the Abdomen and Pelvis?

Joel G. Fletcher, MD*, Naoki Takahashi, MD, Robert Hartman, MD,
Luis Guimaraes, MD, James E. Huprich, MD, David M. Hough, MD,
Lifeng Yu, PhD, Cynthia H. McCollough, PhD

KEYWORDS

- Radiation dose • CT applications • Abdominal CT
- Dual-energy CT • Dual-source CT

Dual-energy CT refers to the use of CT data representing two different energy spectra to display anatomy and pathology in addition to differentiating and classifying tissue composition. Dual-energy CT data can be obtained and viewed using various hardware and software applications capable of material-specific classification and image display.

Dual-source CT refers to the use of two x-ray sources and two detectors mounted on a single x-ray gantry. A dual-source CT system can be used in a dual-energy mode (with each x-ray tube operating using a different polychromatic x-ray spectrum), in a cardiac mode (with both tubes operating at the same tube energy to improve temporal resolution), or in an "obese" dual-source mode (to permit a wider range of tube currents at low or high tube energies).[1,2] Throughout this article we refer to this obese mode (using the same tube energy in both tubes) as dual-source CT.

One principal advantage of both dual-energy and dual-source abdominal CT is the ability to perform lower-kV scanning in a larger number of patients. The CT numbers displayed in CT images are related to the linear attenuation coefficient of a substance, which is a function of its material composition, the photon energies generated by the x-ray tube, and the mass density of the material. This relationship explains why two different materials (such as iodine and calcium) can have the same CT number (**Fig. 1**). Both dual-energy and dual-source CT techniques can consequently use lower x-ray tube potentials (ie, photon energies) to highlight pathologies that become more conspicuous with the use of intravenous iodinated contrast, because the signal of iodine at 80 kV is approximately twice that at 140 kV. The difficulty with the routine use of low-kV CT is increased image noise, which can be minimized using both techniques. With dual-energy CT, the noise of the low-kV data is offset by the decreased noise of the higher-kV data. At dual-source CT, the use of both x-ray tubes extends the dynamic range of tube currents available beyond the system limits of single-source CT systems. The separation of materials can be achieved using only dual-energy CT, wherein CT numbers at each voxel can be compared between two different tube energies. Although the polychromatic spectra of commercial x-ray tubes overlap, the mean energy at different tube energies is unique. By analyzing our

Financial Disclosure: J.G. Fletcher receives grant support from Siemens Medical Solutions and GE Healthcare. Cynthia McCollough receives grant support from Siemens Medical Solutions. Lifeng Yu receives grant support from Xoran Technologies.

Images in the article were obtained using a dual-source CT scanner provided by a grant from Siemens Medical Solutions to Mayo Clinic.

Department of Radiology, Mayo Clinic, 200 First Street SW, Rochester, MN 55905, USA
* Corresponding author.
E-mail address: fletcher.joel@mayo.edu (J.G. Fletcher).

Radiol Clin N Am 47 (2009) 41–57
doi:10.1016/j.rcl.2008.10.003
0033-8389/08/$ – see front matter © 2009 Elsevier Inc. All rights reserved.

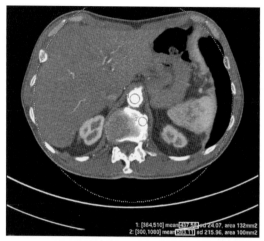

Fig. 1. Using single-source CT two different materials can have the same CT number because they possess different mass densities, a point illustrated by this image from a CT angiogram, in which the CT numbers of the calcium-containing bone overlap with the CT numbers of the aorta, which contains intravenous iodinated contrast.

knowledge of the absorption or properties of different materials at different x-ray energies, materials can be separated. For example, there is a large difference in the linear attenuation coefficients at two energies for iodine but a smaller difference in the linear attenuation coefficients for calcium (**Fig. 2**). Dual-energy CT, therefore, provides an opportunity to separate materials with different effective atomic numbers.

IMPLEMENTATION AND APPROACHES
Dual-Energy Hardware Approaches

There are three primary hardware approaches to dual-energy CT technology: two x-ray sources (in dual-source CT scanner), rapid kV switching (using single-source CT), and a "sandwich" detector. When using a dual-source scanner, each x-ray tube operates at a different energy. With current hardware the x-ray tube operating at a lower kV has a diminished field of view (FOV, 26 cm) compared with the tube operating at the higher energy, which has a 50-cm FOV, because the detector size is limited by the gantry. The advantage of this approach is ample preliminary experience (because dual-source CT technology has been in existence for approximately 2 years) and routine image reconstruction, because images are acquired simultaneously by the two detectors separated by 90° phase. The current weakness of this approach is that the dual-energy processing is performed after image reconstruction (ie, in image space), rather than on projection data before image reconstruction (ie, in projection space), because most data

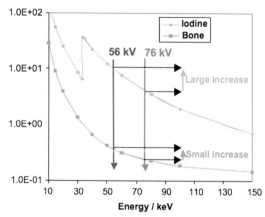

Fig. 2. The separation of materials of different composition can be achieved using dual-energy CT, wherein the CT numbers at each voxel can be compared between two different tube energies. This graph shows the linear attenuation coefficients of iodine (*orange line*) and calcium (*green line*) at 56 kV (the mean photon energy generated from a commercial x-ray tube operating at 80 kV) and 76 kV (the mean photon energy generated from a commercial x-ray tube operating at 140 kV). In this example, there is a large difference in the linear attenuation coefficients of iodine between the two energies, but a much smaller difference in the linear attenuation coefficients for calcium. These unique absorption properties of the two materials permit their material classification at dual-energy CT.

are acquired in helical mode with the two detectors 90° apart. Additionally, there is some slight blurring of mixed-kV image displays when combining the output of the two x-ray tubes.

Another approach is rapid kV switching. In the rapid kV switching paradigm, the x-ray tube is capable of rapid kV and mA modulation, switching from low to high energy at adjacent projections. This switching necessitates doubling the number of projections per rotation to maintain image quality, thereby requiring refinements at the tube and detector levels. The principle advantage of this technique is that it offers the potential to perform dual-energy processing using projection data acquired in both axial and helical modes, theoretically permitting accurate material decomposition and monochromatic CT image display, which should substantially decrease image artifacts. The disadvantage of this technique is that the low- and high-energy scans are limited to the same filtration and hence the spectra separation of the two energies is suboptimal. Another potential disadvantage of this technique is that it may be difficult to change the tube current fast enough during each kV switching, thus yielding mismatched noise level in the two data sets.

A third hardware solution to obtaining dual-energy CT data can be obtained by using a sandwich detector.[3] Low-energy photons are absorbed in the top layers of the sandwich detector while higher-energy photons are absorbed in the lower levels of the detector.

Dual-Energy CT Acquisition

Whatever the hardware approach used by a particular system, the tube current from the two tubes is generally chosen in an attempt to balance image noise between detectors. Tube currents can be chosen in a way that does not increase the radiation dose to the patient. For example, using a dual-source CT scanner, standard abdominal pelvic CT scanning protocols can be converted to dual-energy protocols by maintaining the same volume computed tomography dose index ($CTDI_{vol}$) and splitting the exposure between the two tube energies. Tube currents for each energy are chosen so that, as much as possible, the image sets are noise matched. In practice the 80-kV tube often uses a tube current approximately four to five times as high as the 140-kV tube, to match the noise level to the extent possible (**Fig. 3**). Automatic exposure

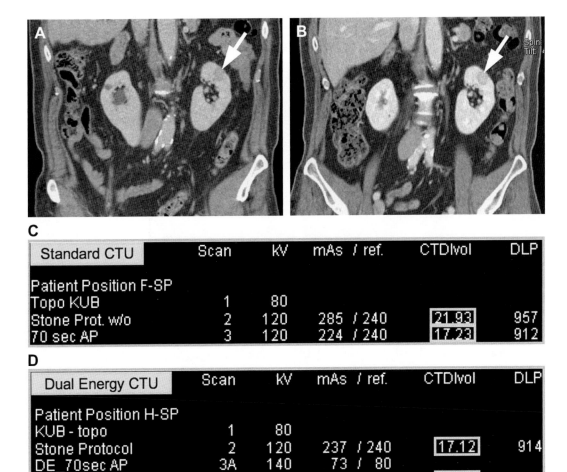

C

Standard CTU	Scan	kV	mAs / ref.	CTDlvol	DLP
Patient Position F-SP					
Topo KUB	1	80			
Stone Prot. w/o	2	120	285 / 240	21.93	957
70 sec AP	3	120	224 / 240	17.23	912

D

Dual Energy CTU	Scan	kV	mAs / ref.	CTDlvol	DLP
Patient Position H-SP					
KUB - topo	1	80			
Stone Protocol	2	120	237 / 240	17.12	914
DE_70sec AP	3A	140	73 / 80		
	3B	80	446 / 340	15.79	814

Fig. 3. Dual-energy CT acquisition protocols can be constructed so there is no increase in radiation dose. (A) Coronal image from a standard CT urogram using 120 kV and showing a mildly enhancing left renal mass in the upper pole of the left kidney (*arrow*), with the corresponding clinically generated dose report (C) showing $CTDI_{vol}$ of 17.23 mGy. (B) Mixed-kV image from a dual-energy CT urogram acquired using a dual-source CT scanner (with tubes operating at 80 and 140 kV) in the same patient, with the corresponding clinically generated dose report (D) showing a slight decline in the $CTDI_{vol}$ to 15.79 mGy and improved image contrast using the dual-energy technique. The tube current of the 80-kV tube was chosen to be roughly four times that of the 140-kV tube (D). Tube currents are chosen at dual-energy CT so that the images created are dose-matched compared with single-source CT acquisition protocols (by adding the $CTDI_{vol}$ of both tubes) and roughly noise matching the images at the two energies.

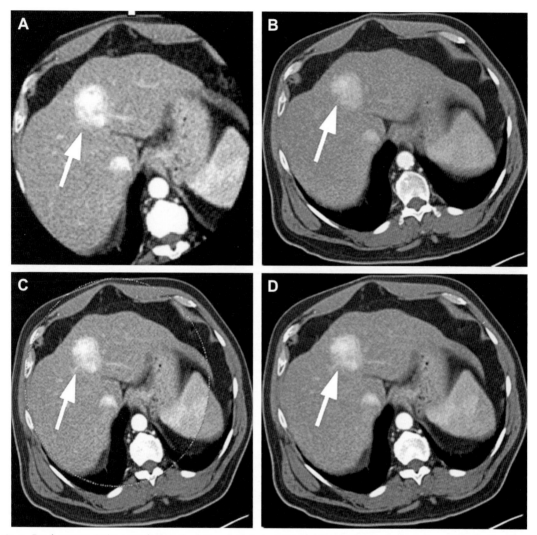

Fig. 4. Dual-energy CT images during the late arterial phase in a patient who had a hepatoma, illustrating linear and sigmoidal blending techniques. *A* and *B* are the outputs of the 80-kV and 140-kV tube, respectively. (*C*) Mixed-kV image using a 0.7 linear blend (with 70% of signal intensity coming from the 80-kV tube), showing improved contrast compared with the 140-kV image, and improved noise compared with the 80-kV image. (*D*) Mixed-kV image created using sigmoidal blending of the output of the two images showing marked improvement in the appearance of the liver parenchyma while preserving the improved contrast in the tumor and small hepatic arteries.

control can be used, but it should be realized that for larger patients, the image quality of the 80-kV tube may be compromised because the system tube currents will be exceeded and the system is not able to provide sufficient radiation dose as desired. Similar considerations apply when acquiring dual-energy CT data with other hardware platforms. As long as the detector input is in the quantum limited region (ie, electronic noise does not predominate), diagnostic images can be obtained while keeping radiation dose constant (see **Fig. 3**). Additionally, to minimize noise in the lower-kV data

set (to expand the technique to larger patients), we widen the minimal collimation (eg, from 32 × 0.60 mm to 14 × 1.2 mm), depending on the desired application.

Dual-Energy Material Classification

Multiple approaches are also possible for the algorithmic separation of different materials and the display of material-specific image data. Commercial dual-energy applications using dual-source CT scanners use a three-material decomposition,

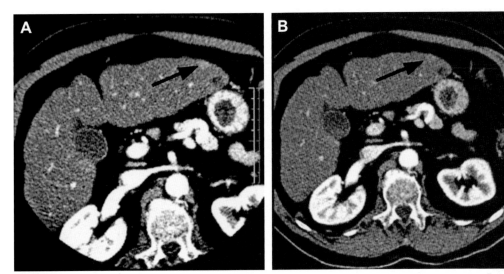

Fig. 5. Improved contrast and improved contrast-to-noise in a patient who had multifocal hepatoma and considering one enhancing focus of tumor (*arrow*), from a late arterial phase dual-energy examination. Using the output of the 80-kV tube (*A*), the tumor nodule (*arrow*) has a mean CT number of 110 ± 21 HU, which is 45 HU above background hepatic parenchyma, and has a contrast-to-noise ratio of 5.2. The 120-kV tube output (*B*) shows the tumor nodule (*arrow*) with a mean CT number of 65 ± 17 HU, which is 21 HU above background hepatic parenchyma and has a contrast-to-noise ratio of 3.8. For small and medium-sized patients, contrast-to-noise ratios will be positive using lower kVs.

which takes the known and unique x-ray absorption properties of three materials into consideration at both the tube energies used during scanning. Each pixel is then classified as being composed of one of these materials or quantified as the concentration of each material. The dual-energy processing in these applications is currently based on the low- and high-energy images reconstructed from the dual-energy scan. It is also possible to perform basis-material decomposition using conventional dual-energy processing methods in projection data space to obtain the material-specific information.[4,5] Once specific materials are identified in specific voxels, corresponding pixels can be highlighted or subtracted from the CT image data set, or superimposed over the grayscale CT image. If the dual-energy processing is performed in projection data space, besides obtaining material-specific information from the dual-energy data, monochromatic images at a preferred energy can also be created, which has a great potential to reduce beam-hardening artifact, improve the image contrast, and provide more quantitative information about the structure.

Dual-Energy Display Methods

Approaches for displaying dual-energy data vary and are evolving, but can primarily be divided into methods for displaying anatomic data in

a single image set versus software and display techniques intended for displaying material-specific information.

For display of anatomic images in a single image stack, the CT number and anatomic detail from the high- and low-energy data must be blended. For contrast-enhanced abdominal CT, the 80-kV data set possesses more contrast and more noise than the 140-kV data set. This impact can be dramatic, with the CT number of iodine at 80 kV being twice that at 140 kV, with resulting improvements in contrast-to-noise ratio for small and medium patients.[6] The decreased image noise of the 140-kV data set has advantages in large patients and organs that are homogeneous (such as the liver).

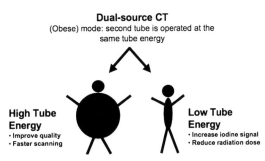

Fig. 6. The use and benefits of dual-source CT depend on patient size.

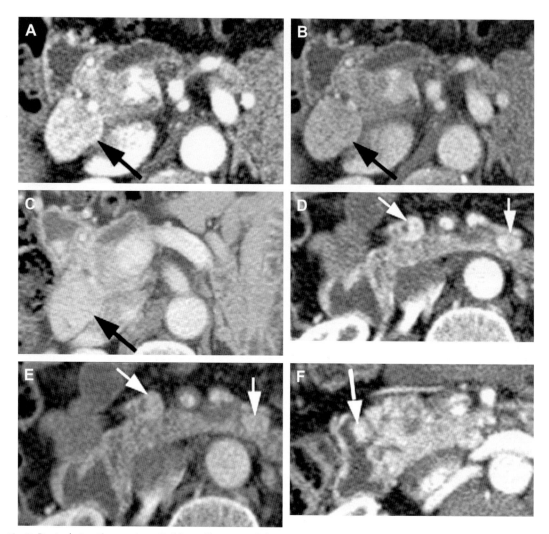

Fig. 7. Duct-obstructing metastatic islet cell tumor of the pancreas using dual-energy CT, demonstrating the improved conspicuity of primary tumor and metastatic periduodenal lymph nodes at 80 compared with 120 kV. (*A, B*) The 80-kV and 120-kV images during the dual-energy pancreatic phase acquisition. The 80-kV data set (*A*) more clearly demonstrates the hypervascular nature of the duct-obstructing primary tumor and large periduodenal metastatic lymph node (*arrow*). (*C*) Similar findings on a prior pancreatic phase image using a single-source CT system at 120 kV. The markedly elevated CT attenuation of small, subcentimeter metastatic preduodenal lymph nodes at 80 kV (*D, arrows*) compared with 120 kV (*E, arrows*) suggested the diagnosis of locally metastatic islet cell tumor of the pancreas. The 80-kV images also demonstrated a focus of duodenal invasion (*F, arrows*), which was confirmed in the resected specimen.

Although 80-kV data offer dramatically increased contrast-to-noise with the smaller patients, the contribution of the higher-energy data becomes progressively important as patient size increases to maintain image quality. Combining the potential advantages of each type of data set is the goal of image blending. Multiple approaches and possibilities exist.[7] Linear blending weights the intensity of all pixels in the image by a constant factor. Nonlinear blending methods, such as sigmoidal blending, in contradistinction, weight the intensity of all pixels by their relative CT number. For example, low CT numbers would preferentially come from the 140-kV data set (so noise is minimized in fat and non-iodinated fluid) and high CT numbers are weighted toward the 80-kV data set (so the CT signal of iodine is displayed maximally; **Fig. 4**). Tunable linear and sigmoidal blending techniques permit optimal contrast selection for any particular patient and organ, with the relative blending of the images being patient and organ dependent.[7]

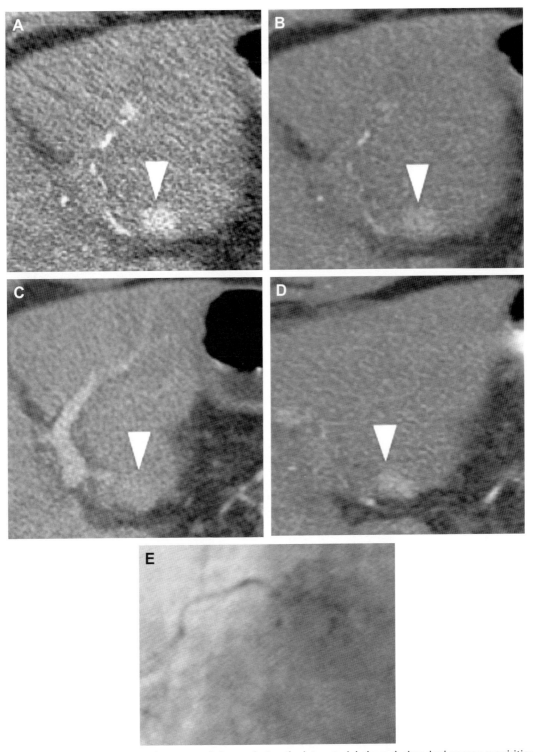

Fig. 8. Hepatocellular carcinoma (*A, B, arrow*) shown during the late arterial phase during dual-energy acquisition is more conspicuous on the output of the 80-kV image (*A*) compared with 140-kV image (*B*). Both the portal phase image at 120 kV (*C*) and the prior late arterial phase at a single-energy 120-kV examination (*D*) show the tumor, but with decreased conspicuity compared with the 80-kV image. Note increased noise in the 80-kV examination (*A*). (*E*) Tumor at chemoembolization shortly after the dual-energy examination.

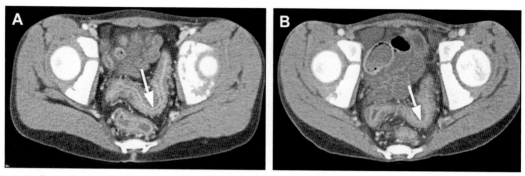

Fig. 9. Pediatric dose reduction using 100 kV (*A*) as opposed to 120 kV (*B*) in the same patient (who had Crohn colitis). Note improved contrast-to-noise and visualization of mural stratification of the 100-kV image (*A, arrow*) despite similar slice thickness and 25% radiation dose reduction.

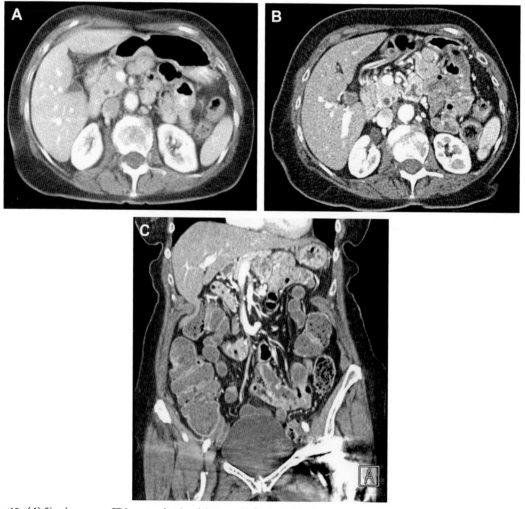

Fig. 10. (*A*) Single-source CT image obtained 8 years before the dual-source examination (*B, C*). Because of compromised intravenous access, contrast could only be injected at a rate of 2 mL/s, prompting the decision to move the patient to a dual-source CT system to perform a dual-source 80-kV CT enterography examination. Axial (*B*) and coronal (*C*) images from the 80-kV dual-source CT enterography examination demonstrate excellent image contrast and sharpness compared with the original study despite a slower injection rate.

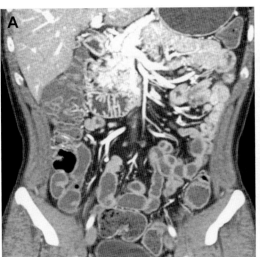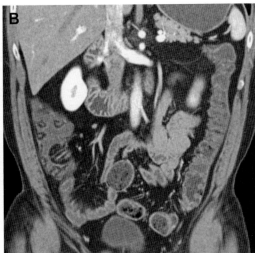

Fig. 11. Comparison of iodine-related signal at CT enterography using same windows and level (400, 40) for routine image display in the same patient undergoing CT enterography using dual-source 80-kV (A) and single-source 120-kV technique (B). The increased signal resulting from 80-kV scanning results in a need to change routine window settings in some patients.

Dual-Source CT Acquisition and Display

For dual-source CT imaging, the tubes are each set at the same kV, with the tube energy chosen based on patient size and the imaging application (improving image quality/speed in large patients, or reducing dose and improving lesion conspicuity in small patients). Not only does 80-kV imaging offer improved iodine signal in appropriate-sized patients, but even taking the increased noise into account, it offers increased contrast-to-noise ratio for smaller patients (**Fig. 5**).[8] In obese patients, the dual-source mode is used to improve image quality and permit faster table speed at higher tube energies. In smaller patients, both tubes are operated at lower kVs to permit an increase in the iodine signal and reduce radiation dose (**Fig. 6**). Because most single-source CT scanners are limited in their ability to image at lower tube energies (because the tube current needed exceeds system limits), one of the principle advantages of dual-source CT is that it extends the dynamic range of tube currents to a wider range of patients. When scanning small and medium-sized patients, we use a cut-off value of 39 cm lateral width as measured from the CT scout to select patients who can undergo dual-source 80-kV imaging without the creation of bothersome artifacts, opting for dual-source 100-kV imaging for larger patients.

The projection data obtained from each of the two sets of detectors at dual-source CT is combined in projection space to yield images that reflect the output of both x-ray tubes. In small and medium-sized patients, the images appear identical to single-source displays. For larger patients, there is a slight but perceptible decline in CT number in the subcutaneous tissues of morbidly obese patients, because this portion of the image is created using only one tube and one detector, as opposed to the inner portion of the image that is created using both tubes and detectors. (Of course even with appropriate selection of single-source CT acquisition parameters there is a generalized decline in CT number throughout the image in a morbidly obese patient because of beam hardening).

APPLICATIONS FOR DUAL-ENERGY AND DUAL-SOURCE CT
Iodine Enhancement

One of the principal advantages for both dual-energy and dual-source CT is in the enhancement of the iodine signal at lower tube energies.[8] Routine contrast-enhanced abdominal CT at 120 or 140 kV of course exploits the tissue and perfusional differences between normal anatomy and pathology because the presence of intravenous iodinated contrast increases the conspicuity of disease, so it comes as no surprise that dual-energy and dual-source CT may potentiate this effect. Organs in which most pathologies are highlighted by intravenous iodine are most susceptible to potential improvements in lesion detection using these techniques. We have found both techniques to be particularly useful in imaging the pancreas (for visualization of hypo- and hypervascular lesions; **Fig. 7**) and small bowel (to increase the identification of hyperenhancement). Because

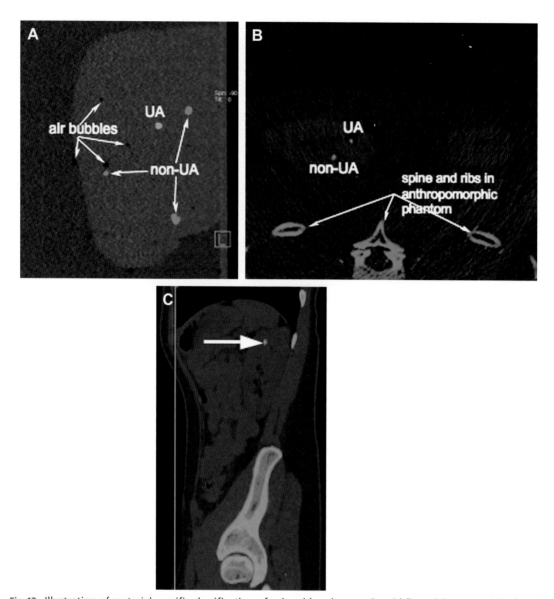

Fig. 12. Illustration of material-specific classification of uric acid and non–uric acid (ie, calcium-containing) renal stones in a phantom (*A, B*) and human (*C*) using a three-material, image space decomposition method. Using this method, pixels are classified as urine (*no color*), uric acid (*red*), or calcium (*blue*). Note that both bones and calcium-containing stone are classified using the same color in the patient examination (*C*).

the liver is a relatively homogeneous organ, the increased noise of a low-kV data set can be problematic when performing hepatic imaging, so we find dual-energy imaging to be particularly beneficial in the liver (for the detection of hepatocellular carcinoma; **Fig. 8**). In each of these clinical applications, detection of suspected pathology depends on the differential iodine content between disease and the background organ during the relevant phase of contrast enhancement. Although one may think that dual-energy scanning may slightly expand the size of patients who can be imaged compared with dual-source low-kV scanning (because of the low-noise 140-kV data set), it must be remembered that the output of the low-energy tube must still generate a relatively artifact-free image, so there is a patient size limitation using either technique.

For dual-energy hepatic and pancreatic imaging, we perform the late arterial and pancreatic phases, respectively, using a dual-energy technique, to maximize the detection of hyper- or hypovascular pathologies, obtaining portal phase imaging using single-source techniques. For

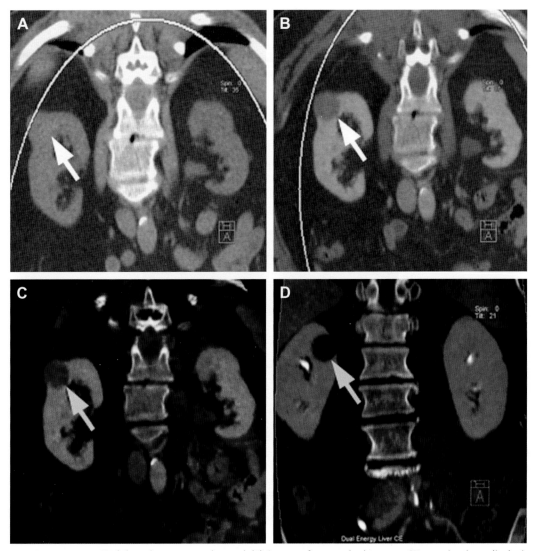

Fig. 13. Noncontrast CT (*A*) and contrast-enhanced (*B*) images from a dual-energy CT examination, displaying mixed-kV 0.3 linear blend images to simulate CT numbers of a 120-kV examination. The noncontrast examination shows the renal mass (*A, arrow*) to have a mean CT number of 28 HU, which increased to 56 HU during the nephrogenic phase (*B, arrow*). Following material classification using dual-energy techniques, iodine overlay images were generated to identify iodine within the renal mass. The corresponding iodine overlay image (*C*) clearly demonstrates iodine within the lesion (*C, arrow*), consistent with the minimally enhancing status of the lesion. (*D*) Iodine overlay image demonstrating lack of iodine (*D, arrow*) within a renal cyst.

enterography examinations we perform only an enteric phase dual-energy acquisition. For interpretation of these examinations, we generally evaluate the mixed-energy data stack only for enterography examinations, but for pancreatic and liver lesion identification, simultaneous display of late arterial phase images (140 kV, 80 kV, mixed kV) and portal phase images (120 kV) is often helpful. Mixed-kV images are created using a commercially available 0.7 linear blend of the 80-kV (70% of image input) and 140-kV (30% of image input) data sets.

Dual-source CT successfully potentiates iodine signal (and consequently, the conspicuity of hyper- or hypovascular lesions) in small and medium-sized patients while preserving image quality. In small patients, the use of lower tube energies may result in improved contrast-to-noise ratios, which can be exploited to achieve radiation dose reduction.[9] We use lower tube energies in pediatric imaging so that we can increase the pitch while maintaining appropriate tube current, permitting improved contrast-to-noise ratio and an approximately 20% to 30% reduction in radiation

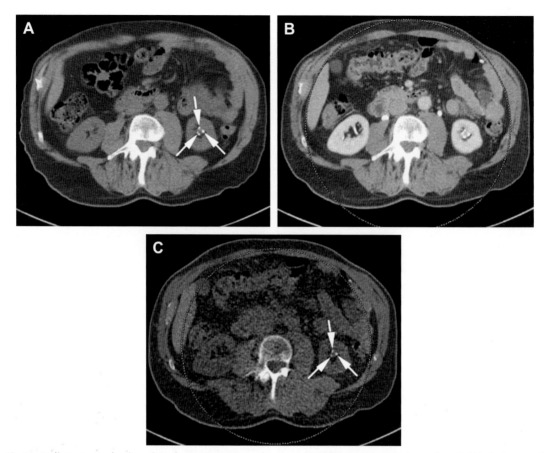

Fig. 14. Iodine removal using virtual noncontrast, as demonstrated by three small stones in a left inferior renal calyx. Unenhanced CT image shows the stones (*arrows*, *A*). During the pyelographic phase (*B*) obtained as part of a dual-energy CT urogram, the mixed-kV image shows high attenuation, which is a mixture of iodinated contrast and the stones, within the left inferior pole calices. Using the high- and low-kV images obtained from the dual-energy examination, iodine classification and removal was performed to yield a virtual noncontrast image (*C*), which also demonstrates the three small stones in the inferior pole calices (*C, arrows*).

dose (**Fig. 9**). We also preferentially use dual-source lower-kV imaging (at 80 or 100 kV) to increase the iodine signal when there is poor IV access and intravenous contrast is injected at a reduced dose or rate. In these circumstances, the improved contrast-to-noise compensates for the suboptimal delivery of intravenous contrast to yield higher-quality images (**Fig. 10**). Because the CT signal intensity related to the iodine signal is dramatic and because both tubes are operating at the lower energy, a change in the routine viewing windows for abdominal CT is often needed, because liver, pancreas, bowel wall, and vessels appear brighter (**Fig. 11**).

Material Classification

Characterization of renal stones
We used a three-material decomposition algorithm (using urine, "pure" calcium-containing stone, or "pure" uric acid stone) to examine the ability of dual energy to differentiate calcium oxylate and hydroxyapatite stones from uric acid stones using various detector configurations, with comparison to micro CT and infrared spectroscopy.[10] For the 40 human renal stones examined, there was 100% accuracy for phantoms simulating average and large patient sizes, but there was diminished performance when phantoms corresponding to morbidly obese patients were scanned with minimal collimation. Others have confirmed our findings[11] and extended this technique to either human studies (**Fig. 12**)[12] or the possible differentiation of different types of calcium stones.[13] A musculoskeletal application of the same technique (to identify uric acid crystals) can be used to identify uric acid crystals in joints, to distinguish tophaceous gout from calcium pyrophosphate dihydrate deposition disease and other arthropathies.

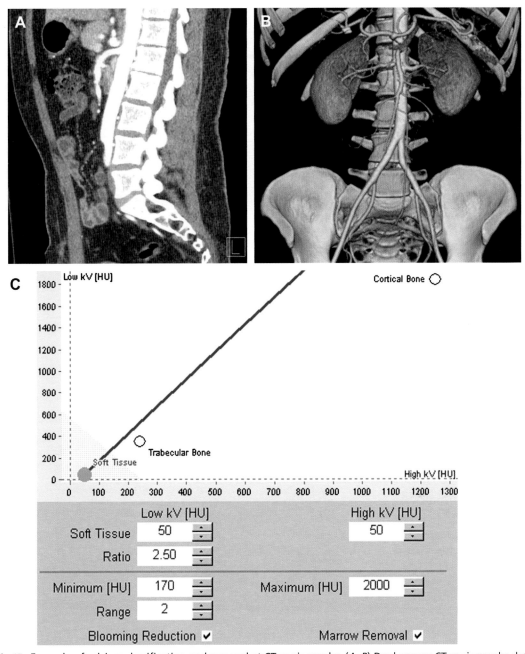

Fig.15. Example of calcium classification and removal at CT angiography. (*A, B*) Dual-energy CT angiography data set using standard two-dimensional sagittal (*A*) and three-dimensional volume-rendered (*B*) displays. (*C*) Initial dual-energy ratio of 2.5 was chosen, which resulted in lack of separation of iodine and calcium (ie, both removed and colored black, *D*). (*E*) Subsequent changing of the dual-energy ratio to 2.0 results in excellent separation, with only calcium-containing pixels colored black (*F*). Unretouched three-dimensional volume-rendered image using the calcium-removed data set in F shows excellent removal of spine (*G*).

Iodine identification

The use of dual-energy CT techniques to highlight pathologies using routine image displays (along with blending techniques) has been previously discussed. The approach for displaying the enhanced iodine signal at dual energy can follow an entirely different paradigm, however, following material-specific classification of iodine-containing pixels, which can then be highlighted using color overlay techniques. We have used dual-energy CT acquisition and material-specific iodine classification and color overlay in the classification of renal

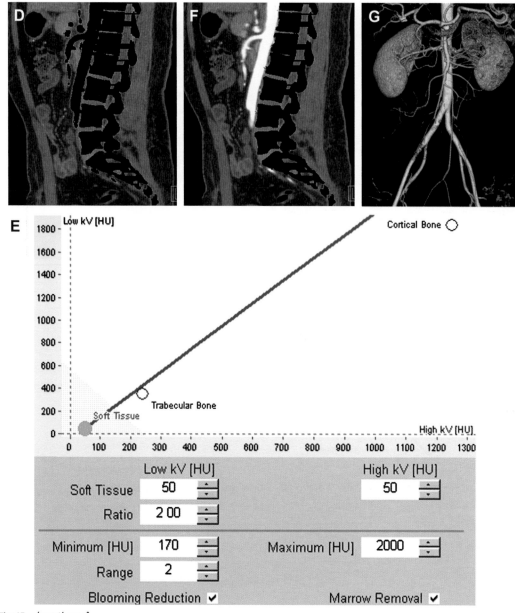

Fig. 15. (continued)

masses.[14] Using single-energy CT, it can be difficult to differentiate between a hemorrhagic cyst versus a papillary renal cell carcinoma, for example. By classifying pixels as containing iodine using dual-energy CT, a single contrast-enhanced pass through a renal mass may be able to clarify the issue of whether a renal lesion has minimal contrast enhancement. In a phantom study mimicking enhancing renal cortex and minimally enhancing renal masses, we found this technique to have 97% sensitivity and 82% specificity for classifying a renal lesion as an enhancing mass. All lesions, ranging in size from 0.5 to 3.0 cm,

with 20 HU or greater enhancement, were correctly classified. We have found dual-energy CT iodine overlay in patients a useful adjunct to the grayscale images when faced with the diagnostic dilemma of differentiating a minimally enhancing renal mass from a hyperdense cyst (Fig. 13).

Iodine identification can also be used to create "virtual noncontrast" images by removing the iodine-containing voxels. Such approaches are in their infancy and seem particularly promising in the evaluation of the kidney and urinary tract. Creation of a virtual noncontrast image set from a contrast-enhanced nephrographic or pyelographic phase data set can potentially lower radiation dose if an unenhanced scan can be avoided, and can be used to identify renal stones from surrounding iodine-containing urine (**Fig. 14**). Current limitations of this approach include the potential for not detecting a small minority of stones less than 3 mm in size, and the necessity for avoiding maximum CT numbers (because of the combination of dense contrast within the collecting system and 80-kV scanning).[15] To avoid maximum CT numbers in the renal collecting system, CT urography protocols can be modified or the lower tube energy can be switched to 100 kV.

Applications that examine liver lesions rely on the integrity of the lower-kV image, which is susceptible to excessive noise artifacts. For applications in which these are less of a concern or situations in which image artifacts are minimized (eg, smaller patients, kidneys) virtual noncontrast remains a viable option that would reduce radiation dose and may eliminate the need for some noncontrast examinations. Virtual noncontrast iodine removal techniques are not adequate to currently replace true noncontrast scans and are undergoing further refinement.[16]

Calcium removal

Postprocessing of CT angiography images can be speeded using dual-energy techniques to remove calcium signal (**Fig. 15**). Such an approach removes bones and calcified plaques. If implemented on a dual-source CT system, however, removal of bone beyond the internal 26-cm FOV still requires manual interaction. Our dual-energy, dual-source CT angiography examination saves 20% to 30% dose over its single-tube counterpart and does so on the basis of the improved iodine signal at 80 kV. Calcium bloom remains a problem (at routine and dual-energy imaging) and can cause overestimation of vascular stenoses. We anticipate dual-energy postprocessing algorithms may be implemented in the future to address this problem.

Lipid identification

Material classification of lipid content may improve adrenal mass characterization beyond the routine noncontrast scan or aid in the characterization of hepatic masses.[17]

OBESE PATIENT SCANNING

In morbidly obese patients adequate image quality using a single-source CT scanner can often be preserved by widening collimation and slice thickness, slowing tube rotation time, and increasing tube current and voltage. Such changes improve image quality at the expense of spatial and temporal resolution and scan time. By extending the dynamic range of tube currents available at high tube voltages, dual-source CT can permit dramatically increased table speeds in morbidly obese patients, while maintaining acceptable image quality and often preserving spatial resolution (**Fig. 16**). Using a dual-source CT system, we can perform multiphasic CT liver, pancreas, and enterography CT scans in even morbidly obese patients without slowing the tube rotation time, and can improve image quality over single-source CT in these patients (**Fig. 17**). Increasing the tube current allows faster pitches while staying in the quantum limited region where image quality is preserved.

SUMMARY AND CHALLENGES

Dual-energy and dual-source CT show great promise in a wide variety of abdominal and pelvic applications. It is likely that dual-energy and dual-source CT could be routinely used in the detection and characterization of liver and pancreatic masses, characterization of renal and adrenal masses, detection of small bowel disease, and classification of renal stones. High-quality, multiphase scanning in obese patients and significant dose savings in smaller patients are additional benefits.

Principle challenges are to identify patients who would benefit from these examinations and to reduce image noise. Reducing the increased image noise seen with low-kV imaging will improve the quality of dual-source and dual-kV images and improve material classification at dual energy. Reducing image noise at dual-source low-kV imaging will also improve contrast-to-noise ratios, permitting further reductions in radiation dose to be achieved. Advances in noise reduction (whether occurring in projection or image space, or during image reconstruction) will enable dual-source low-kV scanning across a wider variety of patient sizes and will likely extend the benefits of low-kV scanning to single-source CT systems. Other advances in dual-energy technology, such as improved separation of tube energies, may improve material classification but have an unclear impact on lesion detection.

The cost of using dual-energy and dual-source scanners into a practice is currently significant, and may be prohibitive for some groups. The cost of a dual-source CT system is considerably higher than that of a single-source scanner, and the increased weight of the machine requires additional structural support, increasing the cost of the installation. In most practices it is difficult to justify purchase of a dual-source system based on abdominal applications alone, and the cardiac

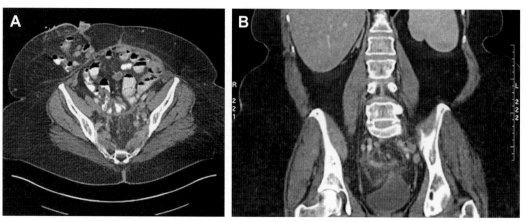

Fig. 16. (*A, B*) Example of dual-source obese mode in a patient who had a prior left colectomy and Hartmann pouch. Using dual-source technique at 140 kV, excellent image quality (without beam hardening) was retained even in the bony pelvis without the need to decrease the tube rotation time or pitch.

applications of the scanner are likely to carry greater importance when considering the purchase. If a dual-source scanner is purchased for its cardiac capability, however, its unique capabilities should be used so that selected abdominal patients can also benefit from being appropriately triaged for dual-source or dual-energy scanning. As dual-energy and dual-source CT systems proliferate and gain increased acceptance of their clinical benefits in abdominal imaging, we

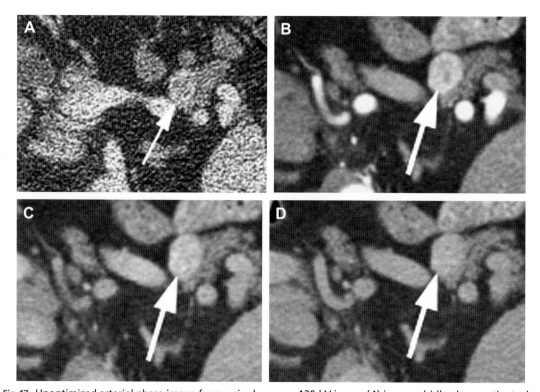

Fig. 17. Unoptimized arterial phase image from a single-source 120-kV image (*A*) in a morbidly obese patient who had suspected pancreatic islet cell neoplasm (*A, arrow*) demonstrates beam hardening and spiral artifacts. Using dual-source 120-kV technique, a bolus-triggered triple phase examination of the liver and pancreas was performed (*B–D*), resulting in marked improvement in image quality and increased conspicuity of the tumor in the arterial and late arterial phases (*arrows, B* and *C*).

anticipate the cost associated with these systems will decline.

Dual-energy applications will continue to expand beyond renal stone classification and renal mass evaluation as new material-specific classification methods are developed and refined and as organ-specific clinical scenarios, such as adrenal imaging, are interrogated. Radiologists should work with industry partners so that appropriate dual-energy and dual-source protocols can be automatically implemented in patients, taking into account patient size and suspected pathology.

Further validation of many dual-energy techniques and their limitations and benefits is needed to understand the clinical scenarios in which such techniques can be used for medical decision making. Current dual-source and dual-energy CT techniques can clearly benefit some patients now, for example, by enhancing iodine signal (to improve lesion detection) in small and moderately-sized patients; by performing dual-source high-kV scanning in morbidly obese patients requiring multiphase scanning, or dual-source low-kV scanning in smaller patients who have compromised renal function or IV access; for problem solving in patients who have indeterminate renal masses; and for noninvasively classifying renal stones greater than 3 mm in size. Dual-energy and dual-source technology remains an ongoing and fruitful source of development for abdominal CT.

REFERENCES

1. Flohr TG, McCollough CH, Bruder H, et al. First performance evaluation of a dual-source CT (DSCT) system. Eur Radiol 2006;16(2):256–68.
2. Schmidt B, Bredenhoeller C, Flohr T. Dual source CT technology. In: Seidensticker PH, Hofman LK, editors. Dual source CT imaging. Heidelberg (Germany): Springer Medizin Verlag; 2008. p. 19–33.
3. Carmi R, Naveh GA, Altman A. Material separation with dual-layer CT. IEEE 2005;M03–367:1876–8.
4. Alvarez RE, Macovski A. Energy-selective reconstructions in X-ray computerized tomography. Phys Med Biol 1976;21(5):733–44.
5. Kalender WA, Perman WH, Vetter JR, et al. Evaluation of a prototype dual-energy computed tomographic apparatus. I. Phantom studies. Med Phys 1986;13(3):334–9.
6. Braeutigam M, Huebner-Steiner U, Pietsch H, et al. Iodinated contrast media: new perspectives with dual source CT. In: Seidensticker P, Hofmann L, editors. Dual source CT imaging. Heidelberg (Germany): Springer Medizin Verlag; 2008. p. 35–47.
7. Holmes DR, FJ, Apel A, et al. Evaluation of non-linear blending in dual-energy computed tomography. Eur J Radiol 2008;68:409–13.
8. Schindera ST, Nelson RC, Mukundan S Jr, et al. Hypervascular liver tumors: low tube voltage, high tube current multi-detector row CT for enhanced detection—phantom study. Radiology 2008;246(1):125–32.
9. Nakayama Y, Awai K, Funama Y, et al. Abdominal CT with low tube voltage: preliminary observations about radiation dose, contrast enhancement, image quality, and noise. Radiology 2005;237(3):945–51.
10. Primak AN, Fletcher JG, Vrtiska TJ, et al. Noninvasive differentiation of uric acid versus non-uric acid kidney stones using dual-energy CT. Acad Radiol 2007;14(12):1441–7.
11. Stolzmann P, Scheffel H, Rentsch K, et al. Dual-energy computed tomography for the differentiation of uric acid stones: ex vivo performance evaluation. Urol Res 2008;36(3–4):133–8.
12. Graser A, Johnson TR, Bader M, et al. Dual energy CT characterization of urinary calculi: initial in vitro and clinical experience. Invest Radiol 2008;43(2):112–9.
13. Matlaga BR, Kawamoto S, Fishman E. Dual source computed tomography: a novel technique to determine stone composition. Urology 2008;72(5):1164–8.
14. Hartman R, Takahashi N, Kawashima A, et al. Dual energy CT iodine overlay images ability to classify renal lesions as a cyst or solid mass. Paper presented at: 94th Scientific Assembly and Annual Meeting, Radiological Society of North America, 2008; Chicago, IL.
15. Takahashi N, Hartman RP, Vrtiska TJ, et al. Dual-energy CT iodine-subtraction virtual unenhanced technique to detect urinary stones in an iodine-filled collecting system: a phantom study. AJR Am J Roentgenol 2008;190(5):1169–73.
16. Scheffel H, Stolzmann P, Frauenfelder T, et al. Dual-energy contrast-enhanced computed tomography for the detection of urinary stone disease. Invest Radiol 2007;42(12):823–9.
17. Graser A, Johnson TR, Chandarana H, et al. Dual energy CT: preliminary observations and potential clinical applications in the abdomen. Eur Radiol 2008; [epub ahead of print].

Advanced Postprocessing and the Emerging Role of Computer-Aided Detection

Anand K. Singh, MD[a], Yoshida Hiroyuki, PhD[a],
Dushyant V. Sahani, MD[b],*

KEYWORDS

- Computed tomography • Three-dimensional imaging
- Postprocessing • Segmentation
- Volume estimation • Virtual endoscopy
- Computer-aided detection

The newer generation multidetector CT (MDCT) scanners have increased the momentum of research on certain important three-dimensional (3D) applications. Thin-section data sets of isotropic voxel resolution have not only improved the quality of simple postprocessing algorithms like maximum intensity projection and volume rendering (VR) but have provided better accuracy and image quality of organ segmentation algorithms and virtual navigation techniques.[1–3] The benefits of advances in CT scanners have also been increasingly used to improve automations in postprocessing by utilizing certain computer-aided postprocessing techniques. Use of certain advanced postprocessing techniques was restricted in the previous decade because of unavailability of thin sections of axial scan data sets of good resolution. With the advent of MDCT, advanced postprocessing applications like virtual endoscopy (VE), segmentation and volumetric estimations, and computer-aided postprocessing methods are gradually becoming an integral component of diagnostic studies.[4] Organ segmentation is basically the first crucial step for performing a virtual fly-through or obtaining the volume of an organ. The result of computer-aided automations in postprocessing also largely depends on the accuracy with which the region of interest is segmented.

POSTPROCESSING MULTIDETECTOR CT DATA

Various studies have highlighted the importance of thin axial sections from 16-channel MDCT in enhancing 3D image quality of brain, cardiac, liver, renal, and aortic CT angiography (CTA) studies.[5,6] The enhancement in image quality of 3D images in cardiac imaging and for simple coronal and sagittal reformations for the abdomen and pelvis has also been highlighted in a study by Singh and colleagues,[7] in which significantly better image quality of reformats obtained from 64-channel MDCT was found in large-sized patients over the reformats obtained from a 16-channel MDCT scanner.

To ensure better accuracy in the results of advanced postprocessing applications like volumetry and viewing on virtual navigation modes, it is important that axial scan data sets available for postprocessing be thin, which can improve lesion definition and its conspicuity. Moreover, such data sets should be devoid of image artifacts. The increasing concern over balancing the radiation dose delivery and still ensuring thin-section

a Department of Three-Dimensional Imaging, Massachusetts General Hospital, Harvard Medical School, 25 New Chardon Street, Suite 400, Boston, MA 02114, USA
b Department of Abdominal Imaging, Massachusetts General Hospital, Harvard Medical School, White 2 270, 55 Fruit Street, Boston, MA 02114, USA
* Corresponding author.
E-mail address: dsahani@partners.org (D.V. Sahani).

Radiol Clin N Am 47 (2009) 59–77
doi:10.1016/j.rcl.2008.11.004
0033-8389/08/$ – see front matter. Published by Elsevier Inc.

scan acquisitions is a surfacing issue for exploring the parameters and dimensions in most postprocessing applications. With the advent of higher generation scanners and availability of sophisticated workstations, axial scan data acquired at 2.5-mm or less usually produce optimal postprocessing results, even with the use of advanced applications like VE, segmentations, and computer-aided detection (CAD). In the present era, in which scanners from 16- to 320-channel and even beyond may provide lucrative opportunities with thin-section data sets, its important to define parameters for their use in postprocessing to optimize radiation dose delivery to patients and to avoid data explosion.[8] With the background and availability of such sophisticated scanners, workstations, and 3D filters, it would be prudent to set the cutoff at a 2.5-mm thickness of axial data sets, greater than which degradations in image postprocessing would become evident. The benefits of thinner scan acquisitions of 1.25 mm or less have been proved for visualizations of subtle arterial variants and arterial abnormalities on 3D CTA images.[9] Recent studies have revealed that postprocessing with CT data sets acquired at 2.5 mm have also produced results with reasonable accuracy for CT venography studies and advanced postprocessing applications like segmentation techniques, virtual bronchoscopy (VB) and colonoscopy, and computer-assisted postprocessing, however.[10]

Recent Advances

The detector rows in the fourth-generation scanners vary in number from 64 to 320, along with differences in width (1.9 and 16 cm). Dual-energy imaging, performed by analyzing the effects of two x-ray signals acquired simultaneously, can offer important new information about tissue properties.[11] Important postprocessing applications of dual-source MDCT include enhanced display of renal stone differentiation patterns and automated bone removal. These newer scanners provide advantages in terms of scan speed and increased range of coverage area in a short time and may point toward valid solutions in cardiac imaging.

The fourth-generation high-definition (HD) scanner improves spatial resolution by using the light-handling properties of a gemstone detector and a software upgrade, which improves resolution of acquired MDCT data sets through reduction of noise. These scanners improve spatial resolution to approximately 230 μm at a 2-mm scan length, which is approximately 300 μm for other fourth-generation scanners. Such upgrades may provide up to 50% improvement in visualization of coronary arteries of the heart and a considerable increase in resolution for visualization of abdominal structures. The gemstone detector, which works on the principle of the superior light-handling properties of garnets, supports material decomposition for the entire 50-cm field of view (FOV) and produces intrinsically sharper and brighter images because of its better optical properties. Because of such inherent properties of the detector material, up to 40% improvement in low-contrast detectability at approximately a 50% lower dose is expected by the HD scan acquisitions. Because of the nuance of this innovation, however, no research data are presently available. With the advent of such scanners, wider applicability of postprocessing applications in the clinical scenario may be expected.

VIRTUAL ENDOSCOPY

VE provides a picture that simulates a view obtained by an invasive endoscopy procedure. Thin sections of artifact-free axial data (0.625–2.5 mm), with optimal distention of the desired lumen to be visualized, are ideal preprocessed data, which ensure generation of high-quality fly-through views.

Technique

To make any navigation possible, segmentation of the structure of interest on CT data sets is the first essential step, after which a virtual navigation path is generated through the lumen of the segmented structure. The segmented volume can be visualized by a surface rendering or VR technique. For creation of a fly-through path, it is essential that a centerline through the tubular lumen be delineated for the purposes of performing the navigation; this is usually simple for structures that are anatomically straight, such as the aorta.[12] The basic requisite is availability of thin-section and artifact-free axial scan data sets. The other important consideration is establishing direct and reliable interpretation of the objects that are encountered while performing the navigation. Especially with respect to screening for precancerous colonic polyps, the present fly-through techniques are significantly accurate for the detection of true polyps, but increasing concern remains over the number of false-positive misrepresentations of various objects, such as colonic folds and fecal material, as polyps.[13]

For generating virtual endoscopic views, it is important that the scan parameters be optimized with appropriate tailoring of the kilovoltage and milliampere settings. Although fast artifact-free scan acquisitions of 0.5-1 mm are now possible with 8- to 64-detector row CT scanners, it is prudent to set the lower limit of acquisition at 2.0 mm, which helps in reducing the radiation dose delivery to the patient. It is important to maintain the spacing at 50% of the prospective scan acquisition or the retrospective reconstruction to ensure optimal overlap between the two data sets and good-quality segmentation.[14] The presence of bright and homogeneous contrast in the vessel lumen is essential to ensure optimal quality of a virtual angioscopy image. Thin-section acquisitions of 0.5 to 1 mm allow optimal postprocessing of data when scan acquisitions are obtained after a 20- to 30-second scan delay after contrast injection.[13] Ensuring a good contrast between the lumen of the structure to be navigated and its wall is one of the most vital prerequisites for successful performance of virtual navigation software. A scan data set devoid of motion artifacts and thin-slice acquisitions from MDCT scanners, which ensure isotropic voxel resolution, are important general requirements for any VE application.

Clinical Applications

Head and neck

The use of VE applications in head and neck imaging has been recognized for guidance of various surgical procedures and diagnosis of foreign bodies in the paranasal sinuses and middle ear, evaluation of the ossicular chain and metallic ear implants, and assessment of the retrobulbar region. Hardening artifacts caused by dental implants may degrade the CT image quality, which is one of the disadvantages of CT data sets over MR imaging, but CT is more useful for assessment of fine bone structures and fibro-osseous lesions in the paranasal sinuses and nasal cavity, where it is at an advantage over MR imaging. VE images generated by means of MDCT provide a reliable assessment of the internal surfaces of the temporal bone. Virtual otoscopy provides a reasonably accurate depiction and outline of the structures in the tympanic cavity and is considered to be complementary to regular axial section CT evaluation.[15] More studies with a large cohort need to be conducted to define the role of otoscopy for evaluation of the ossicular chain and tympanic cavity. Congenital aural atresia is another condition in which the role of virtual CT endoscopy has been investigated.[16] In a recent study performed by Rodt and colleagues,[17] the additive role of 3D CT virtual otoscopy was highlighted in 213 patients suspected of having middle ear pathologic conditions, who were examined using a low-dosage MDCT protocol.

The clinical importance of virtual laryngoscopy has been investigated to assess the extent of laryngeal and hypopharyngeal carcinomas and to visualize laryngeal webs and upper airway stenosis.[18] In a recent study by Firat and colleagues,[19] findings from rigid telescopic videolaryngoscopy and CT virtual laryngoscopy compared well with operative records, with good visualization of lesions on the base of the tongue, pyriform sinus, aryepiglottic folds, and arytenoids by CT virtual laryngoscopy. The additive role that virtual laryngoscopy offers for evaluation of upper airway stenosis over review of axial sections and multiplanar CT reformats has also been proved in a recent study.[20]

Thorax

VB is one of the VE applications that has been extensively investigated (**Fig. 1**A). Effective assessment of tracheal tumors like carcinoids and lung neoplasms, detection of foreign bodies in the pediatric age group, and evaluation of tracheobronchial stenosis are some of the areas in which the usefulness of VB has been established.[21] There is always some loss of surface detail when generating a virtual endoscopic view for the trachea, but VB provides a good way of confirming a suspected mass or lesion along the tracheal wall by simply clicking on it and simultaneously referring to the two-dimensional (2D) scan data sets. The clinical benefits of VB have been shown for confirmation of the location of upper lobe lung tumors along with facilitation of transbronchial lung biopsy.[22] A recent study comparing conventional bronchoscopic findings with those of virtual CT bronchoscopy in 36 patients suspected of having lung cancer found the sensitivity of MDCT VB to be 88%, whereas the specificity was 50%.[23] It has also been recently suggested that virtual positron emission tomography (PET)–CT-bronchoscopy may provide better results than virtual CT-bronchoscopy because of the combination of CT information and molecular or metabolic information on the pathologic process in the former technique.[24] The feasibility of VB with low-dose MDCT protocols has also been investigated for assessing the degree of tracheobronchial narrowing and for suspected foreign body aspiration with considerable success.[25] Virtual mediastinoscopy is currently being studied for its feasibility in showing 3D relations between active lymph nodes and surrounding structures, such as the innominate artery and azygos vein. A small pilot study has shown that virtual mediastinoscopy may make cervical mediastinoscopy and other invasive mediastinal explorations safer and more accurate.[26] Additional roles of VB for diagnosis of tracheal rings and recurrent respiratory papillomatosis

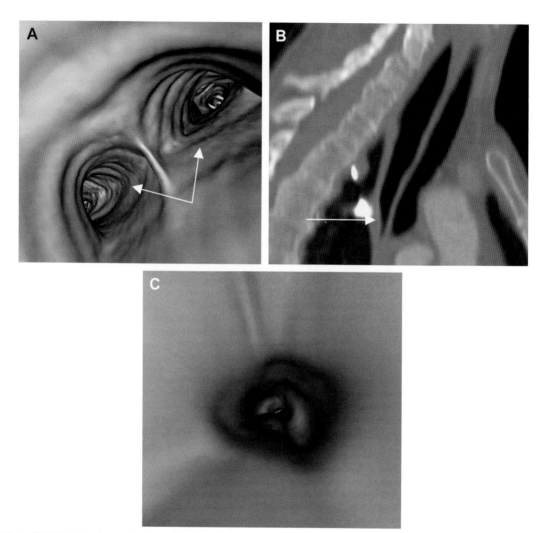

Fig. 1. (*A*) Virtual endoscopic view of tracheal bifurcation and origin of main bronchi (*thin arrows*). (*B*) Sagittal CT reformat of the upper thorax in a 44-year-old man with a history of lye ingestion and dysphagia shows esophageal narrowing (*thin arrow*). (*C*) Virtual CT esophagoscopy confirms a benign stricture with absence of lesions.

and for facilitation of biopsy of lung lesions in sarcoidosis are also under investigation.

Gastrointestinal

Virtual colonoscopy for the detection of precancerous polyps has been the most actively investigated area among existing VE applications. Certain advantages of virtual navigation views generated from MDCT data sets have also been realized for the detection and staging of certain pathologic findings in the esophagus, stomach, and small bowel, however.

In a prospective study performed by Mazzeo and colleagues,[27] the results of CT virtual esophagoscopy compared well with surgical, pathologic, and endoscopic findings in the detection and characterization of esophageal inflammations, benign tumors like leiomyoma, esophageal carcinoma, and stenosis (see **Fig. 1**B, C). Some recent studies have also highlighted the accuracy in tumor, node, metastasis staging of esophageal carcinoma by VE, which was found to be approximately 88% for tumor staging and 70% for nodal staging.[28] Similarly, its usefulness has been better realized for detection of early gastric tumors. A study by Duan and colleagues[29] has proved the effectiveness of virtual CT gastroscopy for the detection of various stomach lesions with greater than 90% accuracy, with the size of the smallest lesion being 1.0 cm × 0.8 cm × 0.5 cm. It is an important complementary technique to endoscopy. In spite of its documented adjunct role in diagnosis of gastric ulcers, polyps, and erosions and assessment of anastomotic sites after gastric bypass surgery, virtual gastroscopy has been found to be most valuable for detection of early gastric cancer. Virtual gastroscopy has been shown to provide similar results as conventional gastroscopy, with an added advantage of the availability of a wider FOV than conventional gastroscopy, which is devoid of blind points, because a retrospective MDCT data set for reconstruction can be used to navigate the areas missed.[30] Virtual CT gastroscopy results have shown significantly higher sensitivity for detection of early gastric carcinoma when compared with regular 2D axial CT data sets.[31] Lack of a wider FOV because of anatomic variations in luminal diameters of the small bowel compared with the stomach has restricted the usefulness of virtual duodenoscopy applications. Some small cohort studies have highlighted the location and extent of carcinoma, but virtual CT duodenoscopy has failed to receive more widespread attention on the research front.[32] Moreover, redundancy and variability in small bowel position may constantly produce challenges for technical advancements in imaging this lengthy structure, and the role of computer-aided techniques for refining this process has yet to be actively investigated.[33]

Virtual colonoscopy

Virtual colonoscopy enables radiologists to perform virtual "fly-through" in the colon, from the rectum to the cecum and back. It has been largely established that virtual colonoscopy is a viable option in screening colonic polyps, with its effectiveness and accuracy is being well established by numerous large clinical trials. CAD in virtual colonoscopy has effectively established greater than 90% per-polyp and per-patient sensitivity for polyps that are less than 6 mm in diameter (**Fig. 2**).[34] CAD for CT colonography (CTC) has proved to be effective so far in detection of tiny colonic polyps, and an update on technical advancements in virtual colonoscopy CAD is provided in subsequent sections of this article.

Optimal bowel preparation and colonic distention have been key elements in generation of a high-quality virtual CT endoscopic view of the colon, wherein a reader navigates through automated generation of the colonic centerline to assess the internal colonic surfaces of colon. Past studies have reported that a combination of dietary fecal tagging by orally administered contrast agents, such as barium, iodine, or Gastrografin (Bracco-diagnostics Inc., Princeton, NJ), and reduced or noncathartic bowel cleansing could be a viable alternative to full cathartic colon cleansing.[35] A more feasible option of mechanical bowel distention by carbon dioxide (CO_2) is a better-tolerated option, because CO_2 is passively absorbed by the colonic mucosa and can be eliminated by expiration. Advantages of new approaches, such as automatic CO_2 insufflation, have been highlighted recently, wherein much better distention of left colon is achieved, especially on supine scans.[36]

Although it is necessary to ensure the best results by acquisition of supine and prone series of CT data, it is important that scan parameters be tailored to keep the radiation dose delivery to a minimum, especially in patients undergoing screening and not diagnosis of a disease.[37] Recent studies have also established that virtual colonoscopy CAD performance for polyp

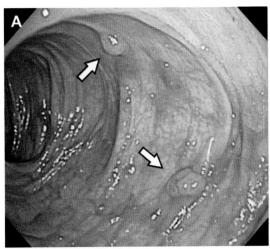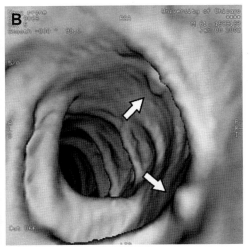

Fig. 2. (A) Screening optical colonoscopy image shows polyps in the colonic lumen (arrows) of a 53-year-old man. (B) Virtual CT colonoscopy image of the same polyps (arrows).

detection largely depends on z-axis spatial resolution and that tube current may not be an influencing factor.[38] Initially, with single-slice CT, collimation of 3 to 5 mm was used. With 8- to 64–detector row CT scanners, however, fast artifact-free scans of 0.5 to 1 mm are possible, which has tremendously enhanced the per-polyp and per-patient sensitivity of detection of polyps.[4] Combined CTC and ^{18}F-fluorodeoxyglucose (FDG) PET studies have been proved effective for the efficient detection of polyps greater than 10 mm, but the role of this combined modality in the detection of smaller polyps needs further validation.[39]

There is existing controversy regarding the clinical importance of flat and depressed colonic polyps in the colon. A high incidence of dysplasia in flat adenomas has been reported in several European and Japanese studies, which necessitates further research.[40]

Hepatobiliary and pancreas

The role of virtual CT endoscopy applications has been comparatively less investigated for the evaluation of diseases in relation to the pancreatic and common bile duct than for those in relation to other luminal structures. A study by Lou and colleagues[41] has highlighted the importance of CT biliary cystoscopy for the diagnosis and management of gallbladder polyps, but further validation is needed to support the findings of that study. Assessment of the pancreatic ductal details by CT–virtual pancreatoscopy has recently been compared with conventional endoscopic retrograde cholangiopancreatography, in which the virtual pancreatoscopy images were found to be of finer quality (Fig. 3).[42] To obtain satisfactory virtual endoscopic images of the pancreatic duct may be a difficult task in the absence of ductal dilatation, which is a major limitation for performing virtual CT pancreatoscopy.

Genitourinary

The evaluation of the urinary bladder by virtual cystoscopy is by far the most well-investigated VE application in the urinary system. The dilatation of the bladder lumen attributable to contrast excretion and the large diameter of the bladder lumen set a conducive platform for the generation of VE images through the bladder lumen. A recent study by Tsampoulas and colleagues[43] performed on MDCT data sets of 50 high-risk patients has highlighted the accuracy of MDCT cystoscopy for the detection of urinary bladder neoplasms by successful identification of lesions as small as 0.5 cm. There are adequate data to prove the effectiveness of CT virtual cystoscopy to follow up bladder tumors and estimation of regions that are inaccessible by endoscope and to differentiate between intravesical and extravesical lesions. CT voiding urethrography (CTVU) coupled with CT urethroscopy has also correlated closely with conventional methods for diagnosis of urethral injuries, strictures, and hypospadias. The smaller diameter of the urethra has restricted the popularity of such studies, however, and usually poses a challenge for the generation of virtual fly-through images. CTVU images used to generate virtual urethroscopy pictures have partially solved this problem. Moreover, CTVU has other advantages over conventional imaging methods, such as better accuracy in measurement of lesions without magnification or distortion and better patient compliance.[44]

The research on CT-pyeloureteroscopy has been restricted because of failure to generate

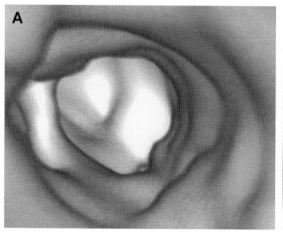 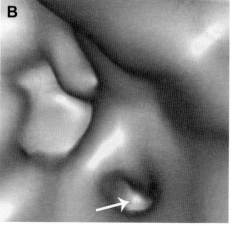

Fig. 3. (A) Virtual CT endoscopy image of a normal main pancreatic duct shows the pancreatic duct lumen. (B) Opening of a side-branch duct (thin arrow) is seen on virtual navigation through the pancreatic duct.

virtual endoscopic images of acceptable quality in normal patients in whom dilatation of the urinary tract is not present. Injection of diuretics before scanning may provide some benefit in achieving a desirable level of ureteric dilatation. It has better results in patients who have some degree of urinary tract dilation (>0.5 cm). With this technique, the sensitivity and specificity for detecting ureteral tumors have been shown to be 81% and 100%, respectively.[45]

An overview of important virtual CT endoscopy applications is given in **Table 1.**

SEGMENTATION AND VOLUMETRY
Technique

Accuracy in segmentation of desired structures is the most important determinant for a reliable generation of volume. Presently, segmentation techniques are becoming increasingly popular in

Table 1
Overview of important virtual CT endoscopy applications

Application	Diagnostic Use	Limitation/ Recommendations[a]	Computer- Aided Detection (±)
Virtual otoscopy	Middle ear pathologic conditions, ossicular chain abnormalities	MDCT acquisitions of 1 mm or less are preferable	−
Virtual fly-through paranasal sinuses	Nasal polyps, tumors, fibro-osseous pathologic conditions	Image degradation is possible with dental prosthesis	
Swallowing should be avoided during scan acquisition	−		
Virtual laryngoscopy	Laryngeal and hypopharyngeal carcinoma staging, vocal cord nodules, stenosis		−
Virtual bronchoscopy	Tracheal/lung tumor, foreign body detection	Ensure suction of secretions in unconscious patients before scan acquisition for better results	+
Virtual esophagoscopy/ gastroscopy	Esophageal strictures, tumors, Barrett's esophagus, gastroesophageal reflux, early gastric tumor/recurrence, ulcers	Optimal gaseous distention of esophageal and gastric lumen is needed for better image quality	−
Virtual colonoscopy	Screening of colonic polyps	Ensure optimal bowel preparation and colonic distention before scan	
Viewing 2D and CAD results for supine and prone scan series is recommended	+[b]		
Virtual cystoscopy and urethroscopy	Detection of small bladder tumors, tumor recurrence, ureteral obstruction/ stricture	CTVU ensures optimal distention of urethra, which is vital for successful generation of virtual navigation	−

[a] MDCT acquisitions devoid of motion/metallic artifacts.
[b] Includes electronic bowel cleansing.

imaging for preoperative planning of transplant surgery and as prognostic indicators of malignancies. Various segmentation techniques exist, namely, manual segmentation, thresholding, edge-based segmentation, region-based segmentation, and automated segmentation.[46] Manual segmentation is basically performing tracing along the borders of the desired structure. This can be on every consecutive or every alternate or third axial section, in which case, the software interpolates all the points between the segmented and unsegmented slices to generate volume results. This method is more reliable in terms of accuracy because it is controlled by an operator. Segmentation based on thresholding is basically assigning a certain Hounsfield unit (HU) range for facilitation of automated recognition by the computer of the desired structure that falls within that HU range. It is increasingly popular in the CAD scenario but has some issues with false-positive detections. Edge-based segmentation works on the principle of recognition of discontinuities in the image data at the border of the desired organ, which, in turn, depends on the difference in pixel values at the border of the organs. This method is not popular in current practice, however, because of technical difficulties. One of the most popular methods is the region-growing method, which is gaining increasing importance for segmentation and is based on the growth from a computer mouse–plotted seed point in the center of the desired structure, such that it grows and includes pixel areas with the same HU value as that of the center point.[47] In this method, a seed point is plotted in the desired organ parenchyma and the growth of the point is then initiated by a mouse click. The point spread is based on identifying similar pixels in the vicinity (HU on CT) and then establishing a growth pattern. This method is much quicker but is only useful for structures that have uniform HU values in their substance, such as free air or fluid, and is not conducive for such organs as the liver and spleen, which present variations in HU values in their parenchyma because of contrast in the vessels. Manual segmentation and the region-growing method are more popular because they allow more operator control, with the latter method being comfortable and automated (**Fig. 4**).

Clinical Applications

For the sole purpose of better visualization, segmentation of the vascular structures has been more popular for visualization of subtle details of the circle of Willis and to assess variants and neoplastic vessel involvement of the liver and of renal

and pancreatic vasculature before surgery. The assessment of aortic aneurysms is by far the most heavily investigated area in which vascular segmentation is reliably used in clinical practice, however, not only for presurgical planning but for visualization of endovascular stents.[48] A region-growing technique is well suited for such vessel segmentations, which display similarity in HU values because of contrast opacification.

CT volumetry in the liver and lung has been by far the most well-investigated area for the role of CT volumetry in clinical applications.[49,50] Some studies have highlighted the importance of quantifying intravertebral cement after kyphoplasty, cerebrospinal fluid in alcoholic subjects, and left ventricular volume, but further validation of such findings with larger cohort studies is still awaited.[51,52] Some researchers have also studied the segmentation of pulmonary arteries and, subsequently, its quantification and importance in subjects who have pulmonary hypertension.[53] The foreseen role of CT volumetry in oncology seems to be promising in the background of numerous recent studies performed on various tumors, of which quantification of liver neoplasms and pulmonary nodules is most popular.

Liver

Estimation of total and partial lobar liver volumes is an important presurgical requisite for preoperative planning of liver transplants, because it is crucial to ensure an optimal liver volume in the donor rather than in the compromised recipient.[54] Estimation of total liver and partial volumes of the right and left lobes of the liver is therefore important for decision making (**Figs. 5** and **6**). The present MDCT protocols for liver donor scanning are more conducive to provide a better 3D display of the vascular maps of liver donors because of the availability of thin-section data acquisitions, and therefore provide better accuracy in segmentation and, subsequently, volume estimations. Recipients with end-stage liver disease need a liver graft volume, which is 1% of the recipient's body mass (calculated by the graft-recipient body weight ratio).[55] The same concept also provides useful clinical information in patients who have end-stage liver disease in whom the remnant liver volume can be estimated and also in recipients in posttransplant settings. For the purposes of volume estimation of the liver, the results of software's interpolations between the manually segmented and unsegmented slices is more accurate if manual segmentation is done on every alternate axial CT slice of 2.5-mm thickness or on every fourth axial CT slice of 1.25-mm thickness, but results from such

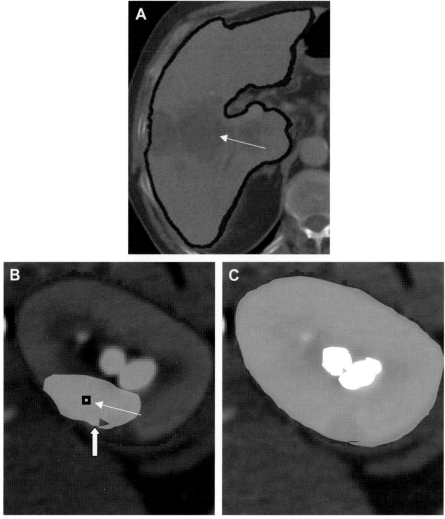

Fig. 4. (*A*) Manual tracing of the liver boundary in a 63-year-old male patient who had hepatocellular carcinoma (*thin arrow*). (*B, C*) Illustration of the region-growing technique for kidney segmentation on CT. Spread of the map to include structures with the same HU attenuation values (*thick arrow* in *B*) occurs from the center point plotted by the computer mouse (*thin arrow* in *B*) and covers the entire kidney (*C*).

computer-assisted postprocessing techniques need further validation.

Kidney

Estimation of kidney volume for transplants is also a promising concept in a transplant setting. Segmentation of the kidney is relatively more simple compared with the liver and seems to be less time-consuming, because the variations in parenchymal HU attenuation are less, thus making it conducive for segmentation by the region-growing method.[56] Previous studies have highlighted the importance of estimating kidney volumes for monitoring of polycystic kidney disease (**Fig. 7**).[57] The difference in CT attenuation values between a cyst and normal renal parenchyma provides

challenges to the region-growing technique, however, because cysts and normal parenchyma may have to be segmented separately. It is appropriate to set the upper limit at 2.5 mm for the thickness of axial slices acquired at a 2.5-mm scan thickness, failing which the resolution may degrade the segmentation process and lead to inaccuracies in volume estimation.

Tumor volumes

Manual segmentation of single tumors on axial slices may be a feasible option when the tumor size is small and the number of tumors is limited. Tumor volumetry requires more automation for purposes of quantification, however, because metastatic liver tumors are often multiple and manual

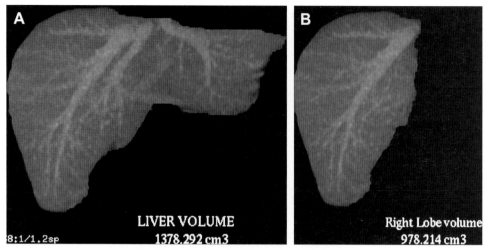

Fig. 5. MDCT segmentation and generation of total liver (*A*) and right liver lobe (*B*) volumes in a 37-year-old male liver donor.

quantification may be time-consuming and unsuitable for a busy radiology workflow. Various computer-aided postprocessing techniques have been developed for automated tumor recognition and subsequent tumor burden quantification.

Volume estimation of primary liver tumors and metastatic lesions, which is used as a monitoring response to chemotherapy and radiotherapy and in the prediction of long-term survival of patients, is one of the most effectively realized applications of volumetry in an oncologic setting.[58] Researchers have also highlighted the superiority of volume estimations of liver tumors over the World Health Organization and Response Evaluation Criteria In Solid Tumors criteria.[59]

Necrosis in liver tumors usually occurs secondary to therapy, the quantification of which is a challenging task considering the uneven distribution of necrotic fluid in the tumor substance. Estimation of renal tumor volume after radiofrequency ablation is another area in which the role of volumetry has recently been investigated.[60] With the availability of the newer generation MDCT scanners, CT data sets of better resolution may add in increasing the pace of progress in further exploring the importance of CT volumetry for evaluation and follow-up of oral cavity carcinomas, primary gastric tumors, gastrointestinal stromal tumors, mediastinal lymphomas, and cervical carcinomas.

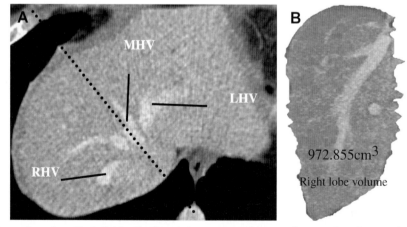

Fig. 6. (*A*) Intervening plane that divides the liver into two parts is created manually using an electronic mouse. This dividing line (*dashed line*) is usually parallel to the right of the middle hepatic vein (MHV), which corresponds to the median fissure that extends from the gallbladder fossa to the inferior vena cava. The right and left lobes are segmented separately using the paint-brush method. LHV, left hepatic vein; RHV, right hepatic vein. (*B*) Right lobe liver volume after segmentation.

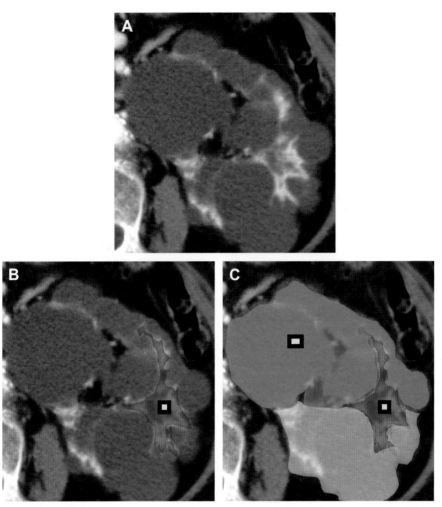

Fig. 7. Region-growing method for polycystic kidney segmentation. (*A*) Axial MDCT image of the left polycystic kidney. (*B*) Image shows partial segmentation of contrast-enhancing areas. (*C*) Images shows complete kidney segmentation after partial segmentation of cystic and contrast-enhancing portions. (*Courtesy of* W. Cai, PhD, Boston, MA.)

An overview of important CT segmentation and volumetry applications is provided in **Table 2**.

COMPUTER-AIDED DETECTION AND POSTPROCESSING

Interpolation tools that calculate the volumes between manually segmented and unsegmented slices and the region-growing tools are semiautomated methods of segmentation and volume estimation, and such algorithms are freely available on newer workstations. The use of computer-aided techniques, which are presently prevalent on a comparatively narrow latitude of clinical practice, is playing an important role in automating advanced postprocessing methods like virtual navigation and volumetry. An increasing demand for good image resolution while developing a CAD algorithm has always existed; therefore,

more preference for MDCT data over MR imaging data sets exists for developing an automated postprocessing algorithm.[61,62] The MDCT data sets from fourth-generation scanners provide artifact-free CT data of superior voxel resolution. This provides clear delineation of a lesion's margins, its conspicuity, and better characterization of tiny lesions, thus ensuring better performance of CAD applications. Some recent study findings for computer-aided postprocessing applications are given in **Table 3**.

Computer-Aided Detection in Imaging of the Thorax

Automated detection and quantification of tumor burden in the lung is one of the most actively investigated computer-assisted advanced postprocessing techniques. A recent study by Larici and

Table 2
Overview of important CT segmentation and volumetry applications

Clinical Application	Recommended Segmentation Technique at Workstations	Recommendations/ Limitation[a]	Computer- Aided Detection (±)
Lung tumor/metastatic burden quantification	Manual with interpolation for single tumor		
CAD for metastatic burden	<2-mm MDCT acquisition for metastatic burden	+	
Liver (transplant/partial lobes and total liver volumes)	Manual with interpolation for single tumor		
(CAD under investigation)	CAD performance for total volume better with precontrast axial data	+	
Kidney (transplant/ polycystic kidney volumes)	Manual with interpolation for polycystic kidney Region-growing method for normal kidney segmentation	When using region-growing tool, coronal and sagittal images should be edited simultaneously with axial images for better results	+
Liver tumor/metastatic burden quantification	Manual with interpolation for single tumor		
CAD for metastatic burden	CAD performance for total volume better with postcontrast axial data	+	

Postprocessing data should include 50% overlap between axial slices.
 [a] MDCT acquisitions devoid of motion/metallic artifacts.

colleagues[63] has highlighted the fact that the best CAD performance depends on scan parameters, such as slice thickness, reconstruction algorithms, and tube current, and is best observed with a slice thickness of 1.25 mm of high spatial resolution.

Computer-aided postprocessing automation is also useful for characterization and quantification of diffuse parenchymal lung disease severity using MDCT, such as assessment of interstitial lung fibrosis burden, and 3D automated approaches for detection and diagnosis of emphysema, fibrosis, honeycombing, and ground-glass haziness are under active consideration.[64]

Computer-Aided Detection in Abdominal Imaging

Colon

CAD has established its role with CTC for detection of colonic polyps because it now automates the essential steps, such as colonic segmentations, virtual navigation, and successful detection of polyps greater than 5 mm in diameter, and it generates electronically cleansed images of the bowel free of fecal matter. For purposes of cleaning the bowel to reduce false-positive CAD detections, electronic bowel cleansing is useful when the residual fecal materials are tagged in the colon by orally administered contrast agents, such as barium, iodine, or Gastrografin, after the bowel preparation and before CTC. The opacified residual solid stool and fluid in the colon can then be removed by an electronic cleansing method, thus improving the accuracy of polyp detection.[65] Most CTC examinations are performed without fecal tagging, with fecal tagging CTC being the second major group, followed by reduced and noncathartic CTC, which is still at an experimental stage. The false-positive interpretations may be caused by the presence of normal structures that resemble polyps or attributable to technical errors with the display.[13] Variable sensitivity for polyp detection

Table 3
Recent updates of computer-aided postprocessing applications

Computer-Assisted Postprocessing Applications	Study Findings
Lung: metastatic tumor burden quantification	Accuracy: 78.26% (18/23) (Goo et al, 2008)
Liver: Total and partial (right and left lobe) liver volumes	Modus 3D CT volumetry: no substantial over- or underestimation (Radtke et al, 2008)
CAD: colonic polyps	CAD per polyp sensitivity: 91% (>10-mm polyps), 82.1% (6–9-mm polyps) (Summers et al, 2008)
Kidney segmentation and volumetry	Correlation coefficients: in vivo = 0.981, ex vivo (volumetry) = 0.973 (Cai et al, 2007)
CAD in emergency settings	
CAD: pulmonary embolus	CAD for embolus: lobar = 87%, segmental = 90%, subsegmental = 77% (Das et al, 2008)
CAD and quantification: pneumothorax	Correlation coefficient of 0.9 between the clinical score and volumetric free air (Cai et al, 2007)
CAD: transition point of small bowel obstructions	CAD sensitivity = 60%, false-positive rate = 3 per patient (Sainani et al, 2007)

across studies, the expertise and time required of the readers for interpreting the CTC images, and the need for full bowel preparation are some surfacing issues that are being actively addressed, however.[66] The use of CAD can be helpful in reducing variability for identifying polyps among readers on CT scans. CAD results need improvement with respect to detection of flat lesions or lesions that are less than 5 mm in diameter, an area that is receiving widespread attention on the research platform because there is no body of large substantial data to prove the high CAD sensitivity for detecting such subtle colonic lesions (**Fig. 8**).

Liver

Computer-aided segmentations of the total liver and the partial liver lobe and quantification of liver tumor burden have been successfully tested and implemented in busy clinical practices.[67] The basic principle is to train the CAD software to detect only the specified range of pixel or voxel values within a specified range of body length on CT data sets while ignoring the rest of the pixels. This principle governs the mapping of the entire liver by CAD or that of metastatic tumors only, which have slightly lower HU values than the liver parenchyma (**Fig. 9**). False-positive

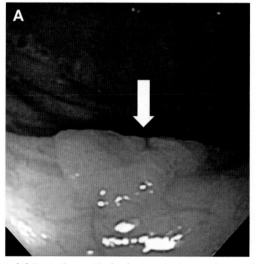 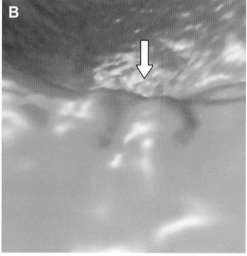

Fig. 8. (*A*) Screening optical colonoscopy image shows a flat lesion in the colonic lumen (*thick arrow*) in a 57-year-old man. (*B*) Depiction of the same lesion (*arrow*) on a virtual CT colonoscopy image. (*From* Taylor SA, Suzuki N, Beddoe G, et al. Flat neoplasia of the colon: CT colonography with CAD. Abdom Imaging. 2008 May 30 [epub ahead of print]; with permission.)

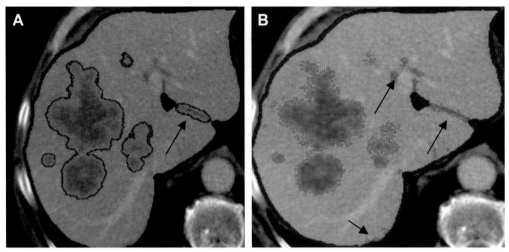

Fig. 9. (A) Automated detection of liver and tumor boundaries by CAD on CT. (B) Automated mapping of tumor content by CAD before generation of the tumor volume. Note the false-positive detections (*thin arrows* in *A* and *B*), which are excluded before tumor volume generation. (*Courtesy of* W. Cai, PhD, Boston, MA.)

detection of surrounding structures and decreased CAD performance to detect margins of hypervascular tumors are two of the issues that need further work, however. Data upgradations and software automations are also available, and they incorporate the results of total liver volume and tumor burden volumes, which are then projected as percentages in respective liver lobes.

Other abdominal applications
Automated segmentation and volume estimations of the kidneys have also been successfully investigated and found to be technically more feasible than CAD of the liver (**Fig. 10**). CAD-based segmentation by the level-set method has been proved to provide quick and automated kidney segmentation.[57] Computer-assisted quantification of abdominal fat accumulation, which is an

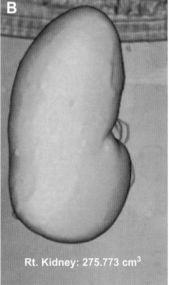

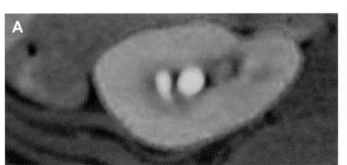

Rt. Kidney: 275.773 cm^3

Fig. 10. Computer-aided segmentation (A) and volume generation (B) of porcine kidney on MDCT. (*Reprinted from* Cai W, Holalkere N-S, Harris G, et al. Dynamic-threshold level set method for volumetry of porcine kidney in CT images: in vivo and ex vivo assessment of the accuracy of volume measurement. Academic Radiology; 14(7):890–6; with permission.)

important cardiovascular risk factor, was found to be technically feasible and effective in 40 subjects, in whom the new method successfully differentiated abdominal fat into subcutaneous and visceral fat components and removed equipment-related artifacts.[68] Some recent studies have provided further validation and strength to this data.[69]

Computer-Aided Detection Applications in Emergencies

Significance
Emergency radiology (ER) contributes to a considerable number of CT scans in radiology, and the development of CAD applications can be important in solving the common problems for diagnosis of life-threatening emergencies. The faster scan speed offered by newer generation CT scanners has decreased the probability of motion artifacts, thus providing solutions to another vital CT data set problem, which may be more relevant to an ER setting, considering the patient status.

Thoracic computer-aided detection applications in emergency radiology
The importance of automated detection and quantification of pneumothorax was recently tested, where assigning a range between −900 and −930 HU for mapping free air in pleura on MDCT data sets of trauma patients revealed a promising accuracy of CAD in quantification of pneumothorax with significant time savings.[70] Computer-aided volumetry revealed a strong correlation coefficient of nearly 0.9 between the clinical score and volumetric free air (**Fig. 11**).

Pulmonary embolism (PE) is a life-threatening emergency and is the only area of the emergency setting in which the use of CAD has been well studied.[71,72] Recent computer-aided detectors have the ability to map tiny clots automatically, even in the sixth-order branches of pulmonary vasculature, with a sensitivity of 85% and a specificity between 90% and 95%. The sensitivity can be further improved to 90%, if CT venography is combined with regular PE protocols on MDCT.

Small bowel obstructions
Use of CAD for locating transition points of small bowel obstructions, such as bowel strictures, has been investigated recently by Sainani and colleagues,[33] where CAD sited at least 60% of surgically confirmed strictures with a false-positive rate of 3 per patient. Of these, 80% of the false-positive findings were easily dismissed as erroneous CAD points in the vessels, abdominal wall, and collapsed large bowel segments (**Fig. 12**).

SUMMARY

Advances in MDCT scanners have increased the pace of development of advanced postprocessing applications, such as VE, segmentation and volumetry, and computer-aided postprocessing methods. Availability of thin-section MDCT data sets of isotropic voxel resolution ensures accuracy in structure segmentation, which is an important initial prerequisite on which the results of such advanced postprocessing applications are based. Although thinner sections provide better results for such advanced postprocessing methods, it is important to set a limit on scan acquisition thickness to 2.5 mm for larger structures and 1.25 mm for small arterial details to prevent excess radiation dose delivery to patients and to avoid issues with data explosion. Moreover, previous studies have provided sufficient data to support such protocol alterations, and results of fourth-generation HD

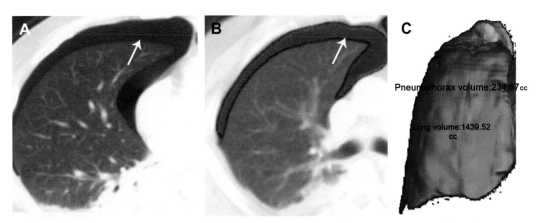

Fig. 11. Process of computer-aided CT quantification of pneumothorax in a 55-year-old man. (*A*) Axial MDCT image shows air in the pleural cavity (*arrow*). (*B*) CAD of pneumothorax (*arrow*). (*C*) Automated generation of pneumothorax and lung volumes. (*Courtesy of* W. Cai, PhD, Boston, MA.)

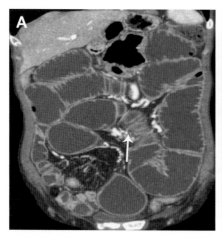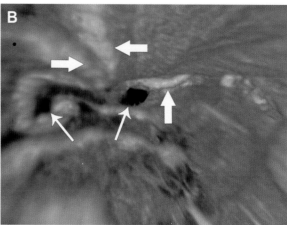

Fig. 12. (A) Small bowel obstruction attributable to mesenteric volvulus in a 39-year-old male patient. The point of obstruction is seen (*thin arrow*). (B) Endoscopy image through the small intestine with CAD points (*thin arrows*) shows luminal narrowing. Convergence of intestinal folds is also seen (*thick arrows*).

CT scanners, which provide better image resolution at less radiation dose, are still awaited.

In addition to image resolution, optimal luminal distention and ensuring the presence of good CT contrast between the lumen and luminal wall are crucial prerequisites for successful generation of high-quality virtual navigation. Virtual CT colonoscopy has received widespread attention and is now a recognized screening tool for detection of premalignant colonic polyps. VB for detection of tracheal pathologic findings, CT cystoscopy for assessment of bladder tumor recurrence, and virtual tympanoscopy for evaluation of middle ear pathologic findings are some of the popular VE applications that are being actively investigated. The role of virtual CT endoscopy has also been proved for detection of pathologic conditions in the paranasal sinuses, larynx, esophagus, stomach, and aorta. Inadequate luminal distention poses some challenge to the generation of good-quality virtual fly-through images for such structures as the common bile duct and pancreatic duct and ureters.

Manual segmentation, thresholding, edge-based segmentation, region-growing segmentation, and automated segmentation are some organ segmentation techniques, of which manual segmentation of organs and region-growing methods are more popular because they allow more operator control and ensure accuracy. Segmentation of organs on MDCT data sets for purposes of volume estimation is useful for estimation of total and partial liver volumes for presurgical planning of liver transplants and partial hepatectomies. Estimation of kidney volumes for monitoring patients who have adult polycystic kidney disease and estimation of single liver tumor volumes are other useful clinical applications of volumetry.

Computer-aided applications segmentation and CT volumetry have proved useful in clinical practice, wherein estimation of multiple structures is needed in less time (eg, estimation of metastatic tumor burden in lungs and liver). Automated calculation of abdominal fat burden and differentiation of fat into subcutaneous and visceral components using the CT data sets have recently become popular in cardiovascular practice. The effective role of CAD of colonic polyps has been well established by numerous large cohort studies, which have also paved the path for technical advancements like electronic cleansing of the large bowel by performing fecal tagging with oral contrast. Automated detection of a pulmonary embolus, quantification of pneumothorax, and automated detection of transition points of small bowel obstructions are some newer advances in CAD applications in an emergency setting, in which active investigation by researchers is expected.

REFERENCES

1. Singh AK, Sahani DV, Kagay CR, et al. Semiautomated MIP images created directly on 16-section multidetector CT console for evaluation of living renal donors. Radiology 2007;244(2):583–90.
2. Vargas R, Nino-Murcia M, Trueblood W, et al. MDCT in pancreatic adenocarcinoma: prediction of vascular invasion and resectability using a multiphasic technique with curved planar reformations. AJR Am J Roentgenol 2004;182(2):419–25.
3. Carrascosa P, Capuñay C, Vembar M, et al. Multislice CT virtual angioscopy of the abdomen. Abdom Imaging 2005;30(3):249–58.
4. Arnesen RB, von Benzon E, Adamsen S, et al. Diagnostic performance of computed tomography

colonography and colonoscopy: a prospective and validated analysis of 231 paired examinations. Acta Radiol 2007;48(8):831–7.

5. Pomerantz SR, Harris GJ, Desai HJ, et al. Computed tomography angiography and computed tomography perfusion in ischemic stroke: a step-by-step approach to image acquisition and three-dimensional postprocessing. Semin Ultrasound CT MR 2006;27(3):243–70.

6. Chen SJ, Lin MT, Liu KL, et al. Usefulness of 3D reconstructed computed tomography imaging for double outlet right ventricle. J Formos Med Assoc 2008;107(5):371–80.

7. Singh AK, Sahani DV, Ouellette-Piazzo K, et al. Comparison of automated CT reconstructions from 64-MDCT with manual reformats from 16-MDCT in emergency radiology setting: an image quality analysis based on patients' body weight and workflow considerations [abstract 093]. In: Abstract Book of American Roentgen Ray Society 107th Annual Meeting, vol. 188, no. 5. Orlando (FL); 2007. p. A28.

8. Sahani DV, Kalva SP, Hahn PF, et al. 16-MDCT angiography in living kidney donors at various tube potentials: impact on image quality and radiation dose. AJR Am J Roentgenol 2007;188(1):115–20.

9. Albrecht T, Meyer BC. MDCT angiography of peripheral arteries: technical considerations and impact on patient management. Eur Radiol 2007;17(Suppl 6):F5–15.

10. Sagawa M, Usuda K, Tsuchihara K, et al. Comparison of the images in virtual bronchoscopy under different conditions. Kyobu Geka 2008;61(2):102–8.

11. Graser A, Johnson TR, Chandarana H, et al. Dual energy CT: preliminary observations and potential clinical applications in the abdomen. Eur Radiol 2008 [epub ahead of print].

12. Sbragia P, Neri E, Panconi M, et al. CT virtual angioscopy in the study of thoracic aortic dissection. Radiologica Medica (Torino) 2001;102(4):245–9.

13. Yoshida H, Näppi J. CAD in CT colonography without and with oral contrast agents: progress and challenges. Comput Med Imaging Graph 2007;31(4–5):267–84.

14. Sun Z, Ferris C. Optimal scanning protocol of multislice CT virtual intravascular endoscopy in pre-aortic stent grafting: in vitro phantom study. Eur J Radiol 2006;58(2):310–6.

15. Trojanowska A, Trojanowski P, Olszanski W, et al. How to reliably evaluate middle ear diseases? Comparison of different methods of post-processing based on multislice computed tomography examination. Acta Otolaryngol 2007;127(3):258–64.

16. Smouha EE, Chen D, Li B, et al. Computer-aided virtual surgery for congenital aural atresia. Otol Neurotol 2001;22(2):178–82.

17. Rodt T, Burmeister HP, Bartling S, et al. 3D-visualisation of the middle ear by computer-assisted post-processing of helical multi-slice CT data. Laryngorhinootologie 2004;83(7):438–44.

18. Walshe P, Hamilton S, McShane D, et al. The clinical usefulness of helical CT multiplanar reformation, three-dimensional reconstruction and virtual laryngoscopy in laryngeal and hypopharyngeal carcinomas. Zhonghua Zhong Liu Za Zhi 2001;23(3):230–3.

19. Firat Y, Aygenç E, Firat AK, et al. Computed tomography virtual laryngoscopy: comparison between radiological and otolaryngological evaluations for laryngeal carcinoma. Kulak Burun Bogaz Ihtis Derg 2006;16(3):97–104.

20. Hoppe H, Thoeny HC, Dinkel HP, et al. Virtual laryngoscopy and multiplanar reformats with multirow detector CT for detection and grading of upper airway stenosis. Rofo 2002;174(8):1003–8.

21. Suter MJ, Reinhardt JM, McLennan G. Integrated CT/bronchoscopy in the central airways: preliminary results. Acad Radiol 2008;15(6):786–98.

22. De Wever W, Bogaert J, Verschakelen JA. Virtual bronchoscopy: accuracy and usefulness—an overview. Semin Ultrasound CT MR 2005;26(5):364–73.

23. Bakir B, Tüzün U, Terzibaşioălu E, et al. The diagnostic efficiency of multislice CT virtual bronchoscopy in detecting endobronchial tumors. Tuberk Toraks 2008;56(1):43–9.

24. Englmeier KH, Seemann MD. Multimodal virtual bronchoscopy using PET/CT images. Comput Aided Surg 2008;13(2):106–13.

25. Heyer CM, Nuesslein TG, Jung D, et al. Tracheobronchial anomalies and stenoses: detection with low-dose multidetector CT with virtual tracheobronchoscopy—comparison with flexible tracheobronchoscopy. Radiology 2007;242(2):542–9.

26. Shiono H, Okumura M, Sawabata N, et al. Virtual mediastinoscopy for safer and more accurate mediastinal exploration. Ann Thorac Surg 2007;84(3):995–9.

27. Mazzeo S, Caramella D, Gennai A, et al. Multidetector CT and virtual endoscopy in the evaluation of the esophagus. Abdom Imaging 2004;29(1):2–8.

28. Panebianco V, Grazhdani H, Iafrate F, et al. 3D CT protocol in the assessment of the esophageal neoplastic lesions: can it improve TNM staging? Eur Radiol 2006;16(2):414–21.

29. Duan SY, Zhang DT, Lin QC, et al. Clinical value of CT three-dimensional imaging in diagnosing gastrointestinal tract diseases. World J Gastroenterol 2006;12(18):2945–8.

30. Kim AY, Kim HJ, Ha HK. Gastric cancer by multidetector row CT: preoperative staging. Abdom Imaging 2005;30(4):465–72.

31. Kim JH, Eun HW, Choi JH, et al. Diagnostic performance of virtual gastroscopy using MDCT in early gastric cancer compared with 2D axial CT: focusing on interobserver variation. AJR Am J Roentgenol 2007;189(2):299–305.

32. Sata N, Endo K, Shimura K, et al. A new 3D-diagnosis strategy for duodenal malignant lesions using

multi-detector row CT, CT virtual duodenoscopy, duodenography and 3D multi-cholangiography. Abdom Imaging 2007;32(1):66–72.

33. Sainani NI, Nappi J, Sahani DV, et al. Computer-aided detection of small bowel strictures in CT enterography (CTE) in an emergency setting: a pilot study. Proceedings of the 93rd Assembly and Annual Meeting of the Radiological Society of North America (RSNA); 2007 Nov 25–30; Chicago, USA. Chicago (IL): RSNA Press; 2007. p. 256.

34. Summers RM, Handwerker LR, Pickhardt PJ, et al. Performance of a previously validated CT colonography computer-aided detection system in a new patient population. AJR Am J Roentgenol 2008; 191(1):168–74.

35. Gryspeerdt S, Lefere P, Herman M, et al. CT colonography with fecal tagging after incomplete colonoscopy. Eur Radiol 2005;15(6):1192–202.

36. Burling D, Halligan S, Taylor S, et al. Polyp measurement using CT colonography: agreement with colonoscopy and effect of viewing conditions on interobserver and intraobserver agreement. AJR Am J Roentgenol 2006;186(6):1597–604.

37. Schopphoven S, Faulkner K, Busch HP. Assessment of patient organ dose in CT virtual colonoscopy for bowel cancer screening. Radiat Prot Dosimetry 2008;129(1–3):179–83.

38. Kim SH, Lee JM, Shin CI, et al. Effects of spatial resolution and tube current on computer-aided detection of polyps on CT colonographic images: phantom study. Radiology 2008;248(2):492–503.

39. Gollub MJ, Akhurst T, Markowitz AJ, et al. Combined CT colonography and 18F-FDG PET of colon polyps: potential technique for selective detection of cancer and precancerous lesions. AJR Am J Roentgenol 2007;188(1):130–8.

40. Fidler J, Johnson C. Flat polyps of the colon: accuracy of detection by CT colonography and histologic significance. Abdom Imaging 2008 Apr 15.

41. Lou MW, Hu WD, Fan Y, et al. CT biliary cystoscopy of gallbladder polyps. World J Gastroenterol 2004; 10(8):1204–7.

42. Sata N, Kurihara K, Koizumi M, et al. CT virtual pancreatoscopy: a new method for diagnosing intraductal papillary mucinous neoplasm (IPMN) of the pancreas. Abdom Imaging 2006;31(3):326–31.

43. Tsampoulas C, Tsili AC, Giannakis D, et al. 16-MDCT cystoscopy in the evaluation of neoplasms of the urinary bladder. AJR Am J Roentgenol 2008;190(3):729–35.

44. Chou CP, Huang JS, Wu MT, et al. CT voiding urethrography and virtual urethroscopy: preliminary study with 16-MDCT. AJR Am J Roentgenol 2005;184(6):1882–8.

45. Prando A. CT-virtual endoscopy of the urinary tract. Int Braz J Urol 2002;28(4):317–22.

46. Abramoff MD, Magelhaesv PJ, Ram SJ. Image processing with Image. J Biophotonics International 2004;11:36–42.

47. Adams R, Bischof L. Seed region growing. IEEE Trans Pattern Anal Mach Intell 2004;16:641–7.

48. Schei TR, Barrett S, Jones D, et al. Automated abdominal aortic aneurysm segmentation using MATLAB. Biomed Sci Instrum 2003;39:53–8.

49. Radtke A, Sotiropoulos GC, Nadalin S, et al. Preoperative volume prediction in adult live donor liver transplantation: 3-D CT volumetry approach to prevent miscalculations. Eur J Med Res 2008; 13(7):319–26.

50. Marten K, Auer F, Schmidt S, et al. Automated CT volumetry of pulmonary metastases: the effect of a reduced growth threshold and target lesion number on the reliability of therapy response assessment using RECIST criteria. Eur Radiol 2007; 17(10):2561–71.

51. Mann K, Opitz H, Petersen D, et al. Intracranial CSF volumetry in alcoholics: studies with MRI and CT. Psychiatry Res 1989;29(3):277–9.

52. Komemushi A, Tanigawa N, Kariya S, et al. Percutaneous vertebroplasty for compression fracture: analysis of vertebral body volume by CT volumetry. Acta Radiol 2005;46(3):276–9.

53. Froelich JJ, Koenig H, Knaak L, et al. Relationship between pulmonary artery volumes at computed tomography and pulmonary artery pressures in patients with and without pulmonary hypertension. Eur J Radiol 2008;67(3):466–71.

54. Tu R, Xia LP, Yu AL, et al. Assessment of hepatic functional reserve by cirrhosis grading and liver volume measurement using CT. World J Gastroenterol 2007;13(29):3956–61.

55. Taner CB, Dayangac M, Akin B, et al. Donor safety and remnant liver volume in living donor liver transplantation. Liver Transpl 2008;14(8):1174–9.

56. Cai W, Holalkere NS, Harris G, et al. Dynamic-threshold level set method for volumetry of porcine kidney in CT images in vivo and ex vivo assessment of the accuracy of volume measurement. Acad Radiol 2007;14(7):890–6.

57. Antiga L, Piccinelli M, Fasolini G, et al. Computed tomography evaluation of autosomal dominant polycystic kidney disease progression: a progress report. Clin J Am Soc Nephrol 2006;1(4):754–60.

58. Pech M, Mohnike K, Wieners G, et al. Radiotherapy of liver metastases: comparison of target volumes and dose-volume histograms employing CT- or MRI-based treatment planning. Strahlenther Onkol 2008;184(5):256–61.

59. Heussel CP, Meier S, Wittelsberger S, et al. Follow-up CT measurement of liver malignoma according to RECIST and WHO vs. volumetry. Rofo 2007; 179(9):958–64.

60. Lee JY, Kim CK, Choi D, et al. Volume doubling time and growth rate of renal cell carcinoma determined by helical CT: a single-institution experience. Eur Radiol 2008;18(4):731–7.

61. Brochu B, Beigelman-Aubry C, Goldmard JL, et al. Computer-aided detection of lung nodules on thin collimation MDCT: impact on radiologists' performance. J Radiol 2007;88(4):573–8.

62. Xu Y, van Beek EJ, Hwanjo Y, et al. Computer-aided classification of interstitial lung diseases via MDCT: 3D adaptive multiple feature method (3D AMFM). Acad Radiol 2006;13(8):969–78.

63. Larici AR, Storto ML, Torge M, et al. Automated volumetry of pulmonary nodules on multidetector CT: influence of slice thickness, reconstruction algorithm and tube current. Preliminary results. Radiologica Medica (Torino) 2008;113(1):29–42.

64. Fetita C, Chang-Chien KC, Brillet PY, et al. Diffuse parenchymal lung diseases: 3D automated detection in MDCT. Med Image Comput Comput Assist Interv Int Conf Med Image Comput Comput Assist Interv 2007;10(Pt 1):825–33.

65. Näppi J, Yoshida H. Adaptive correction of the pseudo-enhancement of CT attenuation for fecal-tagging CT colonography. Med Image Anal 2008; 12:413–26.

66. Petrick N, Haider M, Summers RM, et al. CT colonography with computer-aided detection as a second reader: observer performance study. Radiology 2008;246(1):148–56.

67. Graham KC, Ford NL, MacKenzie LT, et al. Noninvasive quantification of tumor volume in preclinical liver metastasis models using contrast-enhanced x-ray computed tomography. Invest Radiol 2008;43(2): 92–9.

68. Bandekar A, Naghavi M, Kakadiaris I. Performance evaluation of abdominal fat burden quantification in CT. Conf Proc IEEE Eng Med Biol Soc 2005;3:3280–3.

69. Zhao B, Colville J, Kalaigian J, et al. Automated quantification of body fat distribution on volumetric computed tomography. J Comput Assist Tomogr 2006;30(5):777–83.

70. Cai W, Tabbara M, Harris GJ, et al. Automated volumetric measurement of pneumothorax in CT images for trauma patients. Proceedings of the 93rd Assembly and Annual Meeting of the Radiological Society of North America (RSNA); 2007 Nov 25–30; Chicago, USA. Chicago (IL): RSNA Press; 2007. p. 295.

71. Das M, Mühlenbruch G, Helm A, et al. Computer-aided detection of pulmonary embolism: influence on radiologists' detection performance with respect to vessel segments. Eur Radiol 2008;18(7):1350–5.

72. Schoepf UJ, Schneider AC, Das M, et al. Pulmonary embolism: computer-aided detection at multidetector row spiral computed tomography. J Thorac Imaging 2007;22(4):319–23.

The "Post-64" Era of Coronary CT Angiography: Understanding New Technology from Physical Principles

Hansel J. Otero, MD, Michael L. Steigner, MD,
Frank J. Rybicki, MD, PhD*

KEYWORDS
- Computed tomography • Cardiac CT
- Coronary angiography • Temporal resolution
- Spatial resolution • Radiation dose

Multidetector Computed Tomography (MDCT) is now an established modality for noninvasive cardiac imaging. Until recently, 64-slice CT provided state-of-the-art noninvasive coronary imaging. The 64 slices per gantry rotation can be achieved with either 64-detector rows, or 32-detector rows and a strategy to double the slice number by alternating the focal spot of the x-ray source. These "64-generation" scanners offered considerable advantages over earlier technology: superior spatial resolution, temporal resolution, volume coverage, and lower radiation doses for patients. Improving upon these fundamental CT parameters is also the goal of the next generation, or "post-64" era of coronary CT angiography (CTA). This review highlights improvements in the post-64 era of cardiac MDCT.

The newest technology offers significant advantages, but unlike the evolution from 4-to 64-detector row coronary CTA, current CT hardware releases are far from uniform, reflecting different approaches to image acquisition in the post-64 era. No single CT scanner offers the full portfolio of the newest features. This situation underscores the importance of understanding the properties of a cardiac CT scanner. Also, CT vendors continue to eclipse the state-of-the-art from even the recent past. Thus, it is very challenging to accumulate "current" clinical evidence. This reality is reflected in two multi-center 64-era MDCT trials, each of which focused on a single CT platform. The first of these publications,[1] the Assessment by Coronary Computed Tomographic Angiography of Individuals Undergoing Invasive Coronary Angiography (ACCURACY) trial, enrolled United States subjects from predominantly nonacademic (private) centers and found a (patient based) sensitivity, specificity, and positive and negative predictive values to detect >50% or >70% stenosis of 0.95, 0.83, 0.64, and 0.99, respectively, and 0.94, 0.83, 0.48, 0.99, respectively. The second publication,[2] the Coronary Artery Evaluation Using 64-Row Multidetector Computed Tomography Angiography (Core64) study was both international and included predominantly academic centers. This trial had lower test characteristics (patient based detection of >50% stenosis, sensitivity, specificity, and positive and negative predictive

None of the authors received support for collaborating with this manuscript.

Applied Imaging Science Laboratory, Noninvasive Cardiovascular Imaging & Department of Radiology, Brigham and Women's Hospital & Harvard Medical School, 75 Francis Street, Boston, MA 02115, USA

* Corresponding author.

E-mail address: frybicki@partners.org (F.J. Rybicki).

Radiol Clin N Am 47 (2009) 79–90

doi:10.1016/j.rcl.2008.11.001

of 0.85, 0.90, 0.91, 0.83) but showed a similar ability of CT when compared to catheterization to identify, on the basis of obstructive coronary stenoses, patients who underwent revascularization.

The results from the Core64 study call into question the very high negative predictive value,[3] a previously accepted strength of MDCT, namely the exclusion of coronary artery diseases (CAD) in low- and intermediate-risk patients with an exam that is not only much simpler to perform but also has fewer complications than coronary catheterization. With post-64 technology described below, excluding CAD is typically accomplished with radiation doses comparable to, and in many cases lower than, catheterization. The same argument also extends to emergency room imaging; CT can potentially reduce the overall cost of emergency room stays for chest pain patients[4] However, even before the results of multicenter trials can be fully appreciated in the literature, the practice of coronary CT has changed. Specifically, patients in both multicenter studies were scanned with retrospective ECG gating; the current trend in coronary CTA is prospective ECG gating that delivers a lower radiation dose but has fewer phases within the R-R interval to assess the coronary arteries (**Fig. 1**). Thus, the performance of CT cited by each trial must be now confirmed for lower dose, prospectively ECG gated, image acquisitions. The differences and tradeoffs between retrospective and prospective gating are detailed below.

In addition to coronary imaging, cardiac CT enables visualization of the myocardium, the cardiac chambers, the location and patency of coronary bypass grafts, and significant extracardiac disease. Retrospective ECG gating also enables the assessment of cardiac function and valves. Although the high negative predictive value for CAD is now generally accepted, there are other very promising applications with less validation: plaque characterization, the evaluation of myocardial ischemia (perfusion) and scar (myocardial delayed enhancement), and the assessment of coronary artery endothelial shear stress.

The reader who is studying rapidly emerging data should be cautious. Because of its great potential in cardiac diagnoses, the early interpretation of the post-64 era has included speculation, invited by the environment of new technology. Investigators are faced with the challenge of critically evaluating the technology and determining best practice standards for their patients. For imagers and administrators who are acquiring new MDCT technology, it can be challenging to identify and analyze the data. In the authors' experience, the best way to do this is to focus on the physical principles common to cardiac CT. This article has a subsection devoted to each parameter. In addition, the authors individually describe how the choice of one parameter influences other parameters.

This article includes current perspectives from November 2008, before the hardware releases expected at the annual meeting of the Radiological Society of North America (RSNA). In this review, the most recent CT scanner to receive FDA approval is the Siemens Definition AS+ that achieves 128 slices per gantry rotation obtained with 64-detector rows and an x-ray CT source focal spot that alternates between two positions to double the number of slices with respect to the number of detector rows. As discussed in detail in the temporal resolution section, the Siemens Definition (dual-source) 64-slice (32-detector rows × two focal spot positions) scanner features a two x-ray tube and two detector configuration to reduce the temporal resolution to 83 milliseconds.[5] Only days before the Definition AS+ announcement, the General Electric LightSpeed 750HD received FDA approval. Like the AS+, the LightSpeed 750HD is very new, and there are no peer-review publications to date. However, this technology has a proposed improved spatial resolution that will be evaluated in the peer-review literature. This scanner will use the "step and shoot" technique for prospective ECG gating that was introduced with the earlier General Electric LightSpeed VCT64. In November 2007 at the annual meeting of the RSNA, Toshiba introduced the AquilionOne with 320-detector rows and whole heart coverage. This scanner achieves single heartbeat cardiac imaging, including lower-dose imaging with prospective gating.[6] Because the entire cardiac volume is imaged at one time-point, this technology potentially enables myocardial perfusion CT at a single state of iodinated contrast opacification. At RSNA 2007, Philips announced the FDA approval and release of the Brilliance iCT with a 270-millisecond rotation time and 256 slices (128-detector rows × two focal spot positions).

This review of the post-64 era is divided into four parts: spatial resolution; temporal resolution; cranio–caudal volume coverage; and patient radiation. Because coronary imaging is most robustly performed with catheter-based angiography, each part describes particular technologies with catheterization standards in mind. The authors present a set of ideal features of CT, or "what you want" from the perspective of a cardiac imager. The hardware and associated software advances are then framed in the format of "what you can get," keeping in mind that the substantial

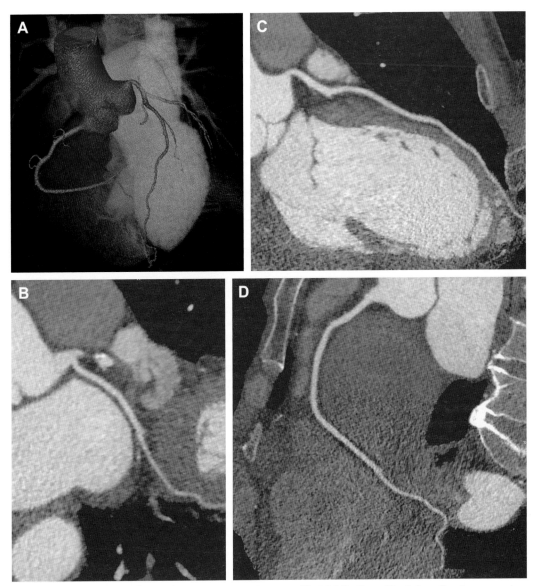

Fig. 1. 48-year-old woman with atypical chest pain and nonspecific ECG findings. Single heartbeat coronary imaging was performed using 320-slice CT (Toshiba AquilionOne, Tochigi-ken, Japan) with 100 kV, 400 mAs, 350 millisecond gantry rotation, and 80 mL of iopamidol 370 mg I/mL (Isovue-370, Bracco Diagnostics, Princeton, NJ). The use of prospective ECG gating (phase window width = 10%) and low kV (patient weight <170 pounds) enabled a 2.6 mSv acquisition. (*A*) 3D volume rendering (Vitrea fx, Vital Images, Minnetonka, MN) of the aortic root, major coronary arteries, and left ventricular cavity. (*B, C, D*) Curved multiplanar reformatted images of the normal coronary arteries.

improvements are still under evaluation and cannot fulfill all expectations.

SPATIAL RESOLUTION
What You Want: 0.1 mm and What You Get: 0.35–0.5 mm

The CT spatial resolution refers to the ability to separate two structures and is scientifically determined by measuring the ability of a CT system to

separate line pairs.[7] There is no systemic comparison of the true spatial resolution capabilities between CT scanners, either in the 64 or post-64 era. The voxel size has become the surrogate parameter for spatial resolution; it is determined by the field of view (FOV), the image matrix, and the section thickness.[8] Because CT applications, including cardiac applications, have demanded characterization of small anatomic structures as well as image post-processing in multiple planes, the spatial resolution has dramatically improved. Even before the 64-era technology matured, most CT image reconstruction algorithms included isotropic voxels. That is, the CT voxels in the x, y, and z dimensions are cubic with equal lengths along each side, for example 0.35 mm^3. This practice is now standard as it facilitates image post-processing.

Because normal coronary arteries have a lumen diameter of approximately 3 mm, a CT scanner with 0.35 mm^3 isotropic voxels will depict the coronary lumen on roughly 9 voxels. Thus, CT can spatially resolve a normal coronary lumen and depict disease, the fundamental basis of coronary CTA. However, the resolution is generally insufficient to perform quantitative assessments of coronary stenosis with high confidence. For example, volume averaging over a single voxel can alter the quantification of stenosis by more than 10%. Thus, stenosis grading should be limited to categories such as <50%, 50%–70%, and >70%. In some practices the categorization is limited to less than 50% versus 50% or greater. The spatial resolution also explains why, to date, the greatest benefit of coronary CTA has been its high negative predictive value. Because of the spatial resolution of cardiac CT, the evaluation of normalcy is simpler and can be made with greater confidence than the assessment of the percentage stenosis.

Typical fluoroscopy tubes have a spatial resolution is approximately 0.16 mm,[9] and thus a normal coronary artery is depicted on roughly 18 pixels. Another important difference is that fluoroscopic images are projections (two-dimensional [2D]), not volumetric as in CT. On one hand, fluoroscopy images do not suffer from volume averaging artifacts inherent to slice thickness. However, CT volumes have a distinct advantage in that lesions can be evaluated from any perspective.

The spatial resolution of sonography is largely determined by the transducer frequency. IntraVascular UltraSound (IVUS) performed with coronary catheterization has frequencies between 20–50 MHz, yielding an axial spatial resolution of 0.15 mm.[10] In addition to the superior spatial resolution, IVUS has good coronary artery contrast resolution, ie, the ability to resolve acoustic differences between calcified, noncalcified, fibrous, mixed, lipid-rich core, and necrotic content plaque. The limitation of IVUS relates to its invasive nature, the large catheter sizes with high rates of complication (3% chance of coronary vasospasm and up to 1% chance of coronary rupture). Also, dense calcification can severely limit the transmission of the high frequency sound waves and thus distort IVUS images.

So, "what do you want?" The spatial resolution of CT would be greatly enhanced if it rivaled catheterization, because a significant limitation in MDCT today is the inability to quantify coronary stenosis. Consider an example of 0.1 mm^3 voxels, recognizing that such a dramatic "improvement" is unrealistic with current technology. With respect to spatial resolution alone, the images would be comparable or superior to coronary catheterization; the lumen of a normal coronary artery would be spanned by 30 voxels, and advanced techniques for measurement of stenoses would become far more robust. However, voxels of this size would present difficulties related to image storage and manipulation with current image post-processing systems. Assuming that the acquisition spans 160 mm in the craniocaudal (z-axis) direction, image reconstruction at a single phase of the R-R interval would include 1600 images. Five reconstructions, currently considered routine, would absorb the memory space of 8000 high-definition images and would overwhelm current data transfer and storage systems.

The signal to noise ratio (SNR) is another important parameter intimately related to spatial resolution. The SNR refers to the amount of signal, or information that can be used for interpretation, divided by the image noise. The noise contains no information; it is akin to an imperfect canvas on which the image data, or signal, is painted. In fact, the image noise is calculated by making Hounsfield unit measurements in air. In general, CT enjoys a healthy SNR, particularly when compared to MRI where low signal can represent a limiting step for both cardiac and noncardiac applications. However, as the CT slice thickness decreases, so does the amount of tissue per slice and hence the signal. This same principle is important to recognize when imaging larger patients who have less signal per unit of photon flux because larger patients have a higher total x-ray CT attenuation. The first step to image this population is to maximize the x-ray CT tube current. However, a significantly higher SNR data set, ie, less noisy images, can be obtained when images are reconstructed at double the slice thickness, for example 0.8 mm instead of 0.4 mm.

It should also be noted that thinner slices are desirable with preserved volume coverage per gantry rotation. The benefits of large volume coverage are discussed in detail later in this article. Thinner slices unchanged in number would result in smaller z-axis coverage per gantry rotation. In turn, this would increase scan time and could compromise image quality by the introduction of breathing artifact. Moreover, longer scan times are generally associated with higher doses of radiation to patients.

Another way to improve the apparent spatial resolution is to increase coronary artery diameter, thus increasing the number of voxels spanning each artery. This is the basis of the near-universal practice of coronary vasodilatation before the CT acquisition. Patients with a contraindication to sublingual nitroglycerine, the agent typically used, can be imaged without it.

TEMPORAL RESOLUTION
What You Want: Less Than 30 ms and What You Get: 83–175 ms

The temporal resolution refers to the time needed to acquire a complete data set for image reconstruction. Superior temporal resolution improves the ability to freeze cardiac motion. Unlike static CT applications, the heart is beating and the gantry of the CT scanner is chasing it. This can result in cardiac motion artifact that compromises image quality. Specifically, severe motion artifact in only a single coronary segment can decrease confidence in rendering a negative examination to the point where additional imaging, typically catheterization, is needed.

The temporal resolution of a single x-ray CT tube and detector system is one half (180 degrees) of the gantry rotation time because image reconstruction requires approximately 180 degrees. The gantry rotation time is the time needed for a complete 360-degree revolution. Paralleling the rapid evolution of multidetector technology have been improved gantry rotation speeds. At the time when each CT vendor reached 64 slices per gantry rotation, the gantry rotation times reached 400 milliseconds or less and are now as low as 270 milliseconds with the Philips Brilliance iCT (**Fig. 2**).

Conventional angiography uses fluoroscopy with acquisition on the order of 30 frames per second. Thus, the temporal resolution (expressed in units of time for image acquisition) is approximately 33 milliseconds, adequate for motion-free cardiac imaging. As an analogy, the temporal resolution of a movie at a theater is 42 milliseconds, or 24 frames per second. At the temporal resolution of all CT applications, motion artifact can be detected, and, in some cases, this problem represents a significant limitation to image quality. Motion artifacts generally become more severe at higher heart rates because CT is unable to "freeze" cardiac motion.[11] Echocardiography has a temporal resolution of between 33–66 milliseconds (15–30 frames per second), effectively freezing cardiac motion, even at high heart rates.[12]

Because motion artifact can compromise CTA studies, there has been substantial effort to improve temporal resolution and effective temporal resolution (defined below). In addition to speeding up the gantry rotation, the temporal resolution can be

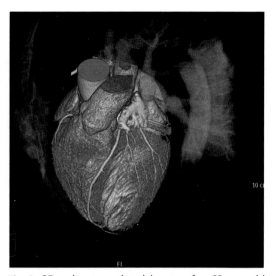

Fig. 2. 3D volume rendered image of a 62-year-old man with chest pain. CT was requested and excluded CAD. The patient was imaged with 256-slice CT, 128 detector rows and an alternating focal spot (Philips Brilliance iCT, Best, The Netherlands). With a scan time of 4 sec, 13 cm of craniocaudal coverage was achieved. (*Courtesy of* Nathan Peled, Carmel Medical Center, Haifa, Israel.)

improved with the introduction of a second x-ray CT source with an independent detector system. Dual-source CT features two x-ray CT sources and detector systems located 90 degrees from one another.[5] Consequently, using both x-ray CT tubes, the temporal resolution is halved from 165 milliseconds (330 milliseconds gantry rotation) to 83 milliseconds, because only one quarter of a gantry rotation is needed for reconstruction (**Fig. 3**).

In general, better temporal resolution improves image quality, decreasing the dependence on heart rate control with beta-blockade. The relationship between image quality, heart rate, and temporal resolution achieved by CT are areas of active investigation, with several investigators testing the hypothesis that routine cardiac CT can be performed without beta-blockade[13] and with reports that beta-blockers are not needed.[14] The benefits of scanning without heart-rate control include: simplified logistics; the ability to scan patients with a contraindication to beta-blockers; and increasing the number of patients scanned per day because of less patient preparation. However, heart-rate control can still be beneficial by reducing beat-to-beat variability; in dual-source CT, data is acquired over multiple R-R intervals. The stack of cardiac slabs, with each slab obtained from one heartbeat, are then visualized together. Thus, variability between heartbeats can degrade image quality.

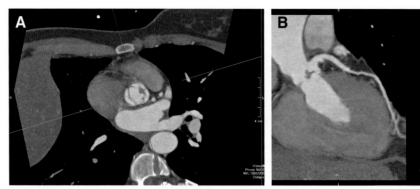

Fig. 3. 55-year-old man with abnormal aortic valve motion by echocardiography. CT was requested to exclude CAD. The patient's heart rate (>100 beats per minute at the time of acquisition) could not be safely lowered because of hypotension. (A) Retrospectively ECG gated dual-source cardiac CT (Siemens Definition, Erlangen, Germany) with 83 milliseconds temporal resolution depicted the vegetation of the aortic valve, as noted on the axial images. (B) Curved multiplanar reformatted image of the LAD also shows the vegetation in addition to demonstrating a normal LAD.

To date there is no established heart rate "cut-off" at which dual-source CT can confidently image; establishing such a limit is challenging. Instead of focusing on imaging without beta-blockade, one can capitalize on dual-source CT by combining the superior temporal resolution with heart-rate control to better eliminate cardiac motion from the list of variables that can compromise an acquisition.

All cardiac CT acquisitions use ECG gating to mitigate motion artifact. Thus, the discussion of temporal resolution inherently includes the two forms of ECG gating: retrospective and prospective. During retrospective gating, the image and ECG data are acquired throughout the cardiac cycle. Therefore, image reconstruction can be performed at any cardiac phase. This was briefly noted in the introduction; all current MDCT data from multicenter trials have been acquired with retrospective gating. Moreover, when retrospective gating is used, the cardiac cycle can be displayed as a cine loop in any projection, enabling myocardial function and valve evaluation. In prospective gating, the scanner uses the ECG to plan the timing of image acquisition and exposes the patient to radiation only during a preselected temporal window of the cardiac cycle. To date, the majority of clinical experience with prospective gating has been acquired with a 64 × 0.625 mm detector row (General Electric LightSpeed VCT64, Waukesha, WI) step-and-shoot technique (**Fig. 4**). In a typical coronary CTA case, imaging will occur over seven heartbeats. Four beats will be used for the prospective data acquisition (the "shoot") and the intervening three beats will be used to move the patient into the updated position within the gantry (the "step").

The preselected temporal window of the cardiac cycle, or "phase window"[15] can be described as a lower and upper bound of the cardiac phases, eg, 65%–75% of the R-R. Alternatively, it can also be described as a "center" phase and a surrounding "pad," eg, 100 milliseconds centered on 75% of the R-R interval.[16] By eliminating patient exposure for the majority of the R-R interval, prospective gating significantly reduces radiation exposure and is now preferred in patients who do not present with a clinical indication for evaluating cardiac function.

A narrower phase window lowers patient radiation dose by shortening the patient exposure time. Initial evidence also suggests that patients with a lower heart rate have a wider range of phases without motion artifact,[15] arguing that beta-blockade will reduce the overall patient radiation dose by increasing the confidence that high quality images will be achieved with a narrow phase window.

Multisegment reconstruction decreases the effective temporal resolution by using CT data from more than one R-R interval to reconstruct a volume.[17] For example, consider a 64 × 0.5 mm detector configuration with 350 milliseconds–gantry rotation. In single-segment reconstruction, 3.2 cm cranio–caudal slabs are reconstructed with 175 milliseconds temporal resolution from one R-R interval. In two-segment reconstruction, the same slab is reconstructed from CT data over two R-R intervals. Thus, only half the data is required per R-R interval, and the effective temporal resolution is reduced to 87.5 (175/2) milliseconds. This strategy decreases motion artifact but has drawbacks. In particular, patients receive

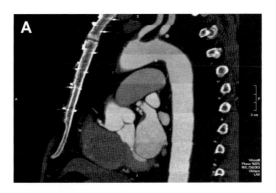

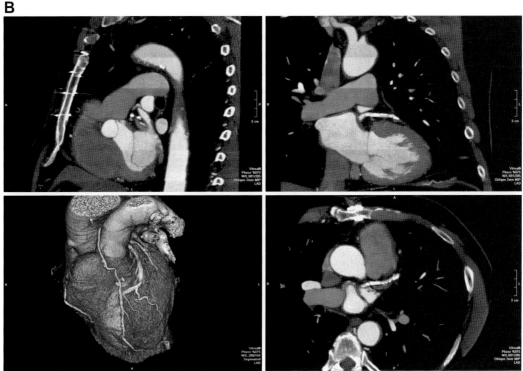

Fig. 4. 72-year-old man status post coronary artery bypass grafting. Because of the large craniocaudal field of view, imaging was performed over 13 heartbeats, 7 beats of data acquisition plus 6 move the patient within the gantry. This "step and shoot" technique significantly decreases the radiation exposure when compared to retrospective ECG gating. (*A*) Left anterior oblique reformation over the entire z-axis FOV shows high image quality. Enhancement pattern in the aorta demonstrates the individual "steps" as described. (*B*) Multiplanar reformatted images as well as 3D volume rendering (*lower left*) focused on the heavily calcified left anterior descending.

more radiation because the exposure time is longer, and as the number of segments increases, so does the length of the exam.

In general, there are two ways to mitigate cardiac motion. The first strategy is to scan faster than the heat beats. The second is to slow the heart rate. Heat rate control can be achieved by using oral or IV beta-blockade, both of which have a very high safety profile,[18] particularly when large doses are avoided. Many large practices, including that of the authors, have no record of an adverse event. In the authors' practice, all patients without

a contraindication receive beta-blockade. The contraindications include: symptomatic hypotension or bradycardia, severe decompensated heart failure, severe chronic obstructive lung disease, and severe peripheral arterial disease. Between 5 and 15 mg of metoprolol tartrate IV typically suffices to lower the heart rate below 65 beats per minute. A first dose of 5 mg can be followed with a second and third dose at 5 min intervals. In patients who are orally premedicated, additional IV beta-blockers can also be used with vital sign monitoring. Oral beta-blockers alone can also be used with a dose that increases in proportion to the patient's heart rate. This protocol is perceived to be safer than intravenous protcols. Efficiency is improved if additional time for IV beta-blockade can be avoided, although the heart rate monitoring required is identical.

CARDIAC COVERAGE PER GANTRY ROTATION
What You Want: Single Gantry Rotation Whole Heart Coverage and What You Get: 1.9 cm–16 cm

Multidector CT expanded the volume coverage per gantry rotation and revolutionized the imaging of many body parts, including the heart. Although the speed of the CT acquisition was enhanced by faster gantry rotation times, the most dramatic advances came from the doubling and continuous re-doubling from single detector slip ring CT to 2-, to 4-, to 8-, and eventually to 64-detector row CT.

Along with the increase in number of detectors, the term "multislice" was introduced and, to a certain extent, was adopted. "Multislice CT" is simpler to say and to write when compared to "multidetector row CT," but there are differences with respect to volume coverage per unit time. As noted in the introduction, an alternating x-ray CT source focal spot doubles the number of slices with respect to the number of detector rows. However, it does not double the volume coverage. As an example, a $128 \times 2 \times 0.625$ mm system (128 detector rows, 2 focal spot positions, and 0.625 mm detector rows) will yield 256 (128×2) slices per gantry rotation while the z-axis coverage is 80 mm (128×0.625 mm).

The first advantage of greater volume coverage is a faster overall CT acquisition. A more rapid acquisition decreases the probability of an irregular cardiac rhythm, typically a premature ventricular contraction, that can severely compromise image quality. A second advantage is the ability to capture the state of iodinated contrast media at a single point in time. The largest volume coverage to date is 320-detector row CT (Toshiba AquilonOne Dynamic Volume CT) that features a 320×0.5 mm configuration, or 16 cm of craniocaudal coverage per gantry rotation. The result is single R-R, or single heartbeat cardiac imaging.

Three-hundred and twenty detector row cardiac CT eliminates "stair-step" artifacts inherent in other forms of cardiac CT in which cardiac subvolumes over multiple gantry rotations are subsequently stacked to create a cardiac volume. In addition, the 16 cm maximum single gantry rotation cranio–caudal coverage decreases the overall exam time to less than one second, and subsecond cardiac CT is expected to reduce artifacts.

This timeframe also potentially reduces radiation exposure by avoiding the oversampling related to helical scanning.

In addition to the ability to perform single heartbeat coronary imaging at doses comparable to diagnostic catheterization, wide area detector coverage enables imaging at multiple points where each entire volume is acquired in a single R-R interval. A craniocaudal field of view that spans the entire heart gives the potential for single heartbeat myocardial perfusion CT, considered to be one of the most important potential applications of post-64 CT technology. An exam that includes accurate perfusion data could, in theory, supplant other technologies such as nuclear imaging and MRI. Myocardial perfusion CT highlights some of the differences between post-64 era technologies. In order to detect ischemia, CT perfusion must be performed under pharmacologic stress, increasing the heart rate. From this perspective alone, dual-source CT would be well suited for perfusion CT since the temporal resolution is 83 milliseconds. However, dual-source CT has relatively poor volume coverage per gantry rotation (1.9 cm) in comparison with 320-detector row CT (16.0 cm). Thus, dual-source CT perfusion would acquire the cardiac volume over approximately eight heartbeats, and the iodinated contrast opacification would be different for each slab. It is likely that accurate delineation of either small or subtle perfusion defects will require that images of the entire myocardial volume are obtained at a single point of iodinated contrast opacification, ie, using 320-detector row CT. However, this scanner has a temporal resolution of 350 milliseconds and thus two-segment reconstruction will be required for the majority of patients so that an effective temporal resolution of 87.5 milliseconds can be achieved (**Fig. 5**). Because the patient will be exposed over two heartbeats instead of one, the radiation will be higher than for single heartbeat imaging. Cardiac CT dose is the topic of the next section.

Myocardial perfusion CT is still experimental and will require first small and then larger validation studies before it could become a routine clinical examination. However, the potential for CT is noteworthy, as it is theoretically possible to use a single bolus of contrast media to acquire anatomic coronary images, followed by myocardial perfusion to detect regions of ischemia, and then myocardial delayed enhancement (MDE) images for the assessment of myocardial scar. MDE images are typically acquired 5–10 min after contrast injection; this acquisition does not require precise timing because iodine remains for some time in the extracellular space surrounding myocardial scar.

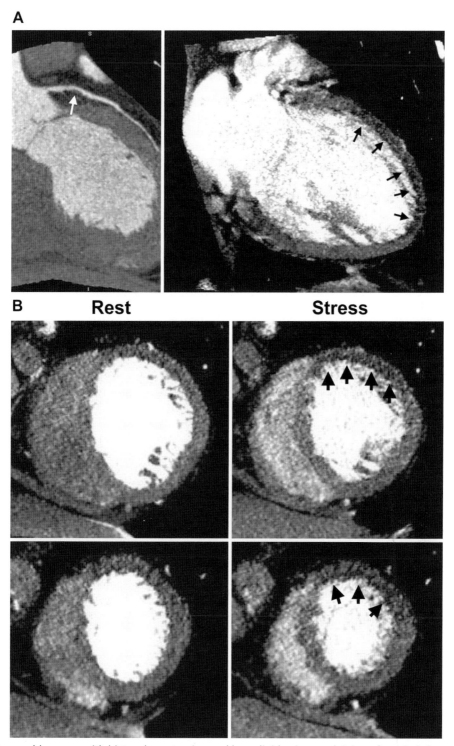

Fig. 5. 57-year-old woman with history hypertension and hyperlipidemia complaining of atypical chest pain. The patient underwent 320-detector row CT (Toshiba AquilionOne, Tochigi-ken, Japan) coronary CTA plus perfusion imaging. (*A*) CTA (*left*) followed by adenosine stress CT perfusion imaging (*right*). CTA shows a noncalcified plaque (*white arrow*) causing a moderate stenosis in the proximal LAD. Stress perfusion imaging (*right*) shows a subendocardial perfusion deficit in the anterior and apical walls (*black arrows*). (*B*) Short axis views reformatted with 3-mm slice thickness. Rest images (*left*) demonstrate very mild hypoattenuation in the anterior wall. Stress CT perfusion images (*right*) show perfusion deficit in the anterior wall at the level of the mid and distal left ventricle. (*Courtesy of* Richard T. George and Joao AC. Lima, Johns Hopkins University, Division of Cardiology.)

CARDIAC CT DOSIMETRY
What You Want: The Minimum Effective Dose to Answer a Specific Clinical Question. What You Get: Dose Estimates, Retrospective vs. Prospective Gating, and ECG Dose Modulation

Medical radiation accounts for a large proportion of the total population exposure. CT is a major contributor; every patient referred for CT requires an evaluation of medical necessity versus radiation risk.[19,20] Because of ECG gating and subsequent image oversampling, cardiac CT is a high radiation dose exam. Image oversampling is discussed below. Although substantial improvements have been made in the last two years, many practices deliver cardiac CT doses on the order of 20 mSv, with reports up to 40 mSv.[21] To place this into a medical imaging perspective, some cardiac CT scans deliver a dose more than 50 times higher than screening mammography.

Some consequences of radiation have an established threshold dose, such as inducing a skin burn.[22] This would require multiple scans over a short period of time. The main concern is induction of a radiation induced fatal neoplasm where cumulative dose is considered to increase risk. The relatively high doses from cardiac CT underscore the need for the imager to understand and be able to estimate dose.

For the radiation levels of diagnostic imaging, there is no data to confirm or refute a radiation "threshold," that is, a level of cumulative effective dose at which the risk of a radiation induced fatal neoplasm is zero. Because data is so scarce, mathematical models are used to estimate risk. These models extrapolate from high-level exposures encountered by Japanese nuclear bomb survivors to much lower levels of medical radiation. Most models use a linear fit to estimate risk and have no threshold. That is, models assume that the risk is linearly proportional to the dose, and risk is present even for the smallest dose. To continue the comparison between the cardiac CT and the mammography patients, both individuals would be at risk for a radiation induced fatal neoplasm (no threshold), and for every one death induced by mammography, 50 people would die from cardiac CT. Because our best estimates are so rough, and because the risk is so low, it is challenging for medical personnel to consider medical radiation risks on a per patient basis. There is also a large potential for miscommunication. However, the cumulative radiation risk to the entire population must be considered, and cardiac CT is appropriately moving towards lower dose acquisitions.

CT has specific parameters to describe radiation dose: the computed tomography dose index (CTDI) and dose length product (DLP). The CTDI uses a 100 mm–long ion chamber and 150 mm–long, 320 mm–diameter cylindrical phantom to measure the radiation dose normalized by the beam width in milliGrays (mGy). Current CTDI estimates also weight the average of the center and peripheral contributions and helical pitch or axial scan spacing to dose. This is referred to as $CDTI_{vol}$. Although the phantom should somehow reflect the attenuation of a human body, the CTDI is not used to make a statement regarding an individual patient's dose but rather as an index of radiation from CT scanning. In contrast to parameters such as the tube current, CTDI values reflect delivered dose because parameters such as the scanner geometry and filtration are considered. In practical terms, the CDTI can be used to compare scanning platforms and individual protocols. The $CTDI_{vol}$ is available from the CT console of all major manufacturers.

The second parameter is the DLP, expressed in mGy × centimeters. The DLP is defined as the product of the $CTDI_{vol}$ and the z-axis FOV. Even though the DLP reflects most closely the radiation dose for a specific CT examination, it is important to keep in mind that the DLP is a function of patient size, ie, how much z-axis coverage is required to complete the CT scan.

$CTDI_{vol}$ and DLP values can be used to characterize the scanner; they do not represent effective dose. The effective dose, with units of milliSevert (mSv), is the weighted sum over the organ doses. Although an estimation because individual organ doses can not be measured directly, the effective dose is the only useful parameter for individual patient risk assessment. The effective dose itself includes estimation because individual organ doses can not be measured directly. A simple estimation is that the effective dose is the product of the DLP and a conversion factor, E_{DLP} that is specific to a body region. For example, for the chest the $E_{DLP} = 0.017$ mSv $\times$ mGy^{-1} $\times$ cm^{-1}.

As an example, suppose a coronary CTA acquisition results in a CTDIvol = 50mGy as stated on the scanner console. If the cranio–caudal extent of the scan is 14 cm (a normal sized heart), the DLP = 50mGy × 14 cm = 700 mGy × cm. Because the heart is in the chest, the appropriate conversion factor is $E_{DLP} = 0.017$ mSv $\times$ mGy^{-1} $\times$ cm^{-1}, and the effective dose for this patient is 50mGy × 14 cm × 0.017mSv × mGy^{-1} × cm^{-1}, or about 12 mSv. At present, there are few centers that include dosimetry in the cardiac CT report. This practice may change over time as the awareness of referring clinicians and patients continues to increase.

There are several strategies to reduce cardiac CT dose. In the "pre-64" era of coronary CTA, all acquisitions used retrospective gating, and the patient exposure was high throughout the R-R interval. This practice continued into the early stages of the 64 era, during which doses began to increase, as did awareness of the high doses. A major step in dose reduction was the introduction of retrospective ECG-dependent tube current modulation.[23] This strategy reduces tube current during systole, that part of the R-R interval least often used for interpretation because of greater coronary motion. The standard tube current is used for a predetermined phase window in diastole where motion is expected to be minimized.

As noted earlier, retrospective ECG gating enables cine evaluations throughout the R-R interval. With ECG-dependent tube current modulation, the images in systole have high noise (low SNR), lending itself to an important tradeoff between dose and image quality. For some applications, such as endocardial tracings to calculate left ventricular function, a relatively lower SNR is acceptable. However, as dose is reduced by further lowering the tube current in systole, the image degradation will eventually render those images not interpretable.

With respect to dose, prospective gating can be considered to be the limit of this tradeoff. As noted earlier, in prospective gating, there is no data acquisition outside the phase window, ie, the tube current is reduced to zero in systole. Coronary calcium scoring uses prospective gating with a very narrow phase window, usually a single phase of the R-R interval. Because there is no data for most of the cardiac cycle, cine evaluations for the myocardium and valves are not available. As the phase window is narrowed, cardiac CT doses become comparable, and in many cases less than, diagnostic cardiac catheterization. However, as this tradeoff is pushed to the limits of a narrower phase window and lower dose, fewer and fewer reconstruction phases are available, and the benefit of very low dose can be negated if every available phase is degraded by motion artifact. There is evidence for single heartbeat imaging that patients with slower heart rates have more phases that contain motion-free images.[15] Thus, beta-blockade will lower the population radiation dose. The phase window should be chosen carefully; there are currently no published guidelines, but lowest dose (eg, single phase) imaging should be reserved for those patients in whom there is very high diagnostic confidence of motion-free images.

The MDCT pitch is a unitless measure for helical CT that describes how much the table feeds per gantry rotation. The pitch determines the amount of overlap between gantry rotations and hence the degree of oversampling for the ECG gated acquisition. For example, for a helical acquisition with a pitch of 0.2, an individual z-axis position of the heart will provide data that is received by 5 (1/0.2) detectors per gantry rotation. The 64-era scanners include software that automatically varies the pitch as a function of the patient's heart rate to optimize image quality and dose. For 320-detector row CT, images are acquired axially and thus the pitch is not a consideration.

One of the simplest methods to lower coronary CTA radiation doses is to limit the z-axis FOV. Scanning as superior as the aortic arch or as inferior as the adrenal glands delivers unnecessary radiation. Also, a complete "x-y", or "skin-to-skin" reconstruction must be obtained, given the high prevalence of extracardiac findings. This does not influence the radiation dose since the larger x-y reconstruction will include only the z-axis FOV acquired to evaluate the coronary arteries.

SUMMARY

The 64-generation scanners added a noninvasive dimension to coronary imaging and have been applied to a large number of patients. Image acquisition has been labor-intensive in comparison to CT of other body parts. In addition, the high radiation levels delivered to the patient using retrospective ECG gating, even though the actual risks are poorly defined, can offset the benefits in comparison with catheterization. The comparison between coronary catheterization and CT is complex, but CT will be forced to measure up to these technical specifications. Thus, imagers and referring clinicians should have a solid understanding of spatial resolution, temporal resolution, volume coverage, and radiation dose.

Noninvasive cardiac imaging now includes the post- 64 era of coronary CTA, and the new hardware incrementally improves on these parameters. The improvement is not uniform. As the technology strives to mirror catheterization benchmarks, the CT vendors have chosen to improve individual parameters. A clear example is the introduction of dual-source and 320-detector row CT. The former has demonstrated improved temporal resolution; the latter has demonstrated whole heart coverage.

Cardiac imaging will continue to define the state-of-the-art in CT. It is safe to predict that the next generation of scanners will again change the way clinicians think about image acquisition. In the meantime, patients today can and should benefit from very high negative predictive value of coronary CTA. Those patients who require coronary imaging but have a low or intermediate probability of CAD can undergo noninvasive diagnostic coronary imaging with radiation levels comparable to catheterization. This group of patients includes uncomplicated patients today who present to the emergency room. Although these patients enjoy a simpler exam to exclude CAD, the newer applications enabled by the post-64 era will be tested.

REFERENCES

1. Budof MJ, Dowe D, Jollis J, et al. Diagnostic Performance of 64-Multidetector Row Coronary Computed Tomographic Angiography for Evaluation of Coronary Artery Stenosis in Individuals Without Known Coronary Artery Disease: Results From the Prospective Multicenter ACCURACY (Assessment by Coronary Computed Tomographic Angiography of Individuals Undergoing Invasive Coronary Angiography) Trial. J Am Coll Cardiol 2008;52:1724–32.

2. Miller JM, Rochitte CE, Dewey M, et al. Diagnostic Performance of Coronary Angiography by 64-Row CT. N Engl J Med 2008;359:2324–36.

3. Achenbach S. Cardiac CT: state of the art for the detection of coronary arterial stenosis. J Cardiovascular Computed Tomography 2007;1:3–20.

4. Hoffmann U, Pena AJ, Cury RC, et al. Cardiac CT in emergency department patients with acute chest pain. Radiographics 2006;26:963–78 [discussion: 979–80].

5. Flohr TG, McCollough CH, Bruder H, et al. First performance evaluation of a dual-source CT (DSCT) system. Eur Radiol 2006;16:256–68.

6. Rybicki FJ, Otero HJ, Steigner ML, et al. Initial evaluation of coronary images from 320-detector row computed tomography. Int J Cardiovasc Imaging 2008;24:535–46.

7. Judy PF. The line spread function and modulation transfer function of a computed tomographic scanner. Med Phys 1976;3:233–6.

8. Sprawls P. AAPM tutorial. CT image detail and noise. Radiographics 1992;12:1041–6.

9. Gershlick AH, de Belder M, Chambers J, et al. Role of non-invasive imaging in the management of coronary artery disease: an assessment of likely change over the next 10 years. A report from the British cardiovascular society working group. Heart 2007;93:423–31.

10. Nissen SE, Yock P. Intravascular ultrasound: novel pathophysiological insights and current clinical applications. Circulation 2001;103:604–16.

11. Dewey M, Teige F, Laule M, et al. Influence of heart rate on diagnostic accuracy and image quality of 16-slice CT coronary angiography: comparison of multisegment and halfscan reconstruction approaches. Eur Radiol 2007;17:2829–37.

12. Goldstein A. Overview of the physics of US. Radiographics 1993;13:701–4.

13. Ropers U, Ropers D, Pflederer T, et al. Influence of heart rate on the diagnostic accuracy of dual-source computed tomography coronary angiography. J Am Coll Cardiol 2007;50:2393–8.

14. Achenbach S, Ropers D, Kuettner A, et al. Contrast-enhanced coronary artery visualization by dual-source computed tomography–initial experience. Eur J Radiol 2006;57:331–5.

15. Steigner ML, Otero HJ, Cai T, et al. Narrowing the phase window width in prospectively ECG-gated single heart beat 320-detector row coronary CT angiography. Int J Cardiovasc Imaging 2009;25:85–90.

16. Earls JP, Berman EL, Urban BA, et al. Prospectively gated transverse coronary CT angiography versus retrospectively gated helical technique: improved image quality and reduced radiation dose. Radiology 2008;246:742–53.

17. Halliburton SS, Stillman AE, Flohr T, et al. Do segmented reconstruction algorithms for cardiac multi-slice computed tomography improve image quality? Herz 2003;28:20–31.

18. Pannu HK, Alvarez W Jr, Fishman EK. {beta}-Blockers for cardiac CT: a primer for the radiologist. Am J Roentgenol. 2006;186:S341–5.

19. Brenner DJ, Hall EJ. Computed tomography–an increasing source of radiation exposure. N Engl J Med 2007;357:2277–84.

20. Cohnen M, Poll L, Puttmann C, et al. Radiation exposure in multi-slice CT of the heart. Rofo 2001;173:295–9.

21. Paul JF, Abada HT. Strategies for reduction of radiation dose in cardiac multislice CT. Eur Radiol 2007;17:2028–37.

22. McNitt-Gray MF. AAPM/RSNA physics tutorial for residents: topics in CT. Radiation dose in CT. Radiographics 2002;22:1541–53.

23. Husmann L, Valenta I, Gaemperli O, et al. Feasibility of low-dose coronary CT angiography: first experience with prospective ECG-gating. Eur Heart J 2008;29:191–7.

Coronary CT Angiography: Applications

Gorka Bastarrika, MD, PhD[a,b], Yeong Shyan Lee, MD[a,c],
Balazs Ruzsics, MD, PhD[a], U. Joseph Schoepf, MD, FAHA[a,d],*

KEYWORDS

- Computed tomography • Multidetector row CT • Heart
- Coronary angiography • Coronary artery disease
- Coronary artery stenosis • Atherosclerosis

Coronary heart disease (CHD) has become an important socio-epidemiologic problem as the main cause of death in developed countries. In 2004, CHD caused one out of every five deaths in the United States. That year, CHD mortality was 451,326 (233,538 males, 217,788 females).[1] Conventional coronary angiography is the invasive reference standard for the diagnosis of coronary artery disease. Nevertheless, nearly half of the coronary angiographies performed every year are done only for diagnostic purposes.

Coronary multidetector-row CT (MDCT) angiography, especially after the introduction of 64-slice MDCT systems into clinical practice, has emerged as a useful technique for noninvasively ruling out CHD.[2–5] This technique is increasingly used for noninvasive detection and grading of coronary artery stenosis. A host of articles demonstrate its usefulness to evaluate the coronary artery wall and assess the atherosclerotic plaque burden.[6–8] Noninvasive MDCT coronary angiography still has some limitations, such as radiation dose and the need of intravenous contrast injection. Evaluation of severely calcified coronary artery lesions (**Fig. 1**) also remains a relative limitation. However,

despite these limitations, the vast potential of this technique to beneficially alter the traditional work-up for CHD is unequivocally recognized. After a decade of feasibility testing, appropriate and useful indications for the use of CT coronary angiography are increasingly emerging. This article describes the more established clinical applications of this test.

CLINICAL INDICATIONS OF CORONARY CT ANGIOGRAPHY

The first major attempt at outlining clinical indications and appropriateness for cardiac computed tomography has been recently published under the auspices of the American College of Cardiology Foundation together with key specialty and subspecialty societies.[9] In this publication, a technical expert panel scored each possible clinical indication based on a numerical scale of 1 to 9, considering the upper range (7 to 9) appropriate and indicated, and the lower range (1 to 3) not appropriate and not recommendable use. The indications presented in this report were selected to cover diverse potential clinical scenarios and common clinical

U.J.S. is a medical consultant for Bayer-Schering, Bracco, General Electric, Medrad, Siemens, and TeraRecon and receives research support from Bayer-Schering, Bracco, General Electric, Medrad, and Siemens.

[a] Department of Radiology and Radiological Science, Medical University of South Carolina, Ashley River Tower, MSC 226, 25 Courtenay Drive, Charleston, SC 29401, USA

[b] Department of Radiology, Clinica Universitaria, Universidad de Navarra, Avenida Pio XII, 36, 31008 Pamplona, Spain

[c] Department of Diagnostic Radiology, Tan Tock Seng Hospital, 11 Jalan Tan Tock Seng, Singapore, 308433

[d] Division of Cardiology, Department of Medicine, Medical University of South Carolina, Ashley River Tower, 25 Courtenay Drive, Charleston, SC 29401, USA

* Corresponding author. Department of Radiology and Radiological Science, Medical University of South Carolina, Ashley River Tower, MSC 226, 25 Courtenay Drive, Charleston, SC 29401.

E-mail address: 29401schoepf@musc.edu (U.J. Schoepf).

Radiol Clin N Am 47 (2009) 91–107
doi:10.1016/j.rcl.2008.10.010

radiologic.theclinics.com

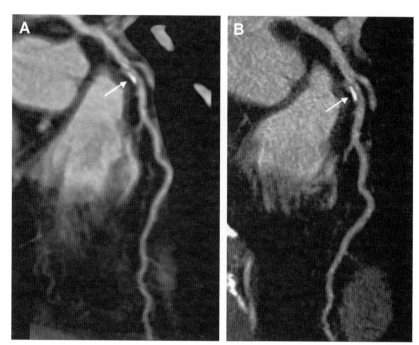

Fig. 1. Calcified plaque (*arrow*) in the mid-segment of left anterior descending coronary artery in a 72-year-old man with atypical chest pain. (*A*) Curved multiplanar reconstruction using a soft tissue kernel (B26f). (*B*) Curved multiplanar reconstruction using a high-resolution kernel (B46f). Note the reduction of blooming artifact in the calcified lesion. The plaque caused nonsignificant coronary artery stenosis.

presentations, including symptoms suggestive of ischemia, cardiovascular risk factors in asymptomatic individuals, and specific scenarios with indices of clinical suspicion. **Box 1** lists appropriate indications for coronary CT angiography as outlined in the appropriateness criteria catalog. Currently, coronary CT angiography is considered most appropriate in symptomatic individuals, especially if symptoms, gender, and age suggest a low to intermediate probability of significant coronary artery stenosis (**Fig. 2**). The usefulness of screening of asymptomatic individuals for occult coronary atherosclerosis with coronary CT angiography is under investigation, but is currently not considered recommendable use because of radiation concerns and unclear benefit.[10] Whether there is a role for coronary CT angiography in providing added value to traditional risk stratification also needs to be determined.

CLINICAL APPLICATIONS OF CORONARY CT ANGIOGRAPHY
Detection of Coronary Anomalies

Coronary artery anomalies are a poorly understood entity in cardiology.[11–13] The prevalence of coronary anomalies is not well known. Autopsy series describe a prevalence of 0.3%,[14] but up to 5.6% prevalence has been reported in actual series using different imaging techniques.[15] Even if uncommon, coronary anomalies may be

a significant cause of chest pain, myocardial ischemia, and sudden cardiac death,[16–18] especially in young athletes.[19] MR imaging plays a key role in identifying coronary anomalies[20] but remains limited when determining the distal course of the coronary vessel. The usefulness of MDCT to demonstrate anomalous coronary arteries has repeatedly been reported.[21,22] For identifying anomalies of the origin and course of the coronary arteries, MDCT has several potential advantages with respect to other imaging modalities. MDCT can demonstrate an anomalous origin in cases in which conventional angiography can mistakenly diagnose vessel occlusion. MDCT can also demonstrate an inter-arterial anomalous coronary course, which has been implicated in decreased myocardial perfusion causing symptoms and sudden cardiac death (**Fig. 3**). Furthermore, preoperative coronary MDCT and demonstration of the course of the artery can be helpful to avoid coronary injury during surgical reimplantation (**Fig. 4**). Usefulness of MDCT to demonstrate morphologic changes in the coronary artery wall have also been demonstrated (**Fig. 5**).

Detection of Coronary Artery Stenosis

The continuous movement of the heart, along with the small caliber and tortuous course of the coronary arteries, make these vessels challenging to

Detection of coronary artery disease

Evaluation of chest pain syndrome in symptomatic subjects

Intermediate pre-test probability of coronary artery disease (CAD)

ECG uninterpretable or unable to exercise

Evaluation of intra-cardiac structures in symptomatic subjects

Evaluation of suspected coronary anomalies

Acute chest pain in symptomatic subjects

Intermediate pre-test probability of CAD

No ECG changes and serial enzymes negative

Detection of CAD with prior test results

Evaluation of chest pain syndrome

Uninterpretable or equivocal stress test (exercise, perfusion, or stress echo)

Structure and function

Morphology

Assessment of complex congenital heart disease, including anomalies of coronary circulation, great vessels, and cardiac chambers and valves

Evaluation of coronary arteries in patients with new onset heart failure to assess etiology

Evaluation of intra- and extra-cardiac structures

Noninvasive coronary arterial mapping, including internal mammary artery before repeat cardiac surgical revascularization

Data from Hendel RC, Patel MR, Kramer CM, et al. ACCF/ACR/SCCT/SCMR/ASNC/NASCI/SCAI/SIR 2006 appropriateness criteria for cardiac computed tomography and cardiac magnetic resonance imaging: a report of the American College of Cardiology Foundation Quality Strategic Directions Committee Appropriateness Criteria Working Group, American College of Radiology, Society of Cardiovascular Computed Tomography, Society for Cardiovascular Magnetic Resonance, American Society of Nuclear Cardiology, North American Society for Cardiac Imaging, Society for Cardiovascular Angiography and Interventions, and Society of Interventional Radiology. J Am Coll Cardiol 2006 Oct 3;48(7):1483.

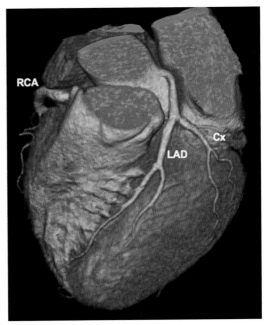

Fig. 2. Normal coronary dual-source CT (DSCT) angiography in a 54-year-old man admitted for atypical chest pain. Volume-rendered image. Currently, coronary CT angiography is considered most appropriate in symptomatic individuals with low to intermediate probability of significant coronary artery stenosis. A normal CT coronary angiogram, as shown in this case, allows to reliably exclude significant coronary artery disease. *Abbreviations*: Cx, circumflex coronary artery; LAD, left anterior descending coronary artery; RCA, right coronary artery.

Coronary CT angiography has proven to be useful for morphologic noninvasive imaging of the coronary arteries and diagnosis of coronary artery disease. In experienced hands, this technique has demonstrated high sensitivity and specificity for the detection of hemodynamically significant stenotic coronary artery disease. The initial publications based on 4-slice MDCT and 16-slice MDCT found sensitivities of up to 80% to 90% for the detection of significant coronary artery stenosis (>50%) when compared with conventional coronary angiography.[4,23] These results were obtained, however, in highly selected patient populations and after exclusion of patients, vessels, or vessel segments that were not assessable because of motion artifacts or calcification.[4,23,24] A recent systematic analysis investigated the sensitivity of coronary CT angiography with 4-slice MDCT and 16-slice MDCT in patients suspected of CAD[25] and found, not surprisingly, that scanners with 16 detectors had higher sensitivities (pooled sensitivity, 91%) than 4-detector MDCT scanners. In this publication, investigators

visualize with any imaging test. A robust technique with high-acquisition speed and high spatial resolution is needed to achieve diagnostic imaging quality.

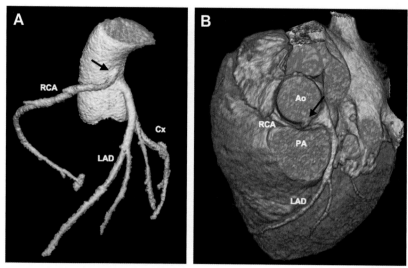

Fig. 3. RCA anomaly in a 22-year-old male. (*A* and *B*) Note the anomalous origin of RCA from the left coronary sinus (*arrow*) and the interarterial course between the aorta (Ao) and the pulmonary artery (PA).

concluded that the sensitivity of 4-detector MDCT and 16-detector MDCT is not yet sufficient to reliably rule out stenosis in patients suspected of CAD.[25]

Relatedly, recent initiatives to curb insurance reimbursement for coronary CT angiography were mainly based on those reported shortcomings of past generation MDCT scanners, and were rescinded after analyzing the performance of more recent generation instruments. Specifically, spatial and temporal resolution of MDCT scanners substantially improved with the development of 64-slice MDCT technology. Recent studies analyzed the accuracy of these last generation scanners for detection of significant coronary stenosis in individuals with suspicion of CAD, in comparison with conventional coronary angiography (**Table 1**).[26–36] Most of the studies included preselected subjects and excluded those with known previous CAD, who were in unstable condition or presented with arrhythmia or renal failure. In these reports, analysis was ordinarily limited to vessel segments with a diameter greater than 1.5 mm or 2 mm. These studies reported sensitivities and specificities of 86% to 99% and 92% to 98%, respectively, for the detection of hemodynamically significant coronary artery stenosis. Most importantly, a very high negative predictive value (ranging from 92% to 100%) was consistently demonstrated, emphasizing the usefulness of current era coronary CT angiography for reliably

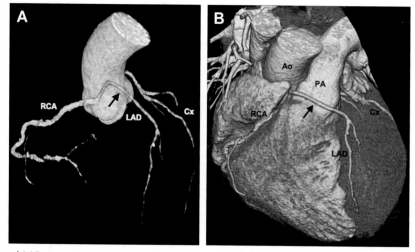

Fig. 4. Incidental LAD coronary artery anomaly in a 57-year-old man with atypical chest pain. (*A* and *B*) Volume rendered images. In this patient, LAD originated from the right coronary sinus and presented an abnormal course (*arrow*), anterior to the pulmonary artery before descending along the anterior interventricular groove.

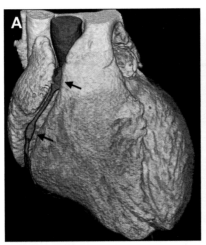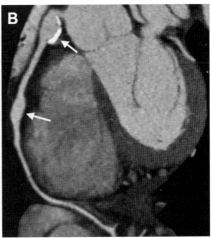

Fig. 5. Right coronary artery aneurysms in a 15-year-old female with Kawasaki disease. (*A*) Volume-rendered image. The right coronary artery, in blue, presented aneurismal dilatations located in the proximal and mid-segments of the vessel (*arrows*). (*B*) Curved multiplanar reformation. Note partial calcification of the proximal aneurysm.

ruling out significant coronary artery stenosis in subjects with clinical suspicion of CAD.

In a systematic analysis by Hamon and colleagues,[37] the diagnostic performance of 16-slice MDCT versus 64-slice MDCT for the diagnosis of CAD was compared. In this analysis, the results for 16-slice MDCT compared with 64-slice MDCT were 95% versus 97% for sensitivity, 69% versus 90% for specificity, 79% versus 93% for positive predictive value, and 92% versus 96% for negative predictive value. Again, not unexpectedly these investigators conclude that for the detection of coronary artery stenosis greater than 50%, 64-slice MDCT has significantly higher specificity

and positive predictive value on a per-patient basis compared with 16-slice MDCT.[37] To date, relatively fewer studies have analyzed the accuracy of coronary CT angiography using dual-source CT (DSCT) to detect significant coronary artery stenosis in comparison with conventional coronary angiography (**Fig. 6**). Because of its inherent high temporal resolution of 83 ms, DSCT allows the obtaining of high diagnostic-quality coronary angiograms within a wide range of heart rates.[38,39] In a recent contribution, Ropers and colleagues[35] evaluated 100 patients using DSCT without pharmaceutic rate control (ie, beta-blockers). The investigators divided their study population

Table 1
Accuracy of 64-slice MDCT and DSCT for detection of coronary stenosis in comparison with conventional coronary angiography (per-segment analysis)

Author	Scanner Type	Number of Patients	Sensitivity (%)	Specificity (%)	PPV (%)	NPV (%)
Ehara[27]	64-MDCT	69	90	94	89	95
Mollet[31]	64-MDCT	52	99	95	76	99
Oncel[32]	64-MDCT	80	96	98	91	99
Raff[33]	64-MDCT	70	86	95	66	98
Ropers[34]	64-MDCT	84	93	97	56	100
Leschka[30]	64-MDCT	67	94	97	87	99
Fine[28]	64-MDCT	66	95	96	97	92
Brodoefel[26]	DSCT	100	91	92	75	97
Ropers[35]	DSCT	100	92	97	68	99
Johnson[29]	DSCT	35	88	98	78	99
Weustink[36]	DSCT	100	95	95	75	99

Abbreviations: NPV, negative predictive value; PPV, positive predictive value.

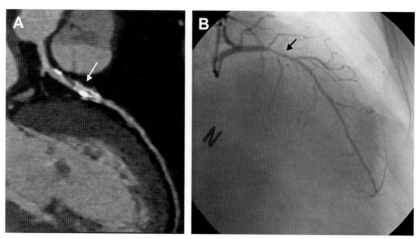

Fig. 6. Significant left anterior-descending coronary artery stenosis in a 67-year-old man with stable angina. (*A*) Curved multiplanar reconstruction of left anterior descending coronary artery showing a mixed plaque causing significant stenosis (*arrow*). (*B*) The conventional coronary angiography confirmed the lesion.

according to heart rate in two groups (heart rate $\geq$65 bpm and heart rate <65 bpm). In 44 patients with heart rates greater than or equal to 65 beats per minute (bpm), they found 566 of 616 (92%) coronary segments evaluable. In 56 patients with heart rates less than 65 bpm, 777 of 778 coronary segments (100%, *P*<.001) were evaluable. When the presence of significant coronary stenoses was validated against invasive coronary angiography as the reference standard, these investigators found no statistically significant differences in per-segment, per-vessel, and per-patient analyses. By classifying nonevaluable segments as positive for stenosis, per-patient sensitivity was 95% for heart rates greater than or equal to 65 bpm and 100% for heart rates less than 65 bpm. The investigators found specificity values of 87% versus 76% and overall diagnostic accuracy of 91% versus 86%.[35]

In a similar study in patients with an intermediate pretest likelihood for coronary artery disease, Leber and colleagues[40] demonstrated that the accuracy to detect patients with coronary stenoses greater than 50% was not significantly different among patients with heart rates greater than or equal to 65 bpm and less than 65 bpm (sensitivity 92% versus 100%; specificity 88% versus 91%). These investigators also found that the concordance of DSCT-derived stenosis quantification showed good correlation (*r* = 0.76; *P*<.001) with quantitative coronary angiography, with a slight trend to overestimate stenosis severity.[40] In 100 symptomatic patients with typical or atypical angina pectoris, or unstable coronary artery disease, Weustink and colleagues[36] reported sensitivity, specificity,

and positive and negative predictive values of DSCT coronary angiography for the detection of significant lesions on a segment-by-segment analysis of 95%, 95%, 75%, and 99%, respectively, when compared with conventional coronary angiography. On a patient-based analysis, these values were 99%, 87%, 96%, and 95%, respectively. In another study performed in 35 patients with known or suspected CAD, Johnson and colleagues[29] reported sensitivity, specificity, positive-predictive, and negative-predictive values of 88%, 98%, 78%, and 99%, respectively for the detection of stenoses greater than 50% on a per-segment basis analysis. Thus, currently there appears to be consensus in the literature that noninvasive coronary CT angiography, using from 64-slice CT technology on upwards, has fair accuracy for stenosis detection and grading, while the negative predictive value for excluding significant stenosis is next to perfect (**Fig. 7**). Accordingly, patient management should mainly be based on this exceedingly high negative predictive value, because significant coronary artery stenosis can be reliably ruled out and further testing avoided when coronary CT angiography shows normal or near normal coronary arteries. The minority of patients where CT angiography shows atherosclerotic disease changes of unclear hemodynamic significance should still undergo physiologic testing to rule out obstructive disease.

Meanwhile, we have left the decade-long phase of feasibility testing and investigators are increasingly addressing more practically relevant questions pertaining to use, cost-effectiveness, and outcome of coronary CT angiography. For

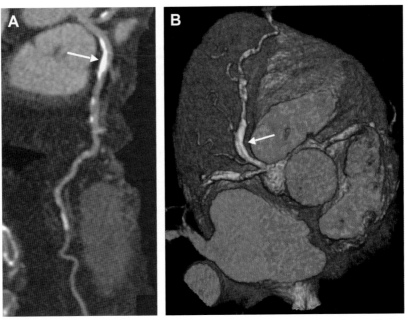

Fig. 7. Severe calcification of the proximal and mid segments of the left anterior descending coronary artery (*arrow*) in a 66-year-old man with atypical chest pain. (*A*) Curved multiplanar reformation. (*B*) Volume-rendered image. The eccentric calcified plaque caused not significant coronary artery stenosis.

example, recent reports have evaluated the prognostic value of 64-slice MDCT during up to 2-year follow-up, with promising results,[41–43] which will most certainly be corroborated by further evidence-based research.

However, coronary CT angiography, even using the latest generation instruments, has limitations and should not be expected to completely replace conventional coronary angiography within the imminent future. The need for intravenous contrast media administration, limitations in spatial and temporal resolution, arrhythmia (ie, atrial fibrillation), and coronary artery calcifications still remain relative limitations for noninvasive coronary CT imaging.

Assessment of Coronary Artery Stents

The successful introduction of coronary stent implantation into clinical practice has significantly increased the use of percutaneous coronary interventions to treat CAD requiring revascularization.[44] Newly introduced drug-eluting stents may further increase the number of patients considered for percutaneous coronary intervention. Although a clear advantage of drug-eluting versus conventional stents remains to be established, these types of stents are marketed based on the notion that they can reduce the risk of in-stent restenosis. Potential noninvasive assessment of coronary artery stent patency and depiction of in-stent

restenosis as an application of coronary CT angiography has been consistently investigated since the introduction of cardiac MDCT in clinical practice.[45,46]

Stent patency may be indirectly inferred by demonstrating the presence of intravenous contrast in the coronary segments distal to the implanted stent, although retrograde filling through collateral vessels in the presence of in-stent occlusion has been discussed as a potential diagnostic pitfall. Conversely, the absence of contrast material in the distal portions of the vessel clearly reflects severe in-stent restenosis[46] or occlusion. The depiction of in-stent intimal hyperplasia remains a challenge for coronary CT angiography, as temporal and spatial resolution of MDCT is still limited. Beam-hardening and streak artifacts caused by metallic stent struts significantly impair the visualization of the coronary artery lumen and make it difficult to diagnose in-stent intimal hyperplasia by means of coronary CT angiography.[47] Artifacts caused by metallic stent struts provoke attenuation defects that may mimic in-stent restenosis.

Several studies have evaluated the usefulness of 16-slice MDCT scanners to assess coronary artery stents and demonstrated low sensitivity (54%–83%) for the detection of in-stent restenosis.[48–50] More recent studies evaluating the usefulness of 64-slice MDCT and DSCT for the assessment of stent patency and in-stent restenosis

Table 2
Accuracy of 64-slice MDCT and DSCT for assessment of stent patency (in-stent restenosis) in comparison with conventional coronary angiography

Author	Scanner Type	Number of Stents	Sensitivity (%)	Specificity (%)	PPV (%)	NPV (%)
Van Mieghem[59,a]	64-MDCT	70	100	91	67	100
Cademartiri[51]	64-MDCT	192	95	93	63	99
Carrabba[52]	64-MDCT	87	84	100	100	97
Rist[57]	64-MDCT	46	75	92	67	94
Oncel[55]	64-MDCT	39	89	95	94	90
Manghat[54]	64-MDCT	103	85	86	61	96
Ehara[53]	64-MDCT	125	92	81	54	98
Rixe[58]	64-MDCT	102	86	98	86	98
Oncel[56]	DSCT	48	100	94	89	100
Pugliese[60]	DSCT	178	94	92	77	98

[a] Left main coronary artery stent.

in comparison with conventional coronary angiography are presented in **Table 2**.[51–60] Van Mieghem and colleagues[59] evaluated 74 patients (27 with 16-slice MDCT and 43 with 64-slice MDCT) scheduled for follow-up coronary CT angiograpy after left main-coronary artery stenting. They found overall sensitivity, specificity, and positive and negative predictive values for detection of in-stent restenosis of 100%, 91%, 67%, and 100%, respectively. Ehara and colleagues[53] analyzed 125 stented lesions in 81 patients. Overall sensitivity, specificity, and positive and negative predictive values for detection of in-stent restenosis were 92%, 81%, 54%, and 98%, respectively. These values increased to 91%, 93%, 77%, and 98%, respectively when they excluded unevaluable segments. In a similar study, Rixe and colleagues[58] evaluated 64-slice MDCT in 64 consecutive patients with previously implanted coronary artery stents (102 stented lesions). In this series, only 59 out of 102 stented lesions (58%) were classified as evaluable by coronary CT angiography. In evaluable stents they found a sensitivity of 86% and a specificity of 98% to detect in-stent restenosis. These investigators conclude that stent type and diameter influence the assessment by 64-slice MDCT, with high accuracy for detection of in-stent restenosis in evaluable stents. A recent meta-analysis designed to define the role of MDCT for the diagnosis of coronary in-stent restenosis using 16-slice MDCT and 64-slice MDCT scanners showed a pooled sensitivity of 0.82 and specificity of 0.92 for studies performed using 16-slice MDCT, and a pooled sensitivity of 0.85 and specificity of 0.91 for the latest-generation scanners.[61] Overall, considering all included studies, Hamon and colleagues[61] found a pooled sensitivity of

0.84 and a specificity of 0.91, concluding that the diagnostic role of coronary CT angiography as an alternative to the conventional catheter-based approach for detection of in-stent restenosis remains limited.

Improved temporal resolution of DSCT may facilitate visualization of coronary artery stents (**Fig. 8**). To date, only a few studies are available evaluating the role of this recent instrument for this purpose. Oncel and colleagues[56] examined

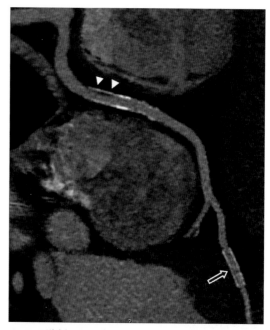

Fig. 8. Mild in-stent restenosis in a right coronary artery stent in 59-year-old man (*arrowheads*). A Curved multiplanar reformation. Note patency of the stent located in the posterior descending artery (*open arrow*).

35 consecutive patients with 48 stents. According to the investigators, all stents were considered assessable for diagnosis. They found sensitivity of 100%, specificity of 94%, positive predictive value of 89%, negative predictive value of 100%, and accuracy of 96% for the detection of in-stent restenosis and occlusion, with excellent intraobserver and interobserver agreement. Pugliese and colleagues[60] evaluated 100 patients with chest pain after coronary artery stent implantation. In stents greater than or equal to 3.5-mm diameter, they found 100% sensitivity and specificity, whereas in stents less than or equal to 2.75 mm, sensitivity and specificity values dropped to 84% and 64%, respectively. The investigators conclude that coronary CT angiography using DSCT reliably rules out in-stent restenosis irrespective of stent size. Nevertheless, further confirmation of these results is needed to demonstrate the potential usefulness of DSCT coronary angiography to exclude in-stent restenosis. Until then, it appears reasonable to restrict the use of coronary CT angiography for the purpose of coronary artery stent-patency assessment to larger stent types in proximal vessels and abstain from attempts to evaluate smaller stents in peripheral vessels.

Assessment of Bypass Grafts

As bypass grafts are larger in diameter and move much less and slower than native coronary arteries, imaging of grafts is less challenging than CT imaging of the coronary arteries proper. Imaging of arterial grafts (internal mammary artery or radial grafts) can be more difficult than visualization of venous grafts because of the smaller vessel lumen, artifacts caused by metal clips, and the small caliber distal anastomosis (**Fig. 9**).

The ability to noninvasively assess patency or occlusion of bypass grafts was already demonstrated using single-slice CT systems, with which sensitivity and specificity values greater than 90% were reported.[62,63] Using 4-slice MDCT scanners, overall sensitivity and specificity of 97% and 98% were reported for the assessment of bypass occlusion. For the assessment of bypass graft stenosis, however, sensitivity and specificity values decreased to 75% and 92%, respectively.[64–66] Studies performed with 16-slice MDCT showed that occlusion and stenoses of bypass grafts could be detected with sensitivity and specificity values of nearly 100%.[67–69] A recent meta-analysis compared 8-slice, 16-slice, and 64-slice MDCT to conventional coronary

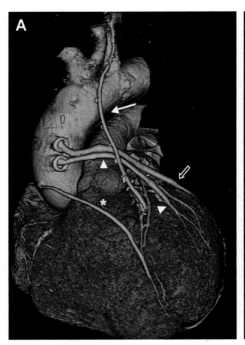
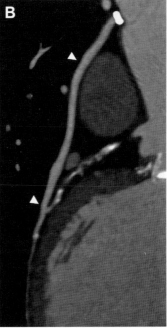

Fig. 9. Bypass study in a 73-year-old man with chest pain. DSCT examination demonstrated patency of bypass grafts without significant stenosis. (*A*) Volume-rendered image. Patency of left internal mammary artery graft to mid-left anterior descending coronary artery (*arrow*) and saphenous vein grafts to the obtuse marginal branch (*open arrow*), first diagonal branch (*arrowhead*), and distal left anterior descending coronary artery (*) was demonstrated. (*B*) Curved multiplanar reformation of a saphenous graft connected to the first diagonal branch (*arrowhead*). The bypass graft was patent, without significant stenosis.

angiography for the assessment of coronary bypass grafts. For assessing occlusion, the included studies showed a pooled sensitivity of 97.6% and specificity of 98.5%, whereas for stenosis assessment, sensitivity was 88.7% and specificity 97.4%.[70]

In **Table 3**, several studies evaluating the accuracy of 64-slice MDCT for the assessment of significant stenosis/occlusion of bypass grafts in comparison with conventional coronary angiography are shown.[71–75] Feuchtner and colleagues[71] compared the diagnostic accuracy of 64-slice MDCT with that of conventional angiography for the detection of bypass graft stenosis of greater than 50% within 2 weeks of coronary artery bypass grafting. They found 75% sensitivity, 95% specificity, positive predictive value of 67%, and negative predictive value of 97% for the detection of 50% to 90% bypass graft stenosis. The investigators conclude that 64-slice MDCT could be used for accurate exclusion of greater than 50% bypass graft stenosis. However, they pointed out that detection of stenosis of the distal anastomosis was limited, with a possible overestimation of the degree of stenosis.[71] Meyer and colleagues[73] investigated the accuracy of 64-slice MDCT in an unselected but symptomatic patient population for detection of stenoses in bypass grafts compared with conventional invasive angiography. In this article the assessment for stenosis or occlusion of bypass grafts resulted in 97% sensitivity, 97% specificity, and 93% and 99% positive and negative predictive values, respectively.

However, in a clinical setting there is also a need to evaluate native coronary arteries distal to the graft anastomoses, which are often difficult to assess by coronary CT angiography because of their small size and extensive calcification.[76] Therefore, noninvasive assessment of bypass grafts with CT will not be completely accepted until these limitations have been overcome. This requires scanners with higher spatial and temporal resolution. Dual-source CT may allow sufficient image quality for this purpose. However, no data are available to date on the accuracy of DSCT for the evaluation of subjects with previous bypass surgery.

Another potential indication of coronary CT angiography in the setting of prior bypass grafting is surgical planning, providing a road-map on anatomic landmarks, graft location, and anastomotic sites before initial or redo coronary artery bypass graft surgery.[64,66,77] Particularly, three-dimensional volumetric reconstruction allows intuitive visualization of the anatomic location of the native vessels, the internal mammary arteries, and their relationship to adjacent mediastinal structures.

Characterization of Coronary Atherosclerotic Plaque

Characterization and quantification of coronary artery atherosclerotic plaque may be useful to improve individualized risk stratification. Several invasive and noninvasive diagnostic techniques allow evaluating the coronary artery wall. Even if invasive and expensive, the standard of reference for this purpose remains intravascular ultrasound (IVUS).[78] Optical coherence tomography[79] has also shown potential for coronary wall tissue characterization, however, with even greater expense and invasiveness than IVUS. Currently, MR coronary angiography is probably the most suitable test for noninvasive characterization of tissue composition and vessel wall structure. This technique is capable of differentiating different stages of atherosclerosis.[80] However, in vivo imaging of the coronary vessels using MR imaging is challenging because of the limited spatial resolution of this technique at the temporal resolutions required for imaging the beating heart and the small caliber of the coronary vessels, so that its use remains reserved to date for research applications and not for actual clinical use.

Table 3
Accuracy of 64-slice MDCT for assessment of significant stenosis/occlusion of bypass grafts in comparison with conventional coronary angiography

Author	Scanner Type	Number of Grafts	Sensitivity (%)	Specificity (%)	PPV (%)	NPV (%)
Feuchtner[71]	64-MDCT	70	75	95	67	97
Meyer[73]	64-MDCT	418	97	97	93	99
Onuma[74]	64-MDCT	146	100	95	85	100
Pache[75]	64-MDCT	96	98	89	90	98
Jabara[72]	64-MDCT	147	93	100	100	98

Contrast-enhanced coronary CT angiography provides an unprecedented combination of temporal and spatial resolution and has shown its potential to visualize the coronary artery wall and delineate calcified (**Fig. 10**) and noncalcified atherosclerotic plaque (**Fig. 11**).[7,8,81] A sensitivity of 80% to 90% has been reported for the detection of coronary atherosclerotic plaque using coronary CT angiography, especially for the detection of calcified plaque.[82–84] Achenbach and colleagues[83] reported sensitivity and specificity values of 78% and 87%, respectively, for the detection of noncalcified plaque in coronary artery segments using 16-slice MDCT. Recent studies suggest that the improved spatial and temporal resolution of 64-slice MDCT may allow more accurate evaluation of the coronary atherosclerotic plaque burden. Based on 64-slice MDCT, Leber and colleagues[85] reported sensitivity of 84% and specificity of 91% for the detection of proximal coronary plaques in comparison to IVUS.

Beyond plaque detection, the accurate, noninvasive characterization of atherosclerotic plaque is a coveted goal. Plaques with high lipid content have been shown to be more vulnerable and prone to rupture, whereas calcified plaques are thought to be more stable. Computed tomography attenuation, value-based atherosclerotic plaque characterization has been shown to be feasible and correlates reasonably well with IVUS[7,81] and histology.[8] Galonska and colleagues evaluated the atherosclerotic plaques of coronary arteries of 30 isolated hearts ex vivo, and compared the plaque attenuation profiles with the corresponding histopathologic sections of the arteries. These investigators found attenuation values between 333 Hounsfield units (HU) and 1,944 HU for calcified plaques, and attenuation values between 26 HU and 124 HU for noncalcified plaques. When noncalcified plaques were further evaluated, lipid-rich plaques with a necrotic core had attenuation values between 26 HU and 67 HU, and fibrous plaques between 37 HU and 124 HU.[86] However, limited spatial resolution of MDCT scanners still prohibits reliable analysis of all atherosclerotic plaque components and significant overlap may be found between different tissues, especially between lipid and fibrous components.

Another factor limiting the validity of measuring attenuation values within atherosclerotic plaques may be the contrast concentration in the coronary lumen,[87] which significantly influences attenuation measurements of the vessel wall. Because of the increasing interest in and potential of noninvasive coronary atherosclerotic plaque characterization, vendors have designed various software algorithms that allow automated detection and quantification of atherosclerotic plaque (**Fig. 12**). With most of these algorithms, the contrast-enhanced lumen, vessel wall, and plaque composition (lipid, fibrous, or calcified) are presented in different

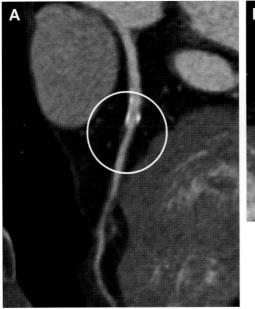
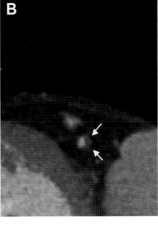

Fig. 10. Mixed plaque in the mid-portion of the circumflex coronary artery in a 62-year-old man with stable angina. (*A*) Curved multiplanar reformation. (*B*) Cross-sectional image. Note the significant positive remodeling with soft tissue component (*arrows*).

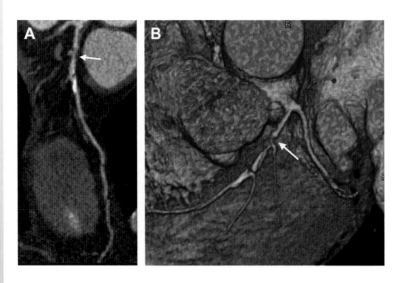

Fig. 11. Significant proximal left anterior descending coronary artery stenosis in a 73-year-old man with atypical chest pain (*arrow*). (*A*) Curved multiplanar reformation. (*B*) Volume-rendered image. A noncalcified atherosclerotic plaque produced this significant stenosis.

colors according to their corresponding CT Hounsfield unit ranges. This intuitive way of presentation allows visually estimating the coronary plaque burden. Furthermore, improved delineation of plaque boundaries permits performing quantitative analyses. A recent study by Sun and colleagues[88] applied a plaque-analysis algorithm in subjects who had undergone coronary CT angiography using 64-slice MDCT. These investigators found sensitivity of 97.4% and specificity of 90.1% for detection of coronary plaques, with a sensitivity of 96.6% for noncalcified plaque, concluding that the increased accuracy compared with previously reported studies may be because of the use of the particular software tool to automatically detect atherosclerotic plaques.[88]

The benefit of improved temporal resolution of DSCT to detect and characterize coronary atherosclerotic plaques in clinical practice has not been evaluated yet. A recent study aimed at quantifying improvements in image quality using DSCT, in comparison to 64-slice MDCT using a moving coronary plaque phantom. In this study, all plaque components could be delineated more clearly with DSCT. This resulted in less volume-averaging and more accurate attenuation measurements. The investigators conclude that, especially for calcified lesions, DSCT may enable improved grading of stenoses.[89] Whether DSCT might improve coronary atherosclerotic plaque characterization in a clinical setting still needs to be evaluated.

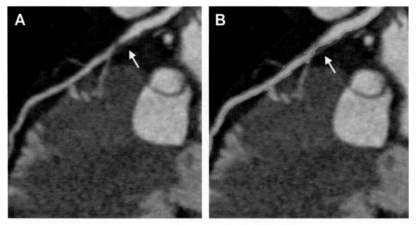

Fig. 12. Software interface designed for automated detection of atherosclerotic plaques. (*A* and *B*) Contrast-enhanced lumen and plaque composition (lipid, fibrous, or calcified) are presented in different colors according to their corresponding CT Hounsfield unit ranges. Lipic components are shown in dark green. Fibrous components are shown in light green. Coronary lumen is shown in orange. Pink color represents calcium.

While there is great interest in using coronary CT angiography for noninvasive plaque detection, quantification, and characterization, and considerable industry resources are devoted to provide the cardiac imaging community with new tools to achieve this goal, the actual rationale of using CT for this purpose deserves some closer examination. Even if coronary CT angiography were able to reliably differentiate stable and unstable plaque, the immediate clinical consequence of a finding of unstable, "vulnerable" plaque would be dubious. Approaches that advocate pre-emptive stenting of nonobstructive lesions that exhibit features of vulnerability do not account for the systemic nature of atherosclerotic disease and are unlikely to become clinically mainstream. Accordingly, the ability to noninvasively detect, quantify, and characterize atherosclerotic plaque may be more realistically applied to improved risk stratification, therapeutic management, and therapeutic response monitoring: that is, rather than striving to identify the "vulnerable" plaque, identifying the vulnerable patient who might benefit from more aggressive risk modification seems like a more realistic and appropriate goal.

Imaging of Ischemic Heart Disease: Dual-Energy CT

In general, clinically available imaging modalities to assess CAD are divided into anatomic and functional techniques, depending on whether they are primarily aimed at visualizing the coronary artery lumen or detecting myocardial perfusion defects or myocardial wall motion abnormalities. To date, no established imaging modality provides anatomic and functional information on coronary artery disease with a single test. So far, attempts to obtain information on myocardial perfusion maps based on anatomic imaging modalities have been of limited success. Few studies report on image registration and fusion of coronary CT angiography with single photon emission computed tomography (SPECT)[90,91] or integrated imaging (ie, SPECT/CT or positron emission tomography or PET/CT)[92] showing promising results. However, these diagnostic approaches involve a significant amount of radiation dose for the patients, are labor intensive and, as in the case of PET/CT, can be prohibitively cost-intensive for widespread use. Thus, a single diagnostic technique that enables both detecting coronary artery stenosis and determining the hemodynamic significance of the lesion for myocardial perfusion, without increasing intravenous contrast volumes, radiation exposure, or cost, would be desirable (**Fig. 13**).

Recently, the ability of dual-energy computed tomography (DECT) to characterize tissue composition and organ perfusion[93] has been demonstrated. Early evidence also supports the potential of DECT for comprehensive cardiac imaging. An initial study suggests that cardiac perfusion-imaging with DECT seems to correlate very well with fixed perfusion defects (ie, perfusion defects at rest imaging) in 99 m-Tc-Sestamibi-SPECT.[94] Furthermore, preliminary experience suggests that DECT, even without the administration of pharmacologic stressors, can detect most of the perfusion defects that are reversible in 99 m-Tc-Sestamibi-SPECT. Thus, the evaluation of myocardial perfusion by DECT promises to complement anatomic evaluation of the coronary arteries by gauging the hemodynamic significance

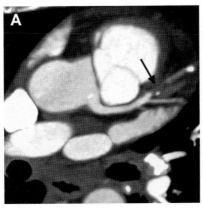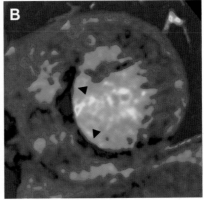

Fig. 13. Dual-energy cardiac CT examination of a 58-year-old female with history of atypical chest pain. (*A*) Multiplanar reformation, spider view. Coronary CT angiography showed occlusion of the LAD coronary artery (*arrow*). (*B*) Dual-energy CT, short-axis view. As a consequence of the significant LAD lesion, anteroseptal perfusion defect was observed at the apical level (*arrowheads*).

of detected stenoses. However, further studies are needed to determine the diagnostic accuracy of perfusion defects detected by DECT, their predictive value, and their impact on patient care.

SUMMARY

The appropriate clinical application of coronary CT angiography remains a topic of intense interest and research. Recent technical developments in MDCT technology increasingly enable obtaining highly diagnostic coronary angiograms in a noninvasive way. The current cornerstone of CT-based patient management is the exceedingly high negative predictive value of a normal or near-normal coronary CT angiogram, allowing the reliable exclusion of significant coronary artery stenosis in a symptomatic patient. With the widespread use of coronary CT angiography, new potential clinical indications are constantly explored. Currently, 64-slice MDCT and DSCT are the benchmark for noninvasive coronary CT angiography; however, new technologies are already on the horizon. While significant obstacles still remain to be overcome, coronary CT angiography is closer than ever to fulfilling its promise of replacing invasive techniques in appropriate patient populations.

REFERENCES

1. AHA Heart Disease and Stroke Statistics—2008 Update. Available at: http://www.americanheart.org/presenter.jhtml?identifier=1928. Accessed August 13, 2008.
2. Achenbach S, Giesler T, Ropers D, et al. Detection of coronary artery stenoses by contrast-enhanced, retrospectively electrocardiographically-gated, multislice spiral computed tomography. Circulation 2001;103(21):2535–8.
3. Hoffmann MH, Shi H, Schmitz BL, et al. Noninvasive coronary angiography with multislice computed tomography. JAMA 2005;293(20):2471–8.
4. Nieman K, Oudkerk M, Rensing BJ, et al. Coronary angiography with multi-slice computed tomography. Lancet 2001;357(9256):599–603.
5. Schoepf UJ, Zwerner PL, Savino G, et al. Coronary CT angiography. Radiology 2007;244(1):48–63.
6. Viles-Gonzalez JF, Poon M, Sanz J, et al. In vivo 16-slice, multidetector-row computed tomography for the assessment of experimental atherosclerosis: comparison with magnetic resonance imaging and histopathology. Circulation 2004;110(11):1467–72.
7. Schroeder S, Kopp AF, Baumbach A, et al. Noninvasive detection and evaluation of atherosclerotic coronary plaques with multislice computed tomography. J Am Coll Cardiol 2001;37(5):1430–5.
8. Becker CR, Nikolaou K, Muders M, et al. Ex vivo coronary atherosclerotic plaque characterization with multi-detector-row CT. Eur Radiol 2003;13(9):2094–8.
9. Hendel RC, Patel MR, Kramer CM, et al. ACCF/ACR/SCCT/SCMR/ASNC/NASCI/SCAI/SIR 2006 appropriateness criteria for cardiac computed tomography and cardiac magnetic resonance imaging: a report of the American College of Cardiology Foundation Quality Strategic Directions Committee Appropriateness Criteria Working Group, American College of Radiology, Society of Cardiovascular Computed Tomography, Society for Cardiovascular Magnetic Resonance, American Society of Nuclear Cardiology, North American Society for Cardiac Imaging, Society for Cardiovascular Angiography and Interventions, and Society of Interventional Radiology. J Am Coll Cardiol 2006 Oct 3;48(7):1475–97.
10. Russo V, Gostoli V, Lovato L, et al. Clinical value of multidetector CT coronary angiography as a preoperative screening test before non-coronary cardiac surgery. Heart 2007;93(12):1591–8.
11. Yamanaka O, Hobbs RE. Coronary artery anomalies in 126,595 patients undergoing coronary angiography. Cathet Cardiovasc Diagn 1990;21:28–40.
12. Baltaxe HA, Wixson D. The incidence of congenital anomalies of the coronary arteries in the adult population. Radiology 1977;122:47–52.
13. Barriales Villa R, Moris C, Lopez Muniz A. Adult congenital anomalies of the coronary arteries described over 31 years of angiographic studies in the Asturias principality: main angiographic and clinical characteristics. Rev Esp Cardiol 2001;54:269–81.
14. Alexander RW, Griffith GC. Anomalies of the coronary arteries and their clinical significance. Circulation 1956;14:800–5.
15. Angelini P, Villason S, Chan AVJ, et al. Normal and anomalous coronary arteries in humans. In: Angelini P, editor. Coronary artery anomalies: a comprehensive approach. Philadelphia: Lippincott Williams & Wilkins; 1999. p. 27–150.
16. Chaitman BR, Lesperance J, Saltiel J, et al. Clinical, angiographic, and hemodynamic findings in patients with anomalous origin of the coronary arteries. Circulation 1976;53(1):122–31.
17. Maron BJ, Epstein SE, Roberts WC. Causes of sudden death in competitive athletes. J Am Coll Cardiol 1986;7(1):204–14.
18. Taylor AJ, Rogan KM, Virmani R. Sudden cardiac death associated with isolated congenital coronary artery anomalies. J Am Coll Cardiol 1992;20(3):640–7.
19. Angelini P, Velasco JA, Flamm S. Coronary anomalies: incidence, pathophysiology, and clinical relevance. Circulation 2002;105(20):2449–54.
20. Taylor AM, Thorne SA, Rubens MB. Coronary artery imaging in grown up congenital heart disease: complementary role of magnetic resonance and x-ray coronary angiography. Circulation 2000;101:1670–8.

21. Gerber TC, Kuzo RS, Safford RE. Computed tomographic imaging of anomalous coronary arteries. Circulation 2002;106(15):author reply e67.

22. Nieman K, Roos-Hesselink JW, de Feyter PJ. Coronary anomaly imaging by multislice computed tomography in corrected tetralogy of Fallot. Heart 2003; 89(6):664.

23. Achenbach S, Ulzheimer S, Baum U, et al. Noninvasive coronary angiography by retrospectively ECG-gated multislice spiral CT. Circulation 2000; 102(23):2823–8.

24. Nieman K, Cademartiri F, Lemos PA, et al. Reliable noninvasive coronary angiography with fast submillimeter multislice spiral computed tomography. Circulation 2002;106(16):2051–4.

25. van der Zaag-Loonen HJ, Dikkers R, de Bock GH, et al. The clinical value of a negative multi-detector computed tomographic angiography in patients suspected of coronary artery disease: a meta-analysis. Eur Radiol 2006;16(12):2748–56.

26. Brodoefel H, Burgstahler C, Tsiflikas I, et al. Dual-source CT: effect of heart rate, heart rate variability, and calcification on image quality and diagnostic accuracy. Radiology 2008;247(2):346–55.

27. Ehara M, Surmely JF, Kawai M, et al. Diagnostic accuracy of 64-slice computed tomography for detecting angiographically significant coronary artery stenosis in an unselected consecutive patient population: comparison with conventional invasive angiography. Circ J 2006;70(5):564–71.

28. Fine JJ, Hopkins CB, Ruff N, et al. Comparison of accuracy of 64-slice cardiovascular computed tomography with coronary angiography in patients with suspected coronary artery disease. Am J Cardiol 2006;97(2):173–4.

29. Johnson TR, Nikolaou K, Busch S, et al. Diagnostic accuracy of dual-source computed tomography in the diagnosis of coronary artery disease. Invest Radiol 2007;42(10):684–91.

30. Leschka S, Alkadhi H, Plass A, et al. Accuracy of MSCT coronary angiography with 64-slice technology: first experience. Eur Heart J 2005;26(15):1482–7.

31. Mollet NR, Cademartiri F, van Mieghem CA, et al. High-resolution spiral computed tomography coronary angiography in patients referred for diagnostic conventional coronary angiography. Circulation 2005;112(15):2318–23.

32. Oncel D, Oncel G, Tastan A, et al. Detection of significant coronary artery stenosis with 64-section MDCT angiography. Eur J Radiol 2007;62(3):394–405.

33. Raff GL, Gallagher MJ, O'Neill WW, et al. Diagnostic accuracy of noninvasive coronary angiography using 64-slice spiral computed tomography. J Am Coll Cardiol 2005;46(3):552–7.

34. Ropers D, Rixe J, Anders K, et al. Usefulness of multidetector row spiral computed tomography with 64- × 0.6-mm collimation and 330-ms rotation for the noninvasive detection of significant coronary artery stenoses. Am J Cardiol 2006;97(3):343–8.

35. Ropers U, Ropers D, Pflederer T, et al. Influence of heart rate on the diagnostic accuracy of dual-source computed tomography coronary angiography. J Am Coll Cardiol 2007;50(25):2393–8.

36. Weustink AC, Meijboom WB, Mollet NR, et al. Reliable high-speed coronary computed tomography in symptomatic patients. J Am Coll Cardiol 2007; 50(8):786–94.

37. Hamon M, Morello R, Riddell JW. Coronary arteries: diagnostic performance of 16- versus 64-section spiral CT compared with invasive coronary angiography–meta-analysis. Radiology 2007;245(3):720–31.

38. Flohr TG, McCollough CH, Bruder H, et al. First performance evaluation of a dual-source CT (DSCT) system. Eur Radiol 2006;16(2):256–68.

39. Achenbach S, Ropers D, Kuettner A, et al. Contrast-enhanced coronary artery visualization by dual-source computed tomography–initial experience. Eur J Radiol 2006;57(3):331–5.

40. Leber AW, Johnson T, Becker A, et al. Diagnostic accuracy of dual-source multi-slice CT-coronary angiography in patients with an intermediate pretest likelihood for coronary artery disease. Eur Heart J 2007;28(19):2354–60.

41. Gilard M, Le Gal G, Cornily JC, et al. Midterm prognosis of patients with suspected coronary artery disease and normal multislice computed tomographic findings: a prospective management outcome study. Arch Intern Med 2007;167(15):1686–9.

42. Min JK, Shaw LJ, Devereux RB, et al. Prognostic value of multidetector coronary computed tomographic angiography for prediction of all-cause mortality. J Am Coll Cardiol 2007;50(12):1161–70.

43. Pundziute G, Schuijf JD, Jukema JW, et al. Prognostic value of multislice computed tomography coronary angiography in patients with known or suspected coronary artery disease. J Am Coll Cardiol 2007; 49(1):62–70.

44. Serruys PW, Kutryk MJ, Ong AT. Coronary-artery stents. N Engl J Med 2006;354(5):483–95.

45. Funabashi N, Komiyama N, Komuro I. Patency of coronary artery lumen surrounded by metallic stent evaluated by three dimensional volume rendering images using ECG gated multislice computed tomography. Heart 2003;89(4):388.

46. Pump H, Mohlenkamp S, Sehnert CA, et al. Coronary arterial stent patency: assessment with electron-beam CT. Radiology 2000;214(2):447–52.

47. Maintz D, Seifarth H, Raupach R, et al. 64-slice multidetector coronary CT angiography: in vitro evaluation of 68 different stents. Eur Radiol 2006;16(4): 818–26.

48. Gilard M, Cornily JC, Pennec PY, et al. Assessment of coronary artery stents by 16 slice computed tomography. Heart 2006;92(1):58–61.

49. Kitagawa T, Fujii T, Tomohiro Y, et al. Noninvasive assessment of coronary stents in patients by 16-slice computed tomography. Int J Cardiol 2006;109(2): 188–94.

50. Gaspar T, Halon DA, Lewis BS, et al. Diagnosis of coronary in-stent restenosis with multidetector row spiral computed tomography. J Am Coll Cardiol 2005;46(8):1573–9.

51. Cademartiri F, Schuijf JD, Pugliese F, et al. Usefulness of 64-slice multislice computed tomography coronary angiography to assess in-stent restenosis. J Am Coll Cardiol 2007;49(22):2204–10.

52. Carrabba N, Bamoshmoosh M, Carusi LM, et al. Usefulness of 64-slice multidetector computed tomography for detecting drug eluting in-stent restenosis. Am J Cardiol 2007;100(12):1754–8.

53. Ehara M, Kawai M, Surmely JF, et al. Diagnostic accuracy of coronary in-stent restenosis using 64-slice computed tomography: comparison with invasive coronary angiography. J Am Coll Cardiol 2007; 49(9):951–9.

54. Manghat N, Van Lingen R, Hewson P, et al. Usefulness of 64-detector row computed tomography for evaluation of intracoronary stents in symptomatic patients with suspected in-stent restenosis. Am J Cardiol 2008;101(11):1567–73.

55. Oncel D, Oncel G, Karaca M. Coronary stent patency and in-stent restenosis: determination with 64-section multidetector CT coronary angiography–initial experience. Radiology 2007;242(2):403–9.

56. Oncel D, Oncel G, Tastan A, et al. Evaluation of coronary stent patency and in-stent restenosis with dual-source CT coronary angiography without heart rate control. AJR Am J Roentgenol 2008;191(1): 56–63.

57. Rist C, von Ziegler F, Nikolaou K, et al. Assessment of coronary artery stent patency and restenosis using 64-slice computed tomography. Acad Radiol 2006;13(12):1465–73.

58. Rixe J, Achenbach S, Ropers D, et al. Assessment of coronary artery stent restenosis by 64-slice multidetector computed tomography. Eur Heart J 2006; 27(21):2567–72.

59. Van Mieghem CA, Cademartiri F, Mollet NR, et al. Multislice spiral computed tomography for the evaluation of stent patency after left main coronary artery stenting: a comparison with conventional coronary angiography and intravascular ultrasound. Circulation 2006;114(7):645–53.

60. Pugliese F, Weustink AC, Van Mieghem C, et al. Dual source coronary computed tomography angiography for detecting in-stent restenosis. Heart 2008; 94(7):848–54.

61. Hamon M, Champ-Rigot L, Morello R, et al. Diagnostic accuracy of in-stent coronary restenosis detection with multislice spiral computed tomography: a meta-analysis. Eur Radiol 2008;18(2):217–25.

62. Tello R, Costello P, Ecker C, et al. Spiral CT evaluation of coronary artery bypass graft patency. J Comput Assist Tomogr 1993;17(2):253–9.

63. Engelmann MG, von Smekal A, Knez A, et al. Accuracy of spiral computed tomography for identifying arterial and venous coronary graft patency. Am J Cardiol 1997;80(5):569–74.

64. Ohtsuka T, Takamoto S, Endoh M, et al. Ultrafast computed tomography for minimally invasive coronary artery bypass grafting. J Thorac Cardiovasc Surg 1998;116(1):173–4.

65. Ropers D, Ulzheimer S, Wenkel E, et al. Investigation of aortocoronary artery bypass grafts by multislice spiral computed tomography with electrocardiographic-gated image reconstruction. Am J Cardiol 2001;88(7):792–5.

66. Yamaguchi A, Adachi H, Ino T, et al. Three-dimensional computed tomographic angiography as preoperative evaluation of a patent internal thoracic artery graft. J Thorac Cardiovasc Surg 2000; 120(4):811–2.

67. Nieman K, Pattynama PM, Rensing BJ, et al. Evaluation of patients after coronary artery bypass surgery: CT angiographic assessment of grafts and coronary arteries. Radiology 2003;229(3):749–56.

68. Martuscelli E, Romagnoli A, D'Eliseo A, et al. Evaluation of venous and arterial conduit patency by 16-slice spiral computed tomography. Circulation 2004;110(20):3234–8.

69. Schlosser T, Konorza T, Hunold P, et al. Noninvasive visualization of coronary artery bypass grafts using 16-detector row computed tomography. J Am Coll Cardiol 2004;44(6):1224–9.

70. Hamon M, Lepage O, Malagutti P, et al. Diagnostic performance of 16- and 64-section spiral CT for coronary artery bypass graft assessment: meta-analysis. Radiology 2008;247(3):679–86.

71. Feuchtner GM, Schachner T, Bonatti J, et al. Diagnostic performance of 64-slice computed tomography in evaluation of coronary artery bypass grafts. AJR Am J Roentgenol 2007;189(3):574–80.

72. Jabara R, Chronos N, Klein L, et al. Comparison of multidetector 64-slice computed tomographic angiography to coronary angiography to assess the patency of coronary artery bypass grafts. Am J Cardiol 2007;99(11):1529–34.

73. Meyer TS, Martinoff S, Hadamitzky M, et al. Improved noninvasive assessment of coronary artery bypass grafts with 64-slice computed tomographic angiography in an unselected patient population. J Am Coll Cardiol 2007;49(9):946–50.

74. Onuma Y, Tanabe K, Chihara R, et al. Evaluation of coronary artery bypass grafts and native coronary arteries using 64-slice multidetector computed tomography. Am Heart J 2007;154(3):519–26.

75. Pache G, Saueressig U, Frydrychowicz A, et al. Initial experience with 64-slice cardiac CT: non-invasive

visualization of coronary artery bypass grafts. Eur Heart J 2006;27(8):976–80.

76. Salm LP, Bax JJ, Jukema JW, et al. Comprehensive assessment of patients after coronary artery bypass grafting by 16-detector-row computed tomography. Am Heart J 2005;150(4):775–81.

77. Gulbins H, Reichenspurner H, Becker C, et al. Preoperative 3D-reconstructions of ultrafast-CT images for the planning of minimally invasive direct coronary artery bypass operation (MIDCAB). Heart Surg Forum 1998;1(2):111–5.

78. Nissen SE, Yock P. Intravascular ultrasound: novel pathophysiological insights and current clinical applications. Circulation 2001;103(4):604–16.

79. Yabushita H, Bouma BE, Houser SL, et al. Characterization of human atherosclerosis by optical coherence tomography. Circulation 2002;106(13):1640–5.

80. Botnar RM, Stuber M, Kissinger KV, et al. Noninvasive coronary vessel wall and plaque imaging with magnetic resonance imaging. Circulation 2000; 102(21):2582–7.

81. Kopp AF, Schroeder S, Baumbach A, et al. Non-invasive characterisation of coronary lesion morphology and composition by multislice CT: first results in comparison with intracoronary ultrasound. Eur Radiol 2001;11(9):1607–11.

82. Becker CR, Knez A, Ohnesorge B, et al. Imaging of noncalcified coronary plaques using helical CT with retrospective ECG gating. AJR Am J Roentgenol 2000;175(2):423–4.

83. Achenbach S, Moselewski F, Ropers D, et al. Detection of calcified and noncalcified coronary atherosclerotic plaque by contrast-enhanced, submillimeter multidetector spiral computed tomography: a segment-based comparison with intravascular ultrasound. Circulation 2004;109(1):14–7.

84. Leber AW, Knez A, Becker A, et al. Accuracy of multidetector spiral computed tomography in identifying and differentiating the composition of coronary atherosclerotic plaques: a comparative study with intracoronary ultrasound. J Am Coll Cardiol 2004; 43(7):1241–7.

85. Leber AW, Knez A, von Ziegler F, et al. Quantification of obstructive and nonobstructive coronary lesions by 64-slice computed tomography: a comparative study with quantitative coronary angiography and intravascular ultrasound. J Am Coll Cardiol 2005; 46(1):147–54.

86. Galonska M, Ducke F, Kertesz-Zborilova T, et al. Characterization of atherosclerotic plaques in human coronary arteries with 16-slice multidetector row computed tomography by analysis of attenuation profiles. Acad Radiol 2008;15(2): 222–30.

87. Cademartiri F, Mollet NR, Runza G, et al. Influence of intracoronary attenuation on coronary plaque measurements using multislice computed tomography: observations in an ex vivo model of coronary computed tomography angiography. Eur Radiol 2005; 15(7):1426–31.

88. Sun J, Zhang Z, Lu B, et al. Identification and quantification of coronary atherosclerotic plaques: a comparison of 64-MDCT and intravascular ultrasound. AJR Am J Roentgenol 2008;190(3):748–54.

89. Reimann AJ, Rinck D, Birinci-Aydogan A, et al. Dual-source computed tomography: advances of improved temporal resolution in coronary plaque imaging. Invest Radiol 2007;42(3):196–203.

90. Hacker M, Jakobs T, Matthiesen F, et al. Comparison of spiral multidetector CT angiography and myocardial perfusion imaging in the noninvasive detection of functionally relevant coronary artery lesions: first clinical experiences. J Nucl Med 2005;46(8): 1294–300.

91. Schuijf JD, Wijns W, Jukema JW, et al. Relationship between noninvasive coronary angiography with multi-slice computed tomography and myocardial perfusion imaging. J Am Coll Cardiol 2006;48(12): 2508–14.

92. Namdar M, Hany TF, Koepfli P, et al. Integrated PET/CT for the assessment of coronary artery disease: a feasibility study. J Nucl Med 2005;46(6):930–5.

93. Johnson TR, Krauss B, Sedlmair M, et al. Material differentiation by dual energy CT: initial experience. Eur Radiol 2007;17(6):1510–7.

94. Ruzsics B, Lee H, Powers ER, et al. Images in cardiovascular medicine. Myocardial ischemia diagnosed by dual-energy computed tomography: correlation with single-photon emission computed tomography. Circulation 2008;117(9):1244–5.

Multimodal CT in Stroke Imaging: New Concepts

Carlos J. Ledezma, MD[a], Max Wintermark, MD[b],*

KEYWORDS

- Acute stroke • Thrombolysis • Penumbra
- Collateral flow • Computed tomography
- CT perfusion • CT-angiography

Imaging has revolutionized acute ischemic stroke diagnosis and management. Previously, anatomic (structural) imaging modalities, typically noncontrast CT, were used to assess the presence or absence of acute ischemic stroke and exclude stroke mimics, such as hemorrhage and neoplasms. With the development of functional (or physiologic) imaging, such as perfusion CT (PCT), stroke has been redefined from an all-or-none process to a dynamic and evolving process. In particular, the advent of efficacious thrombolytic therapies, such as intravenous tissue plasminogen activator (IV-tPA),[1] has served as the impetus to better define the so-called ischemic penumbra or "tissue at risk" and thus better select those patients who would be more amenable to successful therapy. Several studies have suggested favorable clinical outcomes with thrombolytic therapies that were based on imaging criteria.[2–4]

Multimodal CT—noncontrast CT, CT angiography (CTA), and PCT (**Fig. 1**)—has been shown to be fast, reliable, and effective in improving stroke detection in the emergency setting.[5–7] Noncontrast CT can identify intracranial hemorrhage and detect early signs of acute ischemic stroke. CTA can identify the occlusion site, detect arterial dissection, and grade collateral blood flow, whereas PCT can accurately delineate the infarct core and the ischemic penumbra. A multimodal CT stroke protocol might be used to properly select those patients who might be amenable to reperfusion therapy.[2] This article discusses the individual components of multimodal CT and addresses the potential role of a combined multimodal CT stroke protocol in acute stroke therapy.

CONVENTIONAL CT: NONCONTRAST CT

With its widespread availability, short scan time, noninvasiveness, and safety, CT has been the traditional first-line imaging modality for the evaluation of acute ischemic stroke. In the acute ischemic stroke setting, noncontrast CT is typically used to rule out intracranial hemorrhage (a contraindication to thrombolysis) or other stroke mimics (eg, tumor, infection, and so forth) that preclude the use of thrombolytic therapy and to detect early CT signs (ie, scans obtained within 6 hours of the onset of stroke).[8–10] Early noncontrast CT signs of stroke include:

Insular ribbon sign. With proximal middle cerebral artery (MCA) occlusion, blood flow to the insular region is decreased. This region is particularly vulnerable because the insular cortex is the region most distal from the potential anterior and posterior collateral circulation, and as such a watershed arterial zone. When ischemic, the insular region shows loss of definition of the gray-white interface, or loss of the "insular ribbon."[3]

Obscuration of the lentiform nucleus. An obscured outline or partial disappearance of the lentiform nucleus is another early ischemic sign on noncontrast CT.[4] Because the blood supply to the basal ganglia (ie, lenticulostriate branches of the MCA) are end arteries, the basal ganglia are particularly vulnerable to early infarction.[4]

Hyperdense artery sign. An acute thrombus in an intracranial vessel appears as an area of

[a] Morristown Memorial Hospital, Department of Radiology, 100 Madison Avenue, Morristown, NJ 07962, USA
[b] University of California, Department of Radiology, Neuroradiology Section, 505 Parnassus Avenue, L-358, Box 0628, San Francisco, CA 94143-0628, USA
* Corresponding author.
E-mail address: max.wintermark@radiology.ucsf.edu (M. Wintermark).

Radiol Clin N Am 47 (2009) 109–116
doi:10.1016/j.rcl.2008.10.008

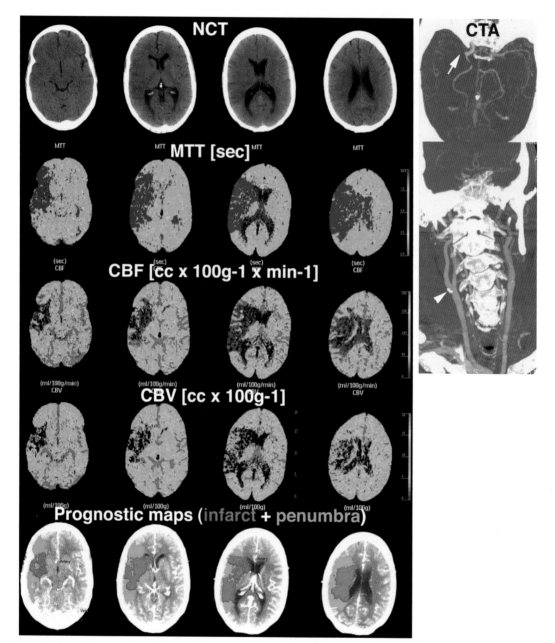

Fig. 1. Modern CT survey in a 57-year-old male patient admitted in our emergency room with a left hemisyndrome, including an unenhanced CT (first row), a PCT (rows 2–5) and a CTA (right column). The unenhanced CT ruled out a cerebral hemorrhage. From the PCT raw data, three parametric maps were extracted, relating to mean transit time (MTT, second row), cerebral blood flow (CBF, third row), and cerebral blood volume (CBV, fourth row), respectively. Application of the concept of cerebral vascular autoregulation led to a prognostic map (fifth row), describing the infarct in red and the penumbra in green, the latter being the target of acute reperfusion therapies. CTA identified an occlusion at the right M1-M2 junction (*arrow*) as the origin of the hemodynamic disturbance demonstrated by PCT. CTA also revealed a calcified atheromatous plaque at the right carotid bifurcation (*arrowhead*).

increased attenuation. This radiologic sign has been called the hyperdense artery sign.[5–11] Contrary to other CT early signs, the hyperdense artery sign represents a thrombotic event, not infarction.[10] Although this sign is highly specific, its sensitivity is poor,[12] and false positives should be excluded, such as those caused by a high hematocrit level or atherosclerotic calcifications, but in such cases the hyperattenuation is usually bilateral.[13] In addition, distal MCA (M2 or M3 branches of MCA) thromboemboli create punctate hyperattenuation, also known as the MCA dot sign.[14,15]

Although these early ischemic changes can be helpful in stroke detection, they are subtle and difficult to detect. They also have limited sensitivity for the hyperacute stage of ischemic stroke, in particular within the first 3 hours after onset of symptoms, a critical window for therapeutic interventions. When compared with diffusion-weighted MR imaging, these signs have a sensitivity of 25%.[9,16–20] Moreover, noncontrast CT cannot reliably differentiate between irreversibly damaged brain tissue and penumbra. Finally, the relationship between early ischemic changes on CT and adverse outcomes after recombinant tPA treatment is not straightforward.[21,22]

In contrast to these early ischemic changes, frank hypoattenuation is highly specific for irreversible tissue damage[23] and its extent is predictive of the risk for hemorrhagic transformation.[24] Nevertheless, it is critical to determine the tissue at risk before irreversible tissue damage occurs and frank hypoattenuation appears; this is essential to prevent hemorrhagic transformation. In the European Cooperative Acute Stroke Study trials, involvement of more than one third of the MCA territory on noncontrast CT was used as the criterion for patient exclusion for reperfusion therapy because of the potential increased risk for hemorrhagic transformation.[25] Subsequent studies using this "one third MCA rule" showed poor interobserver correlation.[26–28] This outcome emphasizes the need for more reliable imaging techniques that can help determine the extent of both irreversibly damaged brain tissue and tissue at risk to avoid unnecessary thrombolytic therapy. In an attempt to provide a more quantitative approach, some authors have attempted to design algorithmic methods to quantitatively assess the extent of cerebral acute ischemia on conventional CT by using a 10-point topographic scoring system called ASPECTS (**Box 1**).[29,30]

CT ANGIOGRAPHY

Although conventional cerebral angiography is considered to be the gold standard for the evaluation of cerebrovascular disease, the advances in multidetector row CT (MDCT) technology have made CTA a valid alternative to conventional catheter-based cerebral angiography.[31,32] CTA is widely available,

---

Box 1
Alberta Stroke Program Early CT Score (ASPECTS) 10-point topographic scoring system for estimating the extent of an ischemic stroke compared with the extent of the middle cerebral artery territory

When three or more of the ASPECTS regions show ischemic changes, the infarct is considered to involve more than one third of the MCA territory.

Caudate nucleus

Lenticular nucleus

Insula

Internal capsule

Inferior anterior MCA territory

Inferior middle MCA territory

Inferior posterior MCA territory

Superior anterior MCA territory

Superior middle MCA territory

Superior posterior MCA territory

Data from Mayer TE, Hamann GF, Baranczyk J, et al. Dynamic CT perfusion imaging of acute stroke. AJNR Am J Neuroradiol 2000;21:1441–9.

---

with fast, thin-section, volumetric spiral CT images acquired during the injection of a time-optimized bolus of contrast material for vessel opacification.[33] With modern multisection CT scanners, the entire region from the aortic arch up to the circle of Willis can be covered in a single data acquisition, with isotropic spatial resolution and acquisition time of less than 5 seconds. Multiplanar reformatted images, maximum intensity projection images, and three-dimensional reconstructions of axial CTA source images provide images comparable to those obtained with conventional angiography.[16,17,34]

CTA allows a detailed evaluation of the intra- and extracranial vasculature.[16,18] Its usefulness in acute stroke lies not only in its ability to detect large vessel thrombi within intracranial vessels and to evaluate the carotid and vertebral arteries in the neck[19,20,26] but also in its potential in guiding therapy. In particular, the exact location (ie, proximal versus peripheral occlusions) and the extent of vascular occlusion have been shown to have prognostic value in the response to thrombolytics and determination of collateral circulation and possible risk for subsequent recanalization.[35] For example, "top of carotid" occlusions, proximal MCA branch occlusions, or significant thrombus burden might be poor candidates for intravenous thrombolytics, and possibly may be better candidates for intra-arterial or mechanical thrombolysis.[36]

PERFUSION CT

Within the last few years, PCT has become the third component in the multimodal CT assessment of acute ischemic stroke. There is considerable literature on the measurement and assessment of cerebral perfusion[37] and a brief review is necessary to understand the parameters and quantitative data that PCT technique provides. In 1981, the landmark study by Jones and colleagues[27] used a primate model to elucidate thresholds for MCA ischemia by restricting blood flow in an awake primate model with pathologic correlation. Their findings form the basis of contemporary human perfusion studies:

15 to 30 minutes of complete ischemia produced only microscopic infarcts.

2 to 3 hours of ischemia produced moderate to severe infarcts.

 Cerebral blood flow (CBF) <23 mL 100 g^{-1} min^{-1} caused reversible paralysis.

 CBF<10–12 mL 100 g^{-1} min^{-1} for 2 to 3 hours, or CBF<17–18 mL 100 g^{-1} min^{-1} permanently, resulted in irreversible paralysis.

Subsequent positron emission tomography[28–30] in humans has corroborated with these earlier finding in primates (in particular, CBF<15 mL 100 g^{-1} min^{-1} has strongly correlated with infarction).[29]

Recently, PCT has been introduced as a simple imaging technique to be used in routine clinical practice.[38,39] The concepts behind this imaging technique were developed about 2 decades ago, but its widespread clinical use has been facilitated by the advent of fast, multidetector CT technology.

PCT involves dynamic acquisition of sequential CT slices on a cine mode during rapid intravenous administration of nonionic iodinated contrast material. PCT allows rapid, noninvasive, quantitative evaluation of cerebral perfusion. Based on the multicompartmental tracer kinetic model, dynamic PCT imaging is performed by monitoring the first pass of an iodinated contrast agent bolus through the cerebral circulation. Because the change in CT enhancement (in Hounsfield units, HU) is proportional to the concentration of contrast, perfusion parameters are calculated by deconvolution from the changes in the density-time curve for each pixel using mathematical algorithms based around the central volume principle.[40,41]

 Mean transit time (MTT) indicates the time difference between the arterial inflow and venous outflow.

 Cerebral blood volume (CBV) indicates the volume of blood per unit of brain mass (normal range in gray matter, 4–6 mL/100 g).

 Cerebral blood flow (CBF) indicates the volume of blood flow per unit of brain mass per minute (normal range in gray matter, 50–60 mL/100 g/min).

 The relationship between CBF and CBV is expressed by the equation CBF = CBV/MTT.

Deconvolution software allows much lower injection rates (5 mL/s as reported above) compared with other software that uses different approaches, such as the maximal slope model.[41] These lower injection rates are more practical and tolerable for patients. They do not impair accuracy, because the deconvolution analysis controls for bolus dispersion by comparing the arterial input time-attenuation curve with that of the tissue.[41]

PCT maps can be generated in a short time at an appropriate workstation.[42] PCT data are analyzed at an imaging workstation. Post–image-collection processing involves semiautomated definition of an input artery and a "vein" (**Fig. 2**). In acute stroke patients, selection of different arterial inputs has been demonstrated to have no significant effect on PCT results for an individual patient.[43] As a result, we routinely use the anterior cerebral artery as the arterial input function, to provide standardization and facilitate intersubject comparison. In patients who have chronic cerebral vascular disease the situation is different, and we select for each vascular territory its own specific arterial input function. The reference "vein" actually needs to be the pixel with the largest area under its contrast-enhancement curve. As such, it must be selected at the center of the largest vascular structure perpendicular to the PCT slices. These requirements are usually met by pixels at the center of the superior sagittal sinus. In some instances, however, other venous structures, or even the supraclinoid internal carotid arteries, can be appropriate "veins" for PCT processing purposes.

MTT maps are more sensitive, whereas CBF and CBV maps are more specific for distinguishing ischemia from infarction.[44,45] PCT distinction of the infarct core from the penumbra is based on the concept of cerebral vascular autoregulation. In the penumbra, autoregulation is preserved, MTT is prolonged, but CBV is preserved because of vasodilatation and collateral recruitment as part of the autoregulation process. In the infarct core, autoregulation is lost, MTT is prolonged, and CBV is down.[39] Using appropriate MTT and CBV thresholds, infarct core and penumbra can thus be distinguished on PCT maps.[46] Direct

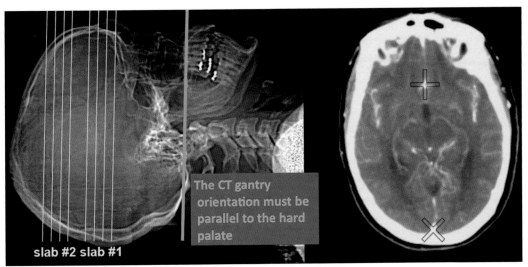

Fig. 2. Representation of the typical location of the two PCT boluses and of the typical selection of the anterior input function (*cross* over the anterior cerebral artery) and of the venous output (*cross* over the superior sagittal sinus).

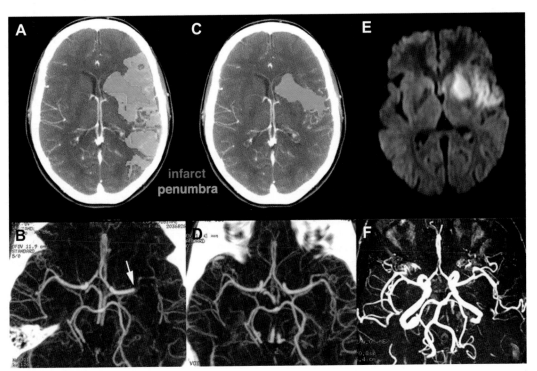

Fig. 3. (*A*) Admission PCT demonstrates mixed infarct and penumbra in the left sylvian territory in a patient who had a right hemisyndrome, whereas (*B*) CTA relates it to an occlusion at the left M1-M2 junction (*arrow*). The patient underwent intravenous thrombolysis and his clinical condition evolved favorably. Twenty-four hours after admission, (*D*) follow-up CTA features recanalization of the left sylvian artery, later confirmed on the MRA (*F*). (*C*) Follow-up PCT shows an almost complete resolution of the penumbra, afforded by the early arterial recanalization. The final PCT infarct has progressed in only a very limited fashion when compared with the admission PCT infarct; its extent closely correlates with that of the abnormality on the delayed diffusion-weighted trace image (*E*).

assessment of an individual patient's ischemic penumbra ("penumbra is brain") may allow more personalized, appropriate selection of candidates for intervention than generalized time criteria ("time is brain"), because individuals may have different timelines for evolution of penumbra into infarct.

PCT provides equivalent results to diffusion/perfusion MR imaging in characterizing the infarct and penumbra (**Fig. 3**),[38,39,46] and also in selection of patients for acute reperfusion therapies.[47] PCT requires a shorter scan time and is usually more widely available in the emergency setting compared with MR imaging. As such, it represents an appealing imaging technique to assess acute stroke patients.[48,49] There are some specific situations (lacunar infarcts, posterior fossa strokes, young patients) in which MR imaging is warranted instead of PCT, however.

The main advantage of PCT is its wide availability and quantitative accuracy.[50] Its main limitation is its inability to image the whole brain because it is limited to a 2- to 4-cm section of brain tissue per bolus. Introduction of 256- and 320-slice CT scanners, offering whole-brain coverage, is likely to overcome this limitation in the near future.[48]

MULTIMODAL CT STROKE PROTOCOL

Multimodal CT allows for the assessment of the four Ps: parenchyma, pipes, perfusion, and penumbra.[51] Noncontrast CT allows one to rule out hemorrhage, CTA identifies intraarterial thrombus, and PCT can differentiate between at-risk (the so-called "penumbra") and irreversibly damaged brain tissue.[52] Multimodal CT offers rapid data acquisition and can be performed with modern CT equipment; a typical multimodal CT stroke protocol is depicted in **Box 2**. PCT is usually performed twice to increase spatial coverage and make it as close as possible to whole-brain coverage.

The advantages of multimodal CT include short protocol time (5–6 minutes) and the availability in the emergency setting. The new generation of portable multislice CT scanners may bring CTP to the patient's bedside in the emergency room or the ICU. The principle disadvantages of this CT-based stroke protocol would be ionizing radiation exposure (recent technological CT advancements, such as dose modulation, have effectively reduced the amount of radiation exposure) and its limited ability to assess ischemia in areas that have a propensity to create so-called "beam-hardening" artifacts (eg, posterior fossa ischemia). We also use lower kV for CTA and PCT to reduce the radiation dose and to improve the signal-to-noise ratio.

Box 2

Summary of multimodal CT imaging acquisition protocol on a 64-slice CT scanner

Series are obtained in this chronologic order, each series being separated from the subsequent one by 2 minutes. PCT is usually performed twice to increase spatial coverage and make it as close as possible to whole-brain coverage

Noncontrast head CT

> 2.5-mm axial cuts from skull base to vertex 120 kVp, 200 mAs

Dynamic CT perfusion (performed two consecutive times)

> 40 mL (300 mg I/mL) iodinated contrast 18- or 20-gauge IV access; 5 mL/s injection rate

> 6-second scan delay, 45-second scan time 80 kVp, 100 mAs

> Cine scan mode, 5-mm slices

CT angiogram

> 40 mL (300 mg I/mL) iodinated contrast 18- or 20-gauge IV access; 5 mL/s injection rate

> Delay calculated based on CT perfusion 100 kV, 250 mAs

> Spiral CT acquisition, 0.625-mm slices, pitch of 1:1

> Coverage from left atrium to vertex

SUMMARY

A multimodal CT protocol provides a comprehensive noninvasive survey of acute stroke patients with accurate demonstration of the site of arterial occlusion and its hemodynamic tissue status. It combines widespread availability with the ability to provide functional characterization of cerebral ischemia and could potentially allow more accurate selection of candidates for acute stroke reperfusion therapy.

REFERENCES

1. The National Institute of Neurological Disorders and Stroke rt-PA Stroke Study Group. Tissue plasminogen activator for acute ischemic stroke. N Engl J Med 1995;333:1581–7.
2. Adams HP Jr, del Zoppo G, Alberts MJ, et al. Guidelines for the early management of adults with ischemic stroke: a guideline from the American Heart

Association/American Stroke Association Stroke Council, clinical cardiology council, cardiovascular radiology and intervention council, and the atherosclerotic peripheral vascular disease and quality of care outcomes in research interdisciplinary working groups: the American Academy of Neurology affirms the value of this guideline as an educational tool for neurologists. Stroke 2007;38:1655–711.

3. Truwit CL, Barkovich AJ, Gean-Marton A, et al. Loss of the insular ribbon: another early CT sign of acute middle cerebral artery infarction. Radiology 1990; 176:801–6.

4. Tomura N, Uemura K, Inugami A, et al. Early CT finding in cerebral infarction: obscuration of the lentiform nucleus. Radiology 1988;168:463–7.

5. Bastianello S, Pierallini A, Colonnese C, et al. Hyperdense middle cerebral artery CT sign. Comparison with angiography in the acute phase of ischemic supratentorial infarction. Neuroradiology 1991;33: 207–11.

6. Launes J, Ketonen L. Dense middle cerebral artery sign: an indicator of poor outcome in middle cerebral artery area infarction. J Neurol Neurosurg Psychiatr 1987;50:1550–2.

7. New PF, Aronow S. Attenuation measurements of whole blood and blood fractions in computed tomography. Radiology 1976;121:635–40.

8. Schuierer G, Huk W. The unilateral hyperdense middle cerebral artery: an early CT-sign of embolism or thrombosis. Neuroradiology 1988;30: 120–2.

9. Schuknecht B, Ratzka M, Hofmann E. The "dense artery sign"—major cerebral artery thromboembolism demonstrated by computed tomography. Neuroradiology 1990;32:98–103.

10. Tomsick TA, Brott TG, Chambers AA, et al. Hyperdense middle cerebral artery sign on CT: efficacy in detecting middle cerebral artery thrombosis. AJNR Am J Neuroradiol 1990;11:473–7.

11. Pressman BD, Tourje EJ, Thompson JR. An early CT sign of ischemic infarction: increased density in a cerebral artery. AJR Am J Roentgenol 1987; 149:583–6.

12. Leys D, Pruvo JP, Godefroy O, et al. Prevalence and significance of hyperdense middle cerebral artery in acute stroke. Stroke 1992;23:317–24.

13. Rauch RA, Bazan C 3rd, Larsson EM, et al. Hyperdense middle cerebral arteries identified on CT as a false sign of vascular occlusion. AJNR Am J Neuroradiol 1993;14:669–73.

14. Barber PA, Demchuk AM, Hudon ME, et al. Hyperdense sylvian fissure MCA "dot" sign: a CT marker of acute ischemia. Stroke 2001;32:84–8.

15. Shetty SK. The MCA dot sign. Radiology 2006;241: 315–8.

16. Prokop M. Multislice CT angiography. Eur J Radiol 2000;36:86–96.

17. Prokop M, Shin HO, Schanz A, et al. Use of maximum intensity projections in CT angiography: a basic review. Radiographics 1997;17:433–51.

18. Lev MH, Farkas J, Rodriguez VR, et al. CT angiography in the rapid triage of patients with hyperacute stroke to intraarterial thrombolysis: accuracy in the detection of large vessel thrombus. J Comput Assist Tomogr 2001;25:520–8.

19. Cumming MJ, Morrow IM. Carotid artery stenosis: a prospective comparison of CT angiography and conventional angiography. AJR Am J Roentgenol 1994;163:517–23.

20. Katz DA, Marks MP, Napel SA, et al. Circle of Willis: evaluation with spiral CT angiography, MR angiography, and conventional angiography. Radiology 1995;195:445–9.

21. Patel SC, Levine SR, Tilley BC, et al. Lack of clinical significance of early ischemic changes on computed tomography in acute stroke. JAMA 2001; 286:2830–8.

22. Roberts HC, Dillon WP, Furlan AJ, et al. Computed tomographic findings in patients undergoing intraarterial thrombolysis for acute ischemic stroke due to middle cerebral artery occlusion: results from the PROACT II trial. Stroke 2002;33:1557–65.

23. von Kummer R, Bourquain H, Bastianello S, et al. Early prediction of irreversible brain damage after ischemic stroke at CT. Radiology 2001;219: 95–100.

24. Larrue V, von Kummer RR, Muller A, et al. Risk factors for severe hemorrhagic transformation in ischemic stroke patients treated with recombinant tissue plasminogen activator: a secondary analysis of the European-Australasian Acute Stroke Study (ECASS II). Stroke 2001;32:438–41.

25. Hacke W, Kaste M, Fieschi C, et al. Intravenous thrombolysis with recombinant tissue plasminogen activator for acute hemispheric stroke. The European cooperative acute stroke study (ECASS). JAMA 1995;274:1017–25.

26. Shrier DA, Tanaka H, Numaguchi Y, et al. CT angiography in the evaluation of acute stroke. AJNR Am J Neuroradiol 1997;18:1011–20.

27. Jones TH, Morawetz RB, Crowell RM, et al. Thresholds of focal cerebral ischemia in awake monkeys. J Neurosurg 1981;54:773–82.

28. Powers WJ, Grubb RL Jr, Darriet D, et al. Cerebral blood flow and cerebral metabolic rate of oxygen requirements for cerebral function and viability in humans. J Cereb Blood Flow Metab 1985;5:600–8.

29. Eastwood JD, Lev MH, Azhari T, et al. CT perfusion scanning with deconvolution analysis: pilot study in patients with acute middle cerebral artery stroke. Radiology 2002;222:227–36.

30. Mayer TE, Hamann GF, Baranczyk J, et al. Dynamic CT perfusion imaging of acute stroke. AJNR Am J Neuroradiol 2000;21:1441–9.

31. Prestigiacomo CJ. Surgical endovascular neuroradiology in the 21st century: what lies ahead? Neurosurgery 2006;59:S48–55 [discussion: S3–13].

32. Wang H, Fraser K, Wang D, et al. The evolution of endovascular therapy for neurosurgical disease. Neurosurg Clin N Am 2005;16:223–9, vii.

33. Vieco PT. CT angiography of the intracranial circulation. Neuroimaging Clin N Am 1998;8:577–92.

34. Lell MM, Anders K, Uder M, et al. New techniques in CT angiography. Radiographics 2006;1(Suppl 26): S45–62.

35. Tan JC, Dillon WP, Liu S, et al. Systematic comparison of perfusion-CT and CT-angiography in acute stroke patients. Ann Neurol 2007;61:533–43.

36. Zaidat OO, Suarez JI, Santillan C, et al. Response to intra-arterial and combined intravenous and intra-arterial thrombolytic therapy in patients with distal internal carotid artery occlusion. Stroke 2002;33: 1821–6.

37. Latchaw RE, Yonas H, Pentheny SL, et al. Adverse reactions to xenon-enhanced CT cerebral blood flow determination. Radiology 1987;163:251–4.

38. Wintermark M, Reichhart M, Cuisenaire O, et al. Comparison of admission perfusion computed tomography and qualitative diffusion- and perfusion-weighted magnetic resonance imaging in acute stroke patients. Stroke 2002;33:2025–31.

39. Wintermark M, Reichhart M, Thiran JP, et al. Prognostic accuracy of cerebral blood flow measurement by perfusion computed tomography, at the time of emergency room admission, in acute stroke patients. Ann Neurol 2002;51:417–32.

40. Latchaw RE, Yonas H, Hunter GJ, et al. Guidelines and recommendations for perfusion imaging in cerebral ischemia: a scientific statement for healthcare professionals by the writing group on perfusion imaging, from the Council on Cardiovascular Radiology of the American Heart Association. Stroke 2003;34:1084–104.

41. Wintermark M, Maeder P, Thiran JP, et al. Quantitative assessment of regional cerebral blood flows by perfusion CT studies at low injection rates: a critical review of the underlying theoretical models. Eur Radiol 2001;11:1220–30.

42. Wintermark M, Sesay M, Barbier E, et al. Comparative overview of brain perfusion imaging techniques. J Neuroradiol 2005;32:294–314.

43. Wintermark M, Lau BC, Chien J, et al. The anterior cerebral artery is an appropriate arterial input function for perfusion-CT processing in patients with acute stroke. Neuroradiology 2007;50(3):227–36.

44. Sparacia G, Iaia A, Assadi B, et al. Perfusion CT in acute stroke: predictive value of perfusion parameters in assessing tissue viability versus infarction. Radiol Med (Torino) 2007;112:113–22.

45. Wintermark M, Fischbein NJ, Smith WS, et al. Accuracy of dynamic perfusion CT with deconvolution in detecting acute hemispheric stroke. AJNR Am J Neuroradiol 2005;26:104–12.

46. Wintermark M, Flanders AE, Velthuis B, et al. Perfusion-CT assessment of infarct core and penumbra: receiver operating characteristic curve analysis in 130 patients suspected of acute hemispheric stroke. Stroke 2006;37:979–85.

47. Wintermark M, Meuli R, Browaeys P, et al. Comparison of CT perfusion and angiography and MRI in selecting stroke patients for acute treatment. Neurology 2007;68:694–7.

48. Wintermark M, Bogousslavsky J. Imaging of acute ischemic brain injury: the return of computed tomography. Curr Opin Neurol 2003;16:59–63.

49. Kaste M. Reborn workhorse, CT, pulls the wagon toward thrombolysis beyond 3 hours. Stroke 2004; 35:357–9.

50. Wintermark M, Thiran JP, Maeder P, et al. Simultaneous measurement of regional cerebral blood flow by perfusion CT and stable xenon CT: a validation study. AJNR Am J Neuroradiol 2001;22:905–14.

51. Rowley HA. The four Ps of acute stroke imaging: parenchyma, pipes, perfusion, and penumbra. AJNR Am J Neuroradiol 2001;22:599–601.

52. Kloska SP, Nabavi DG, Gaus C, et al. Acute stroke assessment with CT: do we need multimodal evaluation? Radiology 2004;233:79–86.

CT Enterography: Concept, Technique, and Interpretation

Sandra Tochetto, MD, Vahid Yaghmai, MD*

KEYWORDS

- CT enterography • Crohn disease
- Gastrointestinal bleeding • Neoplasm
- Small bowel • Computed tomography

The assessment of small bowel abnormalities has traditionally been a challenging task for radiologists and gastroenterologists. Conventional radiologic and endoscopic evaluations are frequently hindered by the length and caliber of small bowel loops.[1] Although, CT in its conventional form has played a significant role in the evaluation of extraenteric manifestations of small bowel disease, it has a limited role for depicting bowel wall and luminal abnormalities.[2] CT enterography, a robust new method for evaluating the small bowel, is a byproduct of the recent advances in multidetector-row CT (MDCT) technology.[3,4] New MDCT scanners, with isotropic image acquisition in a single breath-hold, allow high-resolution multiphasic assessment of the bowel in multiple planes.[4] CT enterography uses this technology to provide a detailed evaluation of the mural features of the gut and its lumen. Additionally, it permits an accurate depiction of the perienteric tissues, thus improving assessment of the disease extension and complications.[5] Multiplanar reformations, obtained from isotropic data sets, allow radiologists to evaluate the entire abdomen in planes that facilitate visualization of the pathology.[6]

In this article, we discuss the advantages of CT enterography over conventional and newer small bowel imaging modalities. Image acquisition and interpretation for the most common indications are also discussed.

CONCEPT

A wide variety of methods are available for the assessment of the small bowel, attesting to the difficulty of evaluating this organ. The current methods of small bowel evaluation include radiologic as well as endoscopic techniques.[7] The radiologic armamentarium includes barium studies (small bowel follow-through [SBFT] and enteroclysis), CT techniques ("routine" CT, CT enterography, and CT enteroclysis), ultrasound, nuclear medicine, and MR (MR enterography and MR enteroclysis). Endoscopic methods include ileoscopy, push enteroscopy, double-balloon endoscopy, and wireless capsule endoscopy.[7] CT enterography and wireless capsule endoscopy are two of the most robust imaging techniques with proven efficacy.[8]

CT enterography combines isotropic-voxel acquisition with the oral intake of large volumes of neutral contrast agents and rapid intravenous administration of iodinated contrast to improve visualization of the small bowel wall and its mural features.[9] Misregistration artifacts due to respiratory motion and small bowel peristalsis are effectively eliminated because data is acquired in a single breath-hold.[6] The acquired data can then be used to perform excellent two- and three-dimensional reformations, producing high-resolution images of the bowel and mesenteric vessels.[10,11] Moreover, the combined use of intravenous and neutral enteric contrast agents optimizes luminal

Department of Radiology, Northwestern University-Feinberg School of Medicine, 676 North Saint Clair, Suite 800, Chicago, IL 60611, USA
* Corresponding author.
E-mail address: v-yaghmai@northwestern.edu (V. Yaghmai).

Radiol Clin N Am 47 (2009) 117–132
doi:10.1016/j.rcl.2008.10.007

distension and depicts attenuation differences among the bowel wall layers, the fluid filled lumen, and the adjacent mesenteric fat.[4,5]

The advantages of CT enterography are its non-invasiveness, its ready availability, and its operator independence. The American College of Radiology Appropriateness Criteria (2005) rates CT enterography as the most appropriate radiologic method in the evaluation of initial presentation or known Crohn disease with acute exacerbation or suspect complications.[12] CT enterography can also play an important role in evaluating obscure gastrointestinal bleeding and in detecting small bowel tumors.[5,13]

CT enterography has several advantages over SBFT study. While SBFT is both operator dependent and limited by deep pelvic and overlapping small bowel loops, CT enterography is not affected by these limitations (Fig. 1). The most distal portion of the terminal ileum is difficult to assess with SBFT but readily evaluated by CT enterography. However, a potential drawback of CT enterography is its higher effective radiation dose when compared with SBFT study.[14]

CT enterography should be distinguished from CT enteroclysis. In CT enterography, the patient drinks a large volume of oral contrast in a short period of time. CT enteroclysis, on the other hand, requires intubation of the descending duodenum or jejunum and administration of enteric contrast material, preferably by a pump, to obtain optimal distension of the small bowel.[15] More reliable distension of the small bowel can be achieved with CT enteroclysis because oral contrast agent is administered by the radiologist.[15] The patient is usually sedated for enteroclysis, leading to increased cost and acquisition time as well as

reduced availability.[4,15] A feasibility study by Wold and colleagues[1] comparing CT enterography to CT enteroclysis did not find significant differences in bowel distension and demonstrated similar accuracy in indentifying active Crohn disease for both methods. However, there are no large studies comparing CT enterography to CT enteroclysis.

Although wireless capsule endoscopy is the most sensitive technique for small bowel mucosal evaluation, it has several limitations.[7,8] Its higher sensitivity compared with CT enterography is accompanied by its lower specificity.[7,16] Solem and colleagues,[16] comparing different imaging modalities to detect active Crohn disease, did not demonstrate significant difference in sensitivity and accuracy in disease diagnosis among CT enterography, wireless capsule endoscopy, ileocolonoscopy, and SBFT. The sensitivity for identification of active disease was 83% for CT enterography, 83% for wireless capsule endoscopy, 74% for ileocolonoscopy, and 65% for SBFT. However wireless capsule endoscopy had lower specificity (53%) and could not be performed in 17% of patients because of an asymptomatic stricture diagnosed by CT enterography.

Wireless capsule endoscopy also has several technical limitations. Retention of the capsule is a serious risk that requires surgical treatment. Cheifetz and colleagues[17] reported a 13% risk for capsule retention in patients with known Crohn disease and 1.6% in those with suspected Crohn disease. The retention rate is 0.7% to 2% in patients with obscure gastrointestinal bleeding.[8,18] Additionally, wireless capsule endoscopy generates several thousand images, requiring long interpretation times. Accurate localization of disease

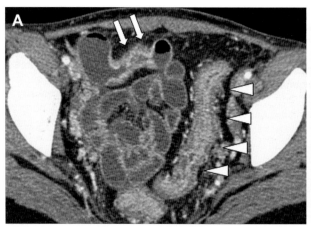
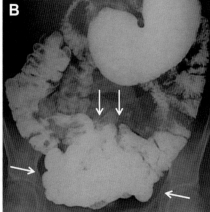

Fig. 1. CT enterography (A) shows segmental mural thickening and hyperenhancement of an ileal loop (arrows) and acute colonic inflammation (arrowheads). SBFT (B) performed in the same patient cannot evaluate the overlapping small bowel loops (small arrows) in the pelvis or the colon.

may be difficult by wireless capsule endoscopy.[19] Also, the evaluation of the small bowel may be incomplete because of fast transit, presence of hemorrhage, or failure to reach the cecum.[8] A patency wireless capsule that dissolves automatically can also be used to ensure safe subsequent usage of wireless capsule endoscopy.

The role of MR in the diagnosis and follow-up of small bowel pathology remains limited at this time. The development of fast imaging sequences has improved the quality of MR imaging. However, MDCT scanners have a superior spatial resolution.[20] In a prospective study comparing CT and MR enteroclysis for the evaluation of Crohn disease, CT showed higher interobserver agreement and superior sensitivity in detecting signs of active disease.[20] Albert and colleagues[21] reported sensitivity of 78% for MR enterography compared with 93% for wireless capsule endoscopy. Masselli and colleagues[22] reported similar performance for MR enterography and MR enteroclysis in Crohn patients. Radiation exposure in CT enterography will likely be a catalyst for further research and acceptance of MR enterography.

TECHNIQUE

When assessing the small bowel with CT enterography, attention to patient preparation and image acquisition techniques is essential. The study should be tailored to answer the question at hand and to optimize visualization of the mural features of the gut. The amount and timing of neutral oral contrast affects the degree of distension. The timing and rate of intravenous contrast administration determines the degree of bowel wall enhancement.[23,24] High spatial resolution and multiplanar reformations are essential for displaying the pathology.[25]

Small Bowel Distension

Adequate bowel distension is of utmost importance in CT enterography. Collapsed or poorly distended bowel loops can obscure pathologic processes and even simulate bowel wall thickness and mucosal hyperenhancement.[25,26] Slow administration of a large volume of oral contrast within a short time is required to achieve bowel distension.[6]

The oral contrast agents used for CT enterography can be categorized into two groups: positive contrast agents and neutral contrast agents.[25] Positive contrast agents, such as iodine solution and barium suspension dilute, have high attenuation values and are routinely used to delineate the intestinal tract in CT.[4] In fact, CT enterography was initially described with the use of positive

contrast agents.[4,27] However, positive contrast agents are not ideal for the evaluation of bowel pathology for several reasons.[5,10,25] They limit the visualization of the mural features of the intestinal tract.[4,5] When assessing for obscure gastrointestinal bleeding, the high attenuation of these contrast agents obscures the source of hemorrhage. Small bowel neoplasms typically enhance with intravenous contrast material. However, this feature cannot be easily assessed when high-density enteric contrast is present.[13] Additionally, positive contrast agents may interfere with the postprocessing techniques and hinder visualization of the mesenteric vessels.[25,28] However, when intravenous contrast material cannot be administered, positive oral contrast is preferable over neutral contrast.

Today, neutral oral contrast agents that have attenuation similar to water (10–30 Hounsfield units [HU]) are routinely used for CT enterography.[4] Their low attenuation combined with intravenous contrast administration allows excellent visualization of the bowel wall and its lumen by maximizing their attenuation differences. The low Hounsfield value of these agents also makes them ideal for CT angiography and positron emission tomography–CT.[29-31]

A variety of neutral contrasts are available, including water, whole milk, methylcellulose solution, polyethylene glycol solution, and low-density barium suspension with sorbitol (0.1% weight per volume barium sulfate suspension).[4,5] Water is a useful contrast agent when used in the upper abdominal CT studies.[6,32] However, it has a slow intestinal transit and is rapidly absorbed through the intestinal wall, resulting in unsatisfactory distension of the jejunal and ileal loops.[4,6] Therefore, water has limited utility for the evaluation of Crohn disease, where the ileum is commonly involved, or of occult gastrointestinal hemorrhage, where the bleeding site may be anywhere in the small bowel.

Water resorption, however, can be slowed with some additives. Neutral oral contrast agents containing osmotic additives, such as polyethylene glycol or sugar alcohols (mannitol and sorbitol), improve small bowel distention significantly and result in superior visualization of its mural features.[5,6,33,34] Megibow and colleagues[6] demonstrated that the low-density barium suspension with sorbitol significantly improved bowel distention in all segments of the gastrointestinal tract when compared with water and methylcellulose solution (**Fig. 2**). Young and colleagues[33] reported better tolerance of low-density barium suspension with sorbitol when compared with polyethylene glycol solution. Another study comparing low-density barium suspension and sorbitol with a solution containing 0.2% of locust bean gum and 2.5%

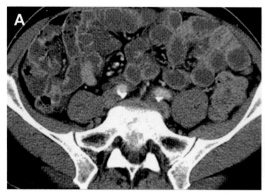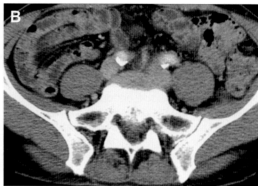

Fig. 2. CT enterography images in the same patient with (*A*) low-density barium suspension with sorbitol and (*B*) with water. Bowel wall detail and distension improve with low-density barium suspension and sorbitol (*A*) when compared with water (*B*).

mannitol demonstrated that both oral agents resulted in better bowel distension than water, but no significant difference was observed between them.[34] A comparison study between milk and low-density barium suspension with sorbitol by Koo and colleagues[28] did not demonstrate significant difference in bowel distension. However, milk may not be well tolerated by many patients and is difficult to store, limiting its use.

There are slight variations in the dosage and timing of oral contrast agent for CT enterography. Kuehle and colleagues,[34] comparing different volumes of the low-density barium suspension with sorbitol, demonstrated that the best bowel distension was achieved with 1350 mL and the result did not improve by increasing the volume to 1800 mL. Moreover, administration of 1800 mL of contrast agent led to lower patient acceptance and higher rate of side effects, such as mild diarrhea and abdominal cramps.[34] In our center, we use 1350 mL of low-density barium suspension with sorbitol. Our protocol is summarized in **Box 1**. Fasting for 6 hours is required to reduce the possibility of misinterpreting ingested hyperdense debris as enhancing lesion or focus of hemorrhage.[4]

Optimal distension of terminal ileum is observed at 45 to 60 minutes after the ingestion of oral contrast, reducing significantly after this period.[10,33] However, the duodenum and proximal jejunum distend early (15–20 minutes after the ingestion), which may be a consideration in the evaluation of pathologic processes involving these segments.[33,34] Patients should be instructed about the importance of continuous intake of the oral contrast and monitored by a nurse or technologist as they ingest the contrast.[34] Noncontinuous intake or poor timing of oral contrast will almost certainly lead to a poor study. In patients who are

debilitated and unable to drink large volumes of the neutral oral contrast, CT enteroclysis may be a better option.[15]

Metoclopramide or glucagon has been used by some investigators to increase gastric and small bowel distension.[9,35] However, their efficacy remains unproven and, thus, their use is not universal.

Administration of Intravenous Contrast Material

The use of intravenous contrast is mandatory in CT enterography.[4,5] Without the use of intravenous contrast material, mural enhancement of the bowel cannot be assessed and intraluminal masses or gastrointestinal hemorrhage may not be visible. Optimal mural enhancement requires rapid intravenous administration of contrast, usually at a rate of 4 to 5 mL/s. Variables, such as cardiac output, weight, and rate of contrast administration, may affect peak enhancement. Therefore, bolus timing

---

Box 1
Enteric contrast material administration protocol for CT enterography

Nothing by mouth for 6 hours before scanning

Oral administration of low-density barium suspension with sorbitol (total of 1350 mL over 60 minutes):

- 450 mL during the first 20 minutes (60–40 minutes before scanning)
- 450 mL during the second 20 minutes (40–20 minutes before scanning)
- 225 mL during the third 20 minutes (20–0 minutes before scanning)
- 225 mL on CT table

techniques may be beneficial in optimizing enteric enhancement.[23,36] When there is a contraindication to iodinated intravenous contrast, CT with positive oral contrast or MR enterography is preferred.[4,37]

CT enterography for the evaluation of inflammatory bowel disease is usually accomplished in a single phase.[10] For the evaluation of suspected or confirmed small bowel tumors, a precontrast phase should be included to distinguish radiodense material in the gut from enhancing masses or contrast extravasation into the lumen.[13]

At our institution, CT enterography for diagnosis or evaluation of inflammatory bowel disease is performed during the enteric phase (45 seconds after initiating intravenous contrast administration). During the enteric phase, mural enhancement is at its maximum and the conspicuity of small bowel mural features is accentuated (**Fig. 3**).[4,9,38] Shindera

and colleagues[23] demonstrated that the peak of small bowel mural enhancement is about 14 seconds after the peak of aortic enhancement or approximately 50 seconds after the start of intravenous contrast administration (starting at 45 seconds and ending at 54 seconds). They also found that during the venous phase (70 seconds after intravenous contrast administration) the enteric enhancement was significantly lower than in enteric phase. Vandenbroucke and colleagues,[39] however, demonstrated no significant difference in the performance of enteric or portal venous phases when assessing Crohn disease activity.

In the evaluation of mesenteric ischemia and small bowel bleeding or neoplasm, a multiphasic study is performed. Huprich and colleagues[13] demonstrated the utility of tri-phasic study in

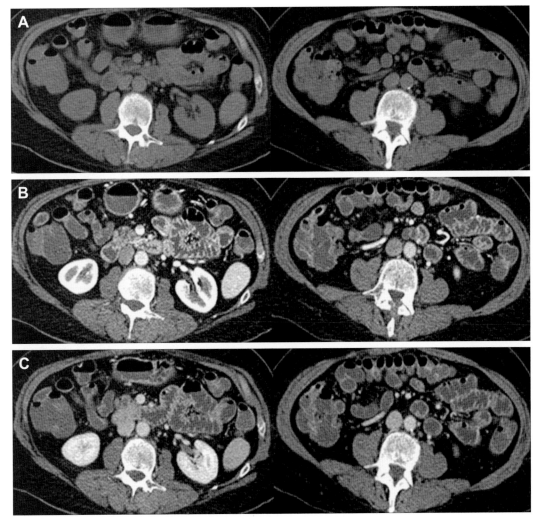

Fig. 3. Effects of scan time on mural enhancement in a normal CT enterography. (*A*) Precontrast phase. (*B*) Enteric phase. (*C*) Portal venous phase. Note optimal mural enhancement during the enteric phase (*B*).

depicting the source of obscure gastrointestinal bleeding. They performed the first phase at the peak of aortic enhancement, the second at enteric phase (20–25 seconds after the beginning of the arterial phase acquisition) and the third at 70 to 75 seconds after the beginning of the arterial phase.[13] In our institution, we perform a multiphasic study that includes an unenhanced phase, followed by arterial and portal venous phases. The unenhanced phase is used to detect radiodense debris that may mimic contrast extravasation. The arterial phase is essential for detection of vascular lesions. The portal venous phase obtained at 70 seconds is useful for the evaluation of neoplastic lesions as well as for contrast extravasation. **Table 1** summarizes the image acquisition timing protocols for different applications of CT enterography in our institution.

Image Acquisition and Display

Scanning is preferably performed on MDCT scanners with 16 or more channels (submillimeter collimation) to improve spatial resolution and to avoid issues related to slow acquisition.[23] To reduce motion artifact, the table speed is adjusted to complete the image acquisition within one breathhold.[10] The images are acquired from the diaphragm to the pubic symphysis and reconstructed with a section thickness of 2 mm (1–3 mm) and reconstruction interval smaller than 2 mm.[9] Dose modulation, when available, should be used to reduce radiation exposure.[4] **Table 2** outlines the acquisition parameters for CT enterography.

INTERPRETATION

Coronal and sagittal reformations are essential when interpreting a CT enterography study. Image reconstructions can be performed at the scanner console or may be obtained from the thin slices on an independent image-processing workstation. Multiplanar images allow better depiction and characterization of enteric and extraenteric abnormalities and are an excellent tool for problem solving.[40,41] **Box 2** summarizes the role of multiplanar reformations in interpretation of CT enterography.

Coronal images display more bowel loops on a single image and are, therefore, useful for quantifying the length of involved segments and improving visualization of the terminal ileum.[42] Sagittal reformations are helpful for evaluation of the rectum and presacral area as well as the mesenteric vessels. Maximum intensity projection images may improve visualization of the mesenteric vascular structures and perienteric fat stranding in the assessment of inflammatory bowel disease or occult gastrointestinal bleeding.

The most common applications of CT enterography include those related to diagnosing and staging Crohn disease, detecting gastrointestinal bleeding, and diagnosing intestinal neoplasms. These applications are reviewed here.

Crohn Disease

Involvement of the bowel in Crohn disease is transmural, segmental, and usually discontinuous. The small bowel is involved in almost 80% of the cases, with ileocecal region affected in 50%. Clinical signs and symptoms vary widely depending on the segment affected and the degree of inflammatory response.[43,44]

Routine CT with positive oral contrast agent is routinely used to evaluate extraenteric complications of Crohn disease.[39,45] CT enterography has the added advantage of depicting mural and luminal abnormalities, thus differentiating acute from

---

Table 1
Timing of image acquisition for CT enterography

Indication	Phases	Timing of Imaging Acquisition	Rate of Contrast
Inflammatory bowel disease	Single phase	Enteric phase (45 s after beginning intravenous administration)	4–5 mL/s
Obscure gastrointestinal bleeding	Multiphasic	Unenhanced phase Arterial phase Portal venous phase (70 s after beginning intravenous administration)	4–5 mL/s
Neoplasm	Multiphasic	Unenhanced phase Arterial phase Portal venous phase (70 s after beginning intravenous administration)	4–5 mL/s

Table 2
Acquisition parameters for CT enterography

Parameter	Measure
Area covered	Diaphragm to the pubic symphysis
Table speed	Scanning the covered area in one breath-hold
Kilovolts	120
Milliampere seconds	Dose modulator
Detector collimation	≤1 mm (16- to 64-channel MDCT)
Slice thickness	2 mm
Interval reconstruction	≤2 mm
Reformatted images	Coronal: 2 × 2 mm; sagittal: 2 × 2 mm
Maximum intensity projection	Coronal recommended: 4 × 2 mm
Reconstruction algorithm	Medium-sharp reconstruction kernel

chronic Crohn disease.[4,9,46] This differentiation is critical because active disease is usually treated medically but chronic disease may require surgical intervention.[5,47]

Active Crohn disease

CT enterography findings of active Crohn disease include mural hyperenhancement, mural stratification, bowel wall thickening, increased attenuation in the perienteric fat, and engorged vasa recta ("comb" sign).[5,9,48]

Mural hyperenhancement refers to segmental hyperenhancement of the small bowel wall when compared with the adjacent small bowel loops.[9,35] The comparison should be made to the loops in the same region because normal jejunal loops enhance to a greater degree than normal ileal loops (**Fig. 4**). It is also important to compare the bowel loops with similar degree of distension because normal collapsed loops exhibit greater attenuation than distended ones do. When assessing nondistended bowel loops, secondary signs of Crohn disease, such as perienteric fat stranding, engorged vasa recta, fistula, and abscess formation, can be used for staging.[5,9]

Mural hyperenhancement is the most sensitive CT finding of active Crohn disease (**Fig. 5**).[9] The degree of bowel wall enhancement correlates with the severity of active inflammation and may be used to monitor anti-inflammatory therapy.[35,38] Hara and colleagues[46] observed that CT enterography findings positively correlated with disease progression or regression.

Quantitative measurement techniques have been used to objectively correlate mural hyperenhancement and wall thickness with disease activity. Using a mural attenuation threshold of 109 HU and an abnormal-to-normal loop enhancement ratio of more than 1.3, CT enterography is highly correlated with histologic findings of active disease. Visual assessment, however, presents higher specificity than do quantitative measurements.[35]

Mural stratification is visualization of the bowel wall layers on CT after intravenous contrast administration.[5,9] Edematous bowel wall usually has a trilaminar appearance on CT enterography ("target" sign): an internal ring of mucosal enhancement, an external ring of serosal and muscular enhancement, and an interposed submucosal layer with decreased attenuation (**Fig. 6**). In chronic inflammatory bowel disease, fat deposition may be seen in the submucosa and should not be

Box 2
Role of multiplanar reformations in interpreting CT enterography

Axial

Usually best for evaluating closely apposed loops of the small bowel and interloop abscesses

Coronal

Allows a global view of the small bowel in its entirety

Helps identify the terminal ileum and quantify length of involved segments

May help identify and localize fistulas

Sagittal

Particularly helpful in evaluating the rectum and in detecting fistulas

Coronal maximum intensity projections

Helpful for visualizing perienteric mesenteric stranding and engorged vasa recta, and for evaluating vascular structures

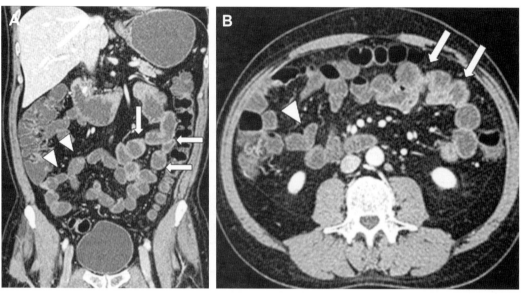

Fig. 4. Normal CT enterography images in coronal plane (*A*) and axial plane (*B*). Note greater enhancement of jejunal loops (*arrows*) when compared with ileal loops (*arrowheads*) in this normal examination.

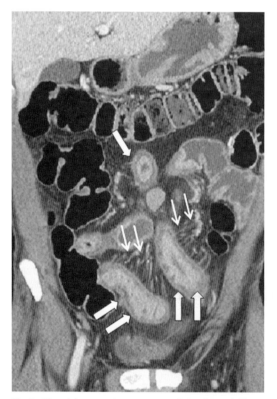

Fig. 5. Mural hyperenhancement of the bowel (*large arrows*) indicates active disease in multiple loops. Also note engorged vasa recta (*small arrows*). The colon is not involved.

confused with the mural stratification that is seen with acute disease (**Fig. 7**).[5,49] In chronic Crohn disease, mural stratification may be absent because of the transmural fibrosis, leading to a homogeneous and less-intense enhancement. Mural stratification is not specific for Crohn disease and may be seen with other small bowel nonneoplastic etiologies, such as ischemia, ulcerative colitis, and radiation enteritis.[50]

Mural thickening refers to wall thickness of greater than 3 mm in a distended bowel loop. It correlates highly with disease activity and, present in up to 82% of patients, it is the most frequently observed CT finding in Crohn disease.[50] When associated with mural hyperenhancement, it is the most sensitive sign of active disease.[9]

Increased attenuation of the mesenteric fat is due to edema and engorgement of the vasa recta. The prominence and engorgement of the vasa recta adjacent to the affected bowel loop is also known as the "comb" sign.[48,50] Increased attenuation of the mesenteric fat in combination with the "comb" sign is the most specific CT finding for active Crohn disease (**Fig. 8**).[38] Colombel and colleagues[38] demonstrated that the perienteric findings of inflammation on CT enterography correlate with the levels of C reactive protein, a marker of disease activity. Lee and colleagues[51] observed that when the "comb" sign is present, the patients were more likely to be admitted to the hospital and to receive aggressive treatment.

Chronic Crohn disease

The long-standing inflammatory process leads to chronic manifestations of Crohn disease. CT

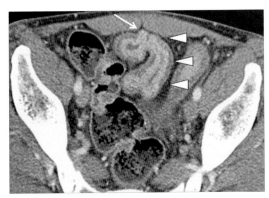

Fig. 6. Mural stratification (*arrowheads*) indicative of active inflammation. CT enterography also shows deep ulcer (*arrow*) extending to the serosal surface.

enterography signs of chronic disease are submucosal fat deposition, sacculations, fibrofatty proliferation, and strictures.[5]

In Crohn disease, the mesenteric border of the bowel is preferentially affected by the inflammatory process. This may result in eventual mural fibrosis and shortening of the wall. Asymmetric fibrosis, combined with the constant increase in intraluminal pressure during the peristaltic movements, results in sacculations of the antimesenteric wall (**Fig. 9**).[3]

Fibrofatty proliferation has been long recognized as a hallmark of Crohn disease. It extends from the mesenteric attachment and partially covers the chronically inflamed loop of bowel, classically the terminal ileum. Recent studies suggest that the hypertrophied mesenteric fat might

have a role—related to the fat's capacity to produce tumor necrosis factor α—in sustaining the inflammatory process in Crohn disease.[52]

Strictures that may occur in patients with active disease are due to inflammatory process and bowel spasm. However, strictures are more frequent with chronic fibrosis.[43,47] CT enterography, similar to SBFT and enteroclysis, has a high sensitivity for diagnosing strictures. A stricture due to acute disease, manifested by bowel wall hyperenhancement, thickening, and mural stratification, is usually treated medically. Lack of enhancement and loss of stratification suggests transmural fibrosis and may require surgical intervention.[47] The findings of acute and chronic Crohn disease are summarized in **Box 3**.

Wireless capsule endoscopy is contraindicated when strictures with a luminal diameter of less than 1 cm are present (**Fig. 10**).[17,53] CT enterography, therefore, assumes an important primary role in the identification of the small bowel strictures.[5,16] Voderholzer and colleagues[53] in a prospective comparison of wireless capsule endoscopy and CT enteroclysis, could not evaluate 27% of their patients with wireless capsule endoscopy because of strictures identified on CT enteroclysis. However, wireless capsule endoscopy has high sensitivity when mild mucosal abnormalities are present and may be useful in the assessment of Crohn disease when both ileocolonoscopy and CT enterography are normal.[53] **Fig. 11** shows the algorithm illustrating our approach to the assessment for Crohn disease.

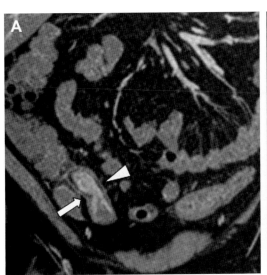
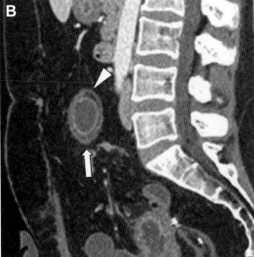

Fig. 7. Coronal (*A*) and sagittal (*B*) CT enterography images demonstrate mucosal thickening and hyperenhancement as well as submusosal edema indicative of active disease (*arrows*). Submucosal fat deposition due to chronic disease is present concurrently (*arrowheads*).

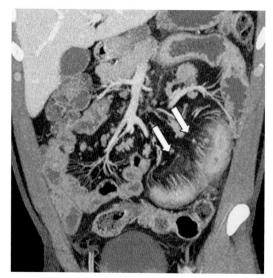

Fig. 8. Engorged vasa recta ("comb" sign) and increased attenuation of the mesenteric fat (*arrows*) adjacent to thickened and hyperenhancing jejunal loop in a patient with relapse of Crohn disease.

CT has an established role in the evaluation of extraenteric complications of Crohn disease. The most common extraenteric complications include fistula, sinus tract, abscess (**Fig. 12**), and flegmon.[2,45,47,54]

CT enterography has a high sensitivity for diagnosing fistulae. A recent study demonstrated that CT enterography correctly identifies the presence or absence of fistulae in 94% of patients.[47]

Multiplanar reformations are particularly useful for detecting fistulae. CT enterography can detect clinically unsuspected fistulae, resulting in changes in treatment regimen.[55]

Other extraenteric manifestations of Crohn disease, such as mesenteric lymphadenopathy, cholelithiasis, nephrolitiasis, sacroiliitis, and primary sclerosing cholangitis, can also be evaluated.[5]

Gastrointestinal Bleeding

Gastrointestinal bleeding may be overt or occult. Overt hemorrhage can be due to active bleeding and may be detected by CT enterography. Yoon and colleagues[56] detected 20 of 22 angiographically confirmed sites of active hemorrhage by CT during the arterial phase. Jaeckle and colleagues[57] reported similar results in a recent study.

The American Gastroenterological Association defines obscure gastrointestinal bleeding as persistent or recurring bleeding of unknown origin after negative upper and lower endoscopies.[58] Following the initial negative studies, a second evaluation with upper and lower endoscopy is performed to identify a possible overlooked lesion. The attention is turned to the small bowel if the second-look examinations are also negative.[58]

The source of obscure gastrointestinal bleeding is the small bowel in approximately 5% to 10% of patients.[59] Various imaging modalities are used for diagnosis, including wireless capsule

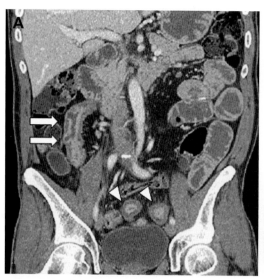

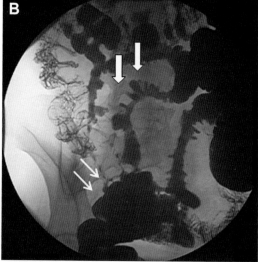

Fig. 9. (*A*) CT enterography shows sacculations along the antimesenteric wall (*arrows*). There is mural hyperenhancement and thickening of the ileal loops in a patient with active disease (*arrowheads*). (*B*) Corresponding SBFT shows sacculations (*arrows*), but overlap of small bowel loops (*small arrows*) in the pelvis limits their evaluation (*small arrows*).

Box 3
Findings of active and chronic Crohn disease on CT enterography

Findings of active inflammation

Mural hyperenhancement, stratification, and thickening

Perienteric fat stranding and engorged vasa recta

Findings of chronic inflammation

Submucosal fat deposition

Mural thickening without enhancement

Perienteric fat hypertrophy

Sacculation of antimesenteric bowel wall

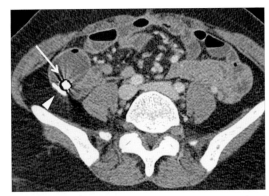

Fig. 10. Axial CT enterography image shows retained capsule endoscope (*arrow*) with an adjacent enterolith (*arrowhead*) in a dilated ileal loop proximal to a stricture (not shown).

endoscopy, push enteroscopy, double-balloon endoscopy, CT enterography, nuclear scan, and SBFT. Currently, wireless capsule endoscopy is the most sensitive examination for detecting the source of occult bleeding with reported sensitivity ranging from 42% to 80%.[60–62] In a meta-analysis by Treister and colleagues[63,64] wireless capsule endoscopy was superior to push enteroscopy and small bowel radiography for detecting small bowel pathology. However, as previously discussed, wireless capsule endoscopy has several disadvantages that may limit its use. SBFT has a limited role in the detection of obscure gastrointestinal bleeding. Its main role is to exclude adhesions and strictures in planning for capsule endoscopy.

The role of CT enterography in the workup of obscure gastrointestinal bleeding is still evolving. CT enterography is an excellent adjunct in the workup of obscure gastrointestinal bleeding. A distinct advantage of CT enterography over wireless capsule endoscopy is its ability to evaluate submucosal and serosal abnormalities.[13] Tew and colleagues[65] reported that MDCT correctly showed the site of bleeding in 7 of 10 patients.

Huprich and colleagues[13] reported that multiphasic CT enterography demonstrated the site of bleeding in 8 of 10 patients. Additionally CT enterography was able to depict abnormalities not identified by wireless capsule endoscopy and colonoscopy.[13]

CT enterography protocols for the evaluation of obscure gastrointestinal bleeding are optimized to detect an abnormal area of enhancement in bowel wall or to demonstrate active bleeding.[13] As described previously, multiple phases are necessary for the detection of gastrointestinal bleeding. Our protocol is summarized in **Table 1**.

The differential diagnosis for obscure gastrointestinal bleeding can be narrowed based on the age of the patient. In the geriatric population, vascular lesions and nonsteroidal anti-inflammatory drug (NSAID) enteropathy are the most common causes of small bowel bleeding.[59] Vascular lesions consist of a variety of different entities with different angiographic and CT appearances.[59,66] Angiodysplasia is the most frequent vascular lesion of the bowel. An early filling vein during the arterial phase may be a clue to the nearby location of this lesion.[66,67] Active small

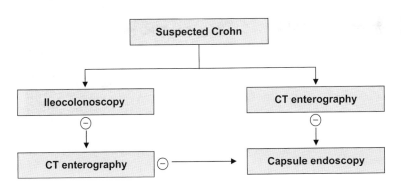

Fig. 11. Algorithm showing authors' approach to the assessment for Crohn disease.

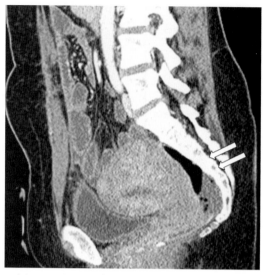

Fig. 12. Presacral abscess (*arrows*) in a patient with Crohn disease. Sagittal reformations are very useful for the evaluation of the presacral space.

bowel bleeding is observed as gradual accumulation of contrast material within the bowel lumen on multiphasic CT enterography (**Fig. 13**).[13] NSAID erosions and ulcers are difficult to distinguish from Crohn disease on wireless capsule endoscopy.[68] NSAID-related weblike strictures in the small bowel are a cause for retained wireless capsule.

In younger adults, Crohn disease, tumors, and Meckel diverticulum are the most frequent sources of occult gastrointestinal bleeding.[59,69]

Small Bowel Neoplasms

Small bowel tumors are uncommon and represent 3% to 6% of all gastrointestinal tumors. The clinical symptoms are frequently nonspecific, resulting in delayed diagnosis.[70] The most common tumors are gastrointestinal stromal tumors (**Fig. 14**), adenocarcinoma, lymphoma, and carcinoid tumors.[71,72] CT enterography may be helpful in detection of polyps in polyposis syndromes. Multiphasic CT enterography, with similar protocol as described for gastrointestinal bleeding, is required to detect many of these neoplasms.[70] Although some tumors are better visualized on the arterial phase, others may be more conspicuous on the portal venous phase (see **Fig. 14**).

Although there are no large published studies on the efficacy of CT enterography for evaluating small bowel tumors, Pilleul and colleagues[70] reported an accuracy of 84.7% in depicting small bowel neoplasms with CT enteroclysis.

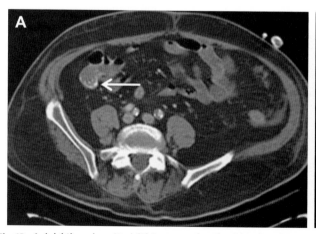
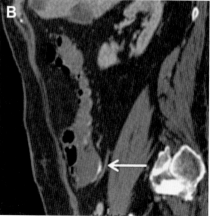

Fig. 13. Axial (*A*) and sagittal (*B*) images of active bleeding in the right colon (*arrows*) due to angiodysplasia.

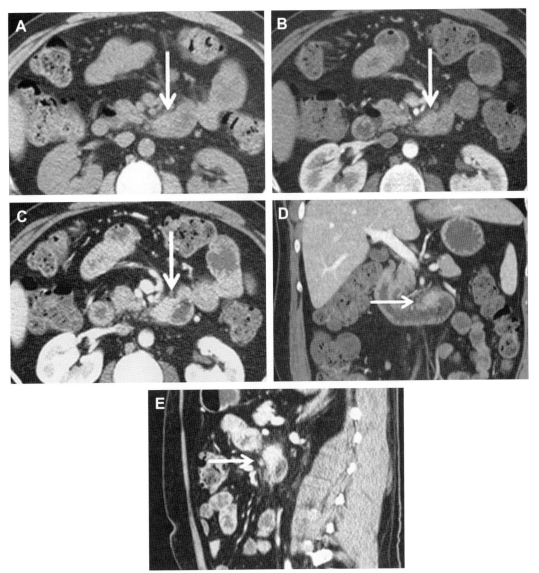

Fig. 14. Gastrointestinal stromal tumor in the duodenum. Multiphasic CT enterography (*A*) precontrast phase, (*B*) arterial phase, and (*C*) portal venous phase show a predominantly subserosal lesion (*arrows*). The tumor is better seen on the portal venous phase images. Coronal (*D*) and sagittal (*E*) images improve localization of the tumor (*arrows*).

SUMMARY

CT enterography is a new imaging modality that has several advantages over conventional CT, wireless capsule endoscopy, and barium examination. CT enterography is noninvasive and allows mapping of disease activity before endoscopy and in cases where the endoscope cannot reach a bowel segment. It is rapid, readily available, operator independent, and allows evaluation of extraenteric complications of small bowel disease. Its role as the first-line modality in the work-up of suspected or known small bowel pathology is evolving.

REFERENCES

1. Wold PB, Fletcher JG, Johnson CD, et al. Assessment of small bowel Crohn disease: noninvasive peroral CT enterography compared with other imaging methods and endoscopy-feasibility study. Radiology 2003;229(1):275–81.
2. Maglinte DD, Hallett RL, Rex D, et al. Imaging of small bowel Crohn's disease: Can abdominal CT replace barium radiography? Emergency Radiology 2001;8:127–33.
3. Paulsen SR, Huprich JE, Hara AK. CT enterography: noninvasive evaluation of Crohn's disease and

obscure gastrointestinal bleed. Radiol Clin North Am 2007;45(2):303–15.

4. Macari M, Megibow AJ, Balthazar EJ. A pattern approach to the abnormal small bowel: observations at MDCT and CT enterography. AJR Am J Roentgenol 2007;188(5):1344–55.

5. Paulsen SR, Huprich JE, Fletcher JG, et al. CT enterography as a diagnostic tool in evaluating small bowel disorders: review of clinical experience with over 700 cases. Radiographics 2006; 26(3):641–57.

6. Megibow AJ, Babb JS, Hecht EM, et al. Evaluation of bowel distention and bowel wall appearance by using neutral oral contrast agent for multi-detector row CT. Radiology 2006;238(1):87–95.

7. Bruining DH, Loftus EV Jr. Technology insight: new techniques for imaging the gut in patients with IBD. Nat Clin Pract Gastroenterol Hepatol 2008; 5(3):154–61.

8. Boriskin HS, Devito BS, Hines JJ, et al. CT enterography vs. capsule endoscopy. Abdom Imaging 2008 [online publication].

9. Booya F, Fletcher JG, Huprich JE, et al. Active Crohn disease: CT findings and interobserver agreement for enteric phase CT enterography. Radiology 2006;241(3):787–95.

10. Fletcher JG. CT enterography technique: theme and variations. Abdom Imaging 2008 [online publication].

11. Hong SS, Kim AY, Byun JH, et al. MDCT of small-bowel disease: value of 3D imaging. AJR Am J Roentgenol 2006;187(5):1212–21.

12. American College of Radiology. ACR Appropriateness Criteria 2005. Available at: www.acr.org.

13. Huprich JE, Fletcher JG, Alexander JA, et al. Obscure gastrointestinal bleeding: evaluation with 64-section multiphase CT enterography—initial experience. Radiology 2008;246(2):562–71.

14. Jaffe TA, Gaca AM, Delaney S, et al. Radiation doses from small-bowel follow-through and abdominopelvic MDCT in Crohn's disease. AJR Am J Roentgenol 2007;189(5):1015–22.

15. Maglinte DD, Sandrasegaran K, Lappas JC, et al. CT enteroclysis. Radiology 2007;245(3):661–71.

16. Solem CA, Loftus EV Jr, Fletcher JG, et al. Small-bowel imaging in Crohn's disease: a prospective, blinded, 4-way comparison trial. Gastrointest Endosc 2008;68(2):255–66.

17. Cheifetz AS, Kornbluth AA, Legnani P, et al. The risk of retention of the capsule endoscope in patients with known or suspected Crohn's disease. Am J Gastroenterol 2006;101(10):2218–22.

18. Cave D, Legnani P, de FR, et al. ICCE consensus for capsule retention. Endoscopy 2005;37(10): 1065–7.

19. Gay G, Delvaux M, Rey JF. The role of video capsule endoscopy in the diagnosis of digestive diseases:

a review of current possibilities. Endoscopy 2004; 36(10):913–20.

20. Schmidt S, Lepori D, Meuwly JY, et al. Prospective comparison of MR enteroclysis with multidetector spiral-CT enteroclysis: interobserver agreement and sensitivity by means of "sign-by-sign" correlation. Eur Radiol 2003;13(6):1303–11.

21. Albert JG, Martiny F, Krummenerl A, et al. Diagnosis of small bowel Crohn's disease: a prospective comparison of capsule endoscopy with magnetic resonance imaging and fluoroscopic enteroclysis. Gut 2005;54(12):1721–7.

22. Masselli G, Casciani E, Polettini E, et al. Comparison of MR enteroclysis with MR enterography and conventional enteroclysis in patients with Crohn's disease. Eur Radiol 2008;18(3):438–47.

23. Schindera ST, Nelson RC, Delong DM, et al. Multidetector row CT of the small bowel: peak enhancement temporal window—initial experience. Radiology 2007;243(2):438–44.

24. Harris JP, Nelson RC. Abdominal imaging with multidetector computed tomography: state of the art. J Comput Assist Tomogr 2004;28(Suppl 1):S17–9.

25. Horton KM, Fishman EK. The current status of multidetector row CT and three-dimensional imaging of the small bowel. Radiol Clin North Am 2003;41(2): 199–212.

26. Horton KM, Eng J, Fishman EK. Normal enhancement of the small bowel: evaluation with spiral CT. J Comput Assist Tomogr 2000;24(1):67–71.

27. Raptopoulos V, Schwartz RK, McNicholas MM, et al. Multiplanar helical CT enterography in patients with Crohn's disease. AJR Am J Roentgenol 1997; 169(6):1545–50.

28. Koo CW, Shah-Patel LR, Baer JW, et al. Cost-effectiveness and patient tolerance of low-attenuation oral contrast material: milk versus VoLumen. AJR Am J Roentgenol 2008;190(5):1307–13.

29. Cohade C, Osman M, Nakamoto Y, et al. Initial experience with oral contrast in PET/CT: phantom and clinical studies. J Nucl Med 2003;44(3):412–6.

30. Prabhakar HB, Sahani DV, Fischman AJ, et al. Bowel hot spots at PET-CT. Radiographics 2007;27(1): 145–59.

31. Antoch G, Kuehl H, Kanja J, et al. Dual-modality PET/CT scanning with negative oral contrast agent to avoid artifacts: introduction and evaluation. Radiology 2004;230(3):879–85.

32. Winter TC, Ager JD, Nghiem HV, et al. Upper gastrointestinal tract and abdomen: water as an orally administered contrast agent for helical CT. Radiology 1996;201(2):365–70.

33. Young BM, Fletcher JG, Booya F, et al. Head-to-head comparison of oral contrast agents for cross-sectional enterography: small bowel distention, timing, and side effects. J Comput Assist Tomogr 2008; 32(1):32–8.

34. Kuehle CA, Ajaj W, Ladd SC, et al. Hydro-MRI of the small bowel: effect of contrast volume, timing of contrast administration, and data acquisition on bowel distention. AJR Am J Roentgenol 2006;187(4): W375–85.

35. Bodily KD, Fletcher JG, Solem CA, et al. Crohn Disease: mural attenuation and thickness at contrast-enhanced CT Enterography—correlation with endoscopic and histologic findings of inflammation. Radiology 2006;238(2):505–16.

36. Bae KT. Peak contrast enhancement in CT and MR angiography: When does it occur and why? Pharmacokinetic study in a porcine model. Radiology 2003; 227(3):809–16.

37. Fidler J. MR imaging of the small bowel. Radiol Clin North Am 2007;45(2):317–31.

38. Colombel JF, Solem CA, Sandborn WJ, et al. Quantitative measurement and visual assessment of ileal Crohn's disease activity by computed tomography enterography: correlation with endoscopic severity and C reactive protein. Gut 2006;55(11):1561–7.

39. Vandenbroucke F, Mortele KJ, Tatli S, et al. Noninvasive multidetector computed tomography enterography in patients with small-bowel Crohn's disease: Is a 40-second delay better than 70 seconds? Acta Radiol 2007;1–9.

40. Jaffe TA, Martin LC, Miller CM, et al. Abdominal pain: coronal reformations from isotropic voxels with 16-section CT–reader lesion detection and interpretation time. Radiology 2007;242(1):175–81.

41. Jaffe TA, Nelson RC, Johnson GA, et al. Optimization of multiplanar reformations from isotropic data sets acquired with 16-detector row helical CT scanner. Radiology 2006;238(1):292–9.

42. Yaghmai V, Nikolaidis P, Hammond NA, et al. Multidetector-row computed tomography diagnosis of small bowel obstruction: Can coronal reformations replace axial images? Emerg Radiol 2006;13(2):69–72.

43. Wills JS, Lobis IF, Denstman FJ. Crohn disease: state of the art. Radiology 1997;202(3):597–610.

44. Stange EF, Travis SP, Vermeire S, et al. European evidence based consensus on the diagnosis and management of Crohn's disease: definitions and diagnosis. Gut 2006;55(Suppl 1):i1–15.

45. Maglinte DD, Gourtsoyiannis N, Rex D, et al. Classification of small bowel Crohn's subtypes based on multimodality imaging. Radiol Clin North Am 2003; 41(2):285–303.

46. Hara AK, Alam S, Heigh RI, et al. Using CT enterography to monitor Crohn's disease activity: a preliminary study. AJR Am J Roentgenol 2008;190(6): 1512–6.

47. Vogel J, da Luz MA, Baker M, et al. CT enterography for Crohn's disease: accurate preoperative diagnostic imaging. Dis Colon Rectum 2007;50(11):1761–9.

48. Meyers MA, McGuire PV. Spiral CT demonstration of hypervascularity in Crohn disease: "vascular jejunization of the ileum" or the "comb sign". Abdom Imaging 1995;20(4):327–32.

49. Jones B, Fishman EK, Hamilton SR, et al. Submucosal accumulation of fat in inflammatory bowel disease: CT/pathologic correlation. J Comput Assist Tomogr 1986;10(5):759–63.

50. Madureira AJ. The comb sign. Radiology 2004; 230(3):783–4.

51. Lee SS, Ha HK, Yang SK, et al. CT of prominent pericolic or perienteric vasculature in patients with Crohn's disease: correlation with clinical disease activity and findings on barium studies. AJR Am J Roentgenol 2002;179(4):1029–36.

52. Desreumaux P, Ernst O, Geboes K, et al. Inflammatory alterations in mesenteric adipose tissue in Crohn's disease. Gastroenterology 1999;117(1): 73–81.

53. Voderholzer WA, Beinhoelzl J, Rogalla P, et al. Small bowel involvement in Crohn's disease: a prospective comparison of wireless capsule endoscopy and computed tomography enteroclysis. Gut 2005; 54(3):369–73.

54. Schwartz DA, Loftus EV Jr, Tremaine WJ, et al. The natural history of fistulizing Crohn's disease in Olmsted County, Minnesota. Gastroenterology 2002;122(4):875–80.

55. Booya F, Akram S, Fletcher JG, et al. CT enterography and fistulizing Crohn's disease: clinical benefit and radiographic findings. Abdom Imaging 2008 [online publication].

56. Yoon W, Jeong YY, Shin SS, et al. Acute massive gastrointestinal bleeding: detection and localization with arterial phase multi-detector row helical CT. Radiology 2006;239(1):160–7.

57. Jaeckle T, Stuber G, Hoffmann MH, et al. Detection and localization of acute upper and lower gastrointestinal (GI) bleeding with arterial phase multi-detector row helical CT. Eur Radiol 2008;18(7):1406–13.

58. AGA technical review on the evaluation and management of occult and obscure gastrointestinal bleeding. Gastroenterology 2000;118:201–21.

59. Lewis BS. Small intestinal bleeding. Gastroenterol Clin North Am 2000;29(1):67–95, vi.

60. Pennazio M, Santucci R, Rondonotti E, et al. Outcome of patients with obscure gastrointestinal bleeding after capsule endoscopy: report of 100 consecutive cases. Gastroenterology 2004;126(3): 643–53.

61. Magnano A, Privitera A, Calogero G, et al. The role of capsule endoscopy in the work-up of obscure gastrointestinal bleeding. Eur J Gastroenterol Hepatol 2004;16(4):403–6.

62. Scapa E, Jacob H, Lewkowicz S, et al. Initial experience of wireless-capsule endoscopy for evaluating occult gastrointestinal bleeding and suspected small bowel pathology. Am J Gastroenterol 2002; 97(11):2776–9.

63. Triester SL, Leighton JA, Leontiadis GI, et al. A meta-analysis of the yield of capsule endoscopy compared to other diagnostic modalities in patients with obscure gastrointestinal bleeding. Am J Gastroenterol 2005;100(11):2407–18.

64. Leighton JA, Triester SL, Sharma VK. Capsule endoscopy: a meta-analysis for use with obscure gastrointestinal bleeding and Crohn's disease. Gastrointest Endosc Clin N Am 2006;16(2):229–50.

65. Tew K, Davies RP, Jadun CK, et al. MDCT of acute lower gastrointestinal bleeding. AJR Am J Roentgenol 2004;182(2):427–30.

66. Huprich JE. Multi-phase CT enterography in obscure GI bleeding. Abdom Imaging 2008 [online publication].

67. Boley SJ, Sprayregen S, Sammartano RJ, et al. The pathophysiologic basis for the angiographic signs of vascular ectasias of the colon. Radiology 1977; 125(3):615–21.

68. Lin S, Rockey DC. Obscure gastrointestinal bleeding. Gastroenterol Clin North Am 2005;34(4):679–98.

69. Elsayes KM, Menias CO, Harvin HJ, et al. Imaging manifestations of Meckel's diverticulum. AJR Am J Roentgenol 2007;189(1):81–8.

70. Pilleul F, Penigaud M, Milot L, et al. Possible small-bowel neoplasms: contrast-enhanced and water-enhanced multidetector CT enteroclysis. Radiology 2006;241(3):796–801.

71. Minardi AJ Jr, Zibari GB, Aultman DF, et al. Small-bowel tumors. J Am Coll Surg 1998 June;186(6):664–8.

72. Horton KM, Kamel I, Hofmann L, et al. Carcinoid tumors of the small bowel: a multitechnique imaging approach. AJR Am J Roentgenol 2004;182(3):559–67.

CT Colonography: Techniques and Applications

Judy Yee, MD

KEYWORDS

- CT colonography • Colorectal carcinoma • Colorectal polyp
- Colonoscopy • Cancer screening • Stool tagging

CT colonography (CTC), also termed virtual colonoscopy, is increasingly accepted at sites throughout the world as a new effective tool for the diagnosis and screening of colorectal carcinoma. The goal of CTC is to identify the benign precursor adenomatous polyp before it has degenerated into adenocarcinoma. The incidence of malignancy in an adenomatous polyp increases with increasing polyp size. Polyps ranging between 10–15 mm in size carry up to a 15% chance of becoming malignant within 10 years whereas polyps between 5–9 mm in size have up to a 5% chance of transforming into a malignancy in 10 years.[1]

Single center studies and multicenter trials using state of the art techniques have shown that CTC has excellent performance for the detection of clinically important polyps with approximately 90%–92% per-polyp sensitivity and 96% specificity for 10 mm and larger polyps.[2–5] The American College of Radiology Imaging Network (ACRIN) National CT Colonography Trial, which is the largest multicenter trial evaluating CTC performance, involved 2531 asymptomatic subjects recruited from 15 sites in the United States. Patients were scanned on 16-row multidetector CT or higher; electronic insufflation of the colon was performed using carbon dioxide; stool and fluid tagging was employed; and qualified readers were included. Results revealed overall per-patient sensitivity and specificity of 90% and 86% respectively for 10 mm or larger neoplasia. with 23% and 99% positive and negative predictive values. The per-polyp sensitivity for large polyps and cancers was 84%.[6]

Meta-analyses have also demonstrated the ability of CTC to detect clinically significant polyps with high sensitivity and specificity. In a meta-analysis by Sosna and colleagues,[7] the results of 14 studies evaluating a total of 1324 patients with 1411 polyps were compiled. All studies used 5 mm collimation and were performed in high-risk patients except for two of the trials. The overall combined per-polyp sensitivity for polyps measuring 10 mm or larger, 6–9 mm, and 5 mm or smaller were 81%, 62% and 43% respectively. The overall combined per-patient sensitivities for polyps measuring 10 mm or larger, 6–9 mm, and 5 mm or smaller were 88%, 84% and 65%, respectively. The overall specificities for detecting polyps 10 mm or larger was 95%. This meta-analysis determined that CTC has high sensitivity and specificity for polyps 10 mm or larger. Halligan and colleagues[8] performed a meta-analysis that included 24 studies with a total of 2610 patients. This study found overall per-patient sensitivity and specificity for 10 mm or larger lesions to be 93% and 97% respectively, which decreased to 86% and 96% respectively for 6–9 mm polyps. Mulhall and colleagues[9] evaluated 33 different studies, which included data on 6393 patients. Heterogeneous sensitivity was found for CTC, which improved with increasing polyp size. The pooled sensitivities for lesions measuring 10 mm or larger, 6–9 mm, and 5 mm or smaller were 85%, 70% and 48%, respectively. The pooled specificities for lesions measuring 10 mm or larger, 6–9 mm, and 5 mm or smaller were 97%, 93% and 92%, respectively. Overall specificity was maintained across different polyp size categories.

University of California, San Francisco, VA Medical Center, 4150 Clement Street, San Francisco, CA 94121, USA
E-mail address: judy.yee@radiology.ucsf.edu

Radiol Clin N Am 47 (2009) 133–145
doi:10.1016/j.rcl.2008.11.002
0033-8389/08/$ – see front Mater. Published by Elsevier Inc.

CT COLONOGRAPHY TECHNIQUE

CT scanner detector configuration, as well as computer hardware and software for CTC, have undergone significant technological evolution and have contributed to the increased ability to obtain diagnostic accuracy. However, the ability of CTC to accurately detect colorectal lesions also depends upon two essential prerequisites. The colon should be optimally cleansed and well distended to ensure the ability of the reader to detect true lesions. The presence of fluid or solid stool remaining in the colon can cause for both missed lesions as well as pseudolesions. A focal area of segmental collapse can also cause polyps to be overlooked and may also mimic an annular carcinoma. Standard CTC protocol requires scanning in two opposing views, typically in supine and prone, so that segments of the colon that have retained material or suboptimal distention on one view may show improved cleansing or distention in the other position.[10,11]

BOWEL CLEANSING

Currently, patients are required to undergo a bowel-cleansing regimen before the CTC that is similar to bowel preparations used for optical colonoscopy. There are two main components of the colonic preparation protocol for CTC. The first component consists of dietary restriction starting the day before the CT scan. Patients are required to avoid solid foods and to maintain a clear liquid diet. The second component is the administration of a cathartic agent that will evacuate remaining contents from the colon. Typical laxatives that are employed for CTC include dry preparation agents or saline cathartics such as magnesium citrate and sodium phosphate. These agents are preferred for CTC because they tend to leave the colon with significantly less residual fluid that may obscure lesions. A wet preparation agent such as polyethylene glycol is commonly ingested in large volumes and is not favored for CTC (**Fig. 1**).

Magnesium Citrate

Magnesium citrate is a saline laxative that is used for CTC. Its mechanisms of action include both prevention of fluid resorption and the stimulation of cholecystokinin. Cholecystokinin acts by stimulating small bowel fluid secretion, enhancing peristalsis and promoting colonic emptying.[12] Magnesium citrate is available in either a powder form that the patient mixes with 8 ounces of water before ingestion or as a liquid in a 10-ounce bottle, which is ready for ingestion. Patients are instructed to drink the magnesium citrate in the late afternoon on the day before the CTC. Onset of action is typically in about one hour. To prevent dehydration patients are encouraged to maintain hydration by ingesting an additional 8 ounces of liquid immediately following ingestion of the magnesium citrate and then every other hour until evacuation is complete. Near bedtime, the patient ingests four 5 mg bisacodyl tablets, which have a relatively long onset of action over 6–12 hours. A 10 mg bisacodyl suppository is administered on the morning of the CTC, which has a short onset of action within one hour. It acts as a contact laxative and stimulates parasympathetic reflexes to increase peristalsis.[13]

Magnesium citrate has the advantage that it does not cause the same severe electrolyte disturbances that have been found associated with other saline cathartics such as sodium phosphate. The sodium content of magnesium citrate is significantly less than sodium phosphate and therefore magnesium citrate may be preferred in patients who are at risk for electrolyte abnormalities. In a study of 506 patients undergoing colonoscopy, 284 patients were randomized to receive magnesium citrate in combination with a low-fiber meal kit and 222 patients received a double-dose of sodium phosphate. The patients who received magnesium citrate were found to have significantly better colon cleansing, with better subject tolerance and willingness to repeat the cathartic preparation.[14] A combination of magnesium citrate with a smaller volume of polyethylene glycol has been used successfully as a cleansing regimen for colonoscopy. This formula was found to improve cleansing and to shorten preparation times.[15]

Sodium Phosphate

Sodium phosphate is a commonly used saline cathartic for bowel cleansing before fiberoptic colonoscopy. It is also used as a colonic cleansing agent before CTC. The osmotic effects of sodium phosphate can cause for large fluid and electrolyte shifts. A single dose of sodium phosphate consisting of an aliquot of 45 mL (1.5 fluid ounces) is typically suggested for CTC. Patients mix 45 mL of sodium phosphate with 4 ounces of water, which is ingested with an additional 8 ounces of water in the late afternoon of the day before the CTC. Onset of action of the laxative effect is in about one hour. Four bisacodyl tablets and a bisacodyl suppository are administered in addition to the sodium phosphate solution as described above for the magnesium citrate regimen.

Saline cathartics such as sodium phosphate result in a relatively dry colon because they leave

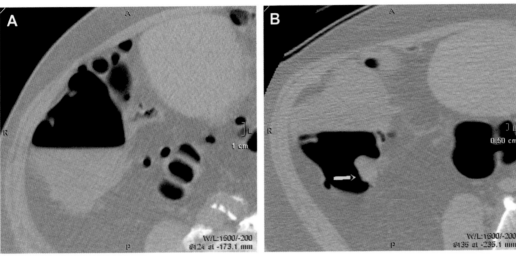

Fig. 1. (*A*) Supine axial image in a patient who received polyethylene glycol lavage solution as a cleansing agent for CTC demonstrates a large amount of residual fluid that obscures about 50% of the lumen. (*B*) Prone axial image in the same patient. The large fluid pool has shifted to reveal a large polyp (*arrow*) that was hidden by it.

minimal fluid in the colon. However, this may then cause small pieces of residual solid material to adhere to the colon wall, which may cause pseudopolyps on CTC. There have been conflicting results in the literature comparing the adequacy of colonic cleansing using sodium phosphate versus polyethylene glycol before colonoscopy. Some studies show no difference between the two agents[16–18] whereas other trials have found sodium phosphate to cleanse the colon more effectively than polyethylene glycol.[19–21] Hsu and colleagues[22] performed a meta-analysis of eight trials that evaluated the adequacy of sodium phosphate versus polyethylene glycol for cleansing the colon before colonoscopy. The quality of bowel cleansing was found to be similar for the two laxatives. The advantages of sodium phosphate were better patient tolerance and a cost savings compared to polyethylene glycol.

The use of sodium phosphate may uncommonly result in serious electrolyte abnormalities. Patients may become dehydrated and develop hypernatremia, hypokalemia, hyperphosphatemia and hypocalcemia.[23,24] Metabolic acidosis, renal failure due to acute phosphate nephropathy, tetany, and death have been reported in patients ingesting more than the 45 mL dose and/or in patients at medical risk.[25,26] Sodium phosphate administration is contraindicated in patients with renal insufficiency, history of electrolyte disturbances, congestive heart failure, ascites, ileus, colitis and bowel obstruction or perforation.[27] Patients taking diuretics, angiotensin-converting enzyme (ACE) inhibitors or other medications

such as nonsteroidal anti-inflammatory drugs (NSAIDS) that affect electrolytes or renal function should also avoid sodium phosphate. The U. S. Food and Drug Administration has published a warning to physicians stating the potential adverse events of sodium phosphate.[28]

STOOL AND FLUID TAGGING

There is increasing experience with the use of oral tagging agents to label residual stool and fluid. The interest in developing tagging regimens is related to potentially improving patient experience by decreasing or eliminating the need for a cathartic. Stool and fluid tagging may also help improve the sensitivity and specificity of CTC for polyp detection. Solid particles that are tagged should be more easily differentiated from the soft tissue density of polyps. Tagged fluid can allow easier discrimination of soft tissue polyps that may be submerged within it (**Fig. 2**). Software is available that allows the electronic subtraction of tagged material from the colon.

Tagging protocols employing barium by itself have been reported to be effective.[29–31] Other studies have demonstrated that iodinated contrast ingested alone may also be used to tag residual material in the colon with the added advantage of an induced osmotic effect that will result in some catharsis.[32–34] A large multicenter trial has successfully used a combination of oral barium and iodinated contrast material for tagging.[6] Typically, barium is ingested to label any solid stool remaining in the colon and iodinated contrast material is taken

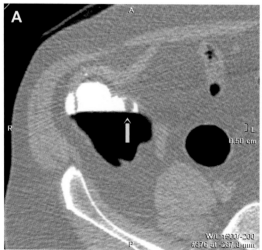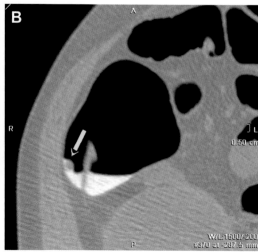

Fig. 2. (*A*) Prone axial image demonstrates a rounded soft tissue density polyp (*arrow*) submerged within a pool of tagged fluid. (*B*) Supine axial image in a different patient reveals easy identification of the soft tissue density polyp (*arrow*) adjacent to a pool of homogeneously tagged fluid.

to tag residual fluid pools with the goal being to obtain homogeneous labeling of all residual material. In the ACRIN National CT Colonography Trial, subjects were restricted to a clear liquid diet the day before the CT scan and underwent colonic cleansing using one of three standardized bowel preparations (ie, magnesium citrate, sodium phosphate, or polyethylene glycol).[6] A total volume of 40 mL of high density 40% weight/volume barium (Tagitol V; Lake Success, NY) was administered orally the day before the CT scan in three doses (20 mL at 8 AM, 10 mL at 11 AM, 10 mL at 2PM). A total volume of 60 mL of iodinated contrast material (Gastrografin 37% organically bound iodine) was administered in three aliquots of 20 mL each starting the evening before the CT scan. Each dose of iodinated contrast material was mixed with 8 ounces of water and then ingested. Modifications of the tagging protocol from another large trial include bowel cleansing with either magnesium citrate or sodium phosphate. Subjects received a single dose of 250 mL of low density 2.1% barium at 6–8 PM for stool tagging and a single dose of 60 mL of diatrizoate meglumine and diatrizoate sodium (Gastrografin) at 9–11 PM for fluid tagging on the evening before the CTC.[35] Although these studies were performed with the use of tagging, a full bowel cleansing regimen was followed. The use of reduced cathartic and noncathartic regimens combined with tagging is currently being investigated. Early studies examining polyp detection in the setting of tagging without cathartic preparation or with reduced cathartic preparation have reported favorable results.[36–38]

BOWEL DISTENTION

Optimal colonic distention is a key prerequisite for obtaining a CTC examination that allows detection of lesions on both two- and three-dimensional (3D) views (**Fig. 3**). A portion of the colon that is poorly distended or collapsed may mimic an annular carcinoma particularly on the 3D endoluminal view. Poor distention can also cause folds to appear thicker or more bulbous in appearance so that they simulate polyps. Suboptimal distention may also cause for missed lesions.

Insufflation of the colon requires placement of a small caliber, flexible rectal tube typically with the patient in a right side down decubitus position. Insertion of the rectal tube is performed by trained personnel according to local guidelines. Initially, there is filling of the rectosigmoid and descending colon. Rotating the patient into the supine position allows filling of the transverse colon and then the right colon. Often a minimum of three liters of gas is required to distend the colon adequately. Additional gas is administered if the patient has difficulty with gaseous retention. The rectal balloon may be inflated with approximately 10–15 mL of room air to aid in gaseous and tube retention. A digital rectal examination is suggested to examine the rectal vault for any lesions before rectal balloon inflation and to help avoid the possibility of causing perforation or significant bleeding. It should be noted that adequate distention is often obtained without the need to inflate the rectal balloon.

Personnel are trained to assess the patient for optimal colonic distention by evaluating for

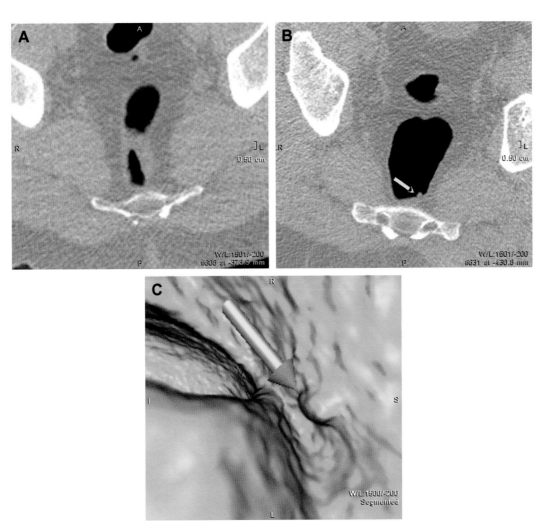

Fig. 3. (*A*) The rectum is nearly collapsed on this supine axial image. (*B*) A small rectal polyp (*arrows*) is identified along the posterior wall with better distention in the prone position. (*C*) Better distention also allows visualization of the small polyp on the 3D endoluminal view.

maximum patient tolerance or inquiring when the patient feels a sense of fullness or mild discomfort in the right abdomen. The sense of fullness is an indicator that gas has moved retrograde sufficiently to distend the right colon and then a CT scout view is acquired. Following the supine CT data acquisition, the patient is moved into the prone position and another scout image is obtained. Additional gas may be administered if there are any colon segments that are not optimally distended. Lifting the torso of the patient off of the CT scanner table in the prone position will aid in improved distention of the transverse colon.

Although room air may be used for distention of the colon for CTC, many sites have converted to the use of electronic insufflation of the colon with carbon dioxide (CO_2). Studies have found that there is improved patient comfort when CO_2 is used for colonic distention. Carbon dioxide has higher lipid solubility and a higher partial pressure gradient compared with room air, which allows increased resorption across the colon wall. Patients will then exhale the resorbed CO_2 through the lungs. Burling and colleagues[39] compared adequacy of colonic distention and patient experience in 47 patients who received automated carbon dioxide insufflation and 94 patients who received manual carbon dioxide insufflation for CTC. Automated carbon dioxide insufflation was found to significantly improve colonic distention with the most benefit in the distal colon with the patient in a supine position. Kim and colleagues[40] performed a study on 36 patients with severe luminal narrowing due to carcinoma who received carbon dioxide insufflation for CTC. Results demonstrated that automated pressure-controlled CO2 insufflation is as efficient for colonic distention in colorectal carcinoma patients with severe luminal narrowing as it is in patients without narrowing.

The electronic insufflator device for CTC allows administration of CO_2 at a fixed rate of 3 L/minute and up to a maximum pressure of 25 mm Hg. Typically a total of approximately 4 L of CO_2 is administered to obtain adequate colonic distention. If there is a segment of the colon that is compromised because of poor distention and/or cleansing on both supine and prone images, a limited rescan of the particular segment may be obtained with the patient in a decubitus position. Additionally, a full rotation of the patient on the CT scanner table may be helpful for redistributing gas and residual material in the colon.

Glucagon

An antispasmodic agent may be administered before CTC to reduce spasm, decrease motion artifacts from peristalsis, and increase patient comfort. Glucagon hydrochloride has been used for CTC although its benefits have not been clearly demonstrated. Patients may uncommonly experience adverse reactions to glucagons, such as nausea, vomiting and headache. Nausea was reported in 4% of patients who received intravenous glucagon before CTC.[41] Contraindications to the use of glucagon include: patients who have insulinoma, pheochromocytoma, poorly controlled diabetes, and known glucagon hypersensitivity. Hyoscine butylbromide (Buscopan) has been found to be effective for improving colonic distention for CTC although it is not approved for use in the United States.[42]

Several studies have been published evaluating the effectiveness of glucagon for CTC. Yee and colleagues[43] studied 60 patients undergoing CTC who received manual air insufflation of the colon. One milligram of glucagon was administered intravenously immediately before the CT scan to 33 patients in the glucagon group. There were no statistically significant differences between the glucagon and nonglucagon groups for segmental as well as overall colonic distention scores in the supine, prone, and combined supine–prone positions. Morrin and colleagues[41] evaluated 74 patients who received intravenous glucagon before CTC. Mean distention scores for the glucagon and nonglucagon groups were similar. The use of glucagon has not been found to improve polyp detection on CTC in an initial study.[44]

The routine administration of glucagon for CTC is not suggested. However, glucagon may be administered when the patient experiences significant abdominal discomfort or if there is persistent spasm or poor distention that is not improved by dual positioning.

MULTIDETECTOR CT PROTOCOL

Multidetector CT scanners are preferred for CTC; they allow thinner slices, shorter scan times, reduced radiation dose and the ability to maintain length of coverage through the abdomen and pelvis so that the entire colorectum can be imaged. The acquisition of thin sections decreases partial volume averaging and improves image quality of the multiplanar reformatted views and the 3D endoluminal images. Lui and colleagues[45] evaluated various slice thicknesses at CTC and demonstrated improved specificity using thin sections. The CTC data from 25 patients were reconstructed using 1.25 mm sections reconstructed every 1.0 mm and using 5.0 mm sections reconstructed every 2.0 mm. Although no significant difference was found in sensitivity for polyp detection comparing thin and thick sections, the number of false positive findings was significantly lower for thin sections compared with thick sections.

Multidetector CT scanners allow narrower collimation for CTC. When using a 64-row multidetector CT scanner, the collimation typically ranges between 0.5–0.625 mm. Other CT scan parameters include: an effective mAs = 50; kV = 120; rotation time = .5 seconds; and reconstructions = 1–1.25 mm. Acquisition times in each position will be less than 10 seconds (**Table 1**). Evaluation of the extracolonic structures using thicker reconstructions of 2.5–5.0 mm is more time efficient. The American College of Radiology Practice Guidelines for the Performance of CTC suggest a collimation of ≤ 3 mm with a reconstruction interval of ≤ 1.5 mm.[11] Increased tube current (mAs) is needed for obese patients or when intravenous contrast is administered for CTC.

Low-dose techniques for screening CTC should be employed. Increasing collimation or decreasing tube current or voltage will decrease radiation dose. However, the diagnostic ability for target-size polyps must be maintained. In a study of 105 patients who underwent four-row multidetector CTC, low-dose technique was used, which consisted of 4 × 1 mm detector collimation, 120 kV, 0.5 second gantry rotation period, and effective mAs of 50. The effective doses for CTC for males and females were 5.0 mSv and 7.8 mSv, respectively, while maintaining 93% sensitivity and 97.7% specificity for large polyps.[46] The radiation exposure of various 64-row multidetector

Table 1 Sample 64-row MDCT colonography protocol	
Collimation (mm)	0.5–0.625
Pitch	0.98–1.4
Feed (mm/sec)	25–48
Effective mAs	50
kV	120
Rotation Time (sec)	0.5
Reconstructions (mm)	1–1.25
Scan Time (sec)	5–7

CTC protocols was evaluated using a phantom.[47] Protocols using 50 mAs and 120 kV with collimation of 20 × 1.2 mm and 64 × 0.6 mm resulted in male and female doses of 3.8/4.2 mSv and 4.2/4.5 mSv, respectively. Liedenbaum and colleagues[48] evaluated 34 research institutions performing CTC and they found that the median effective dose per institution was 5.7 mSv (2.8 mSv supine and 2.5 mSv prone). There is the potential to further decrease dose without compromising the accuracy for polyp detection. Van Gelder and colleagues[49] performed a feasibility study in 15 patients using doses ranging from 0.05 mSv to 12 mSv. Overall sensitivity for polyps 5 mm or larger decreased slightly but remained at 74% or higher down to 1.6 mAs (0.2 mSv).

Shorter scan times have the benefit of a more tolerable breath-hold for the patient, which minimize respiratory and motion artifacts. Hara and colleagues[50] performed a study comparing single-detector and multidetector CTC in 237 patients. Mild respiratory artifacts were identified in 61% of patients who were scanned on single-detector CT compared with only 16% of patients who underwent multidetector CT. Results also showed that there were more patients with suboptimal colonic distention using single-detector CT in 52% of examinations compared with only 16% of multidetector CTC.

INTERPRETATION METHODS

Interpretation of CTC requires two-dimensional (2D) axial images, multiplanar reformats (MPR) and 3D renderings using specific computer software. Readers should be proficient in both 2D and 3D techniques to achieve high accuracy and time-efficient study interpretation. Often either 2D or 3D is chosen as a primary interpretation technique with the complementary view used secondarily for solving problems.

Primary 2D interpretation uses the supine and axial images, which are viewed dynamically by scrolling through them using high contrast window settings (width =1,400, level = -350) when searching for colonic lesions. Polyps appear as ovoid or rounded, homogeneous soft tissue density structures that are fixed in location on supine and prone images (Fig. 4) This is in contrast to residual stool, which is typically heterogeneous density and mobile (Fig. 5). Stool may have a linear or irregular shape. A common pitfall is a pedunculated polyp, which may trap air underneath it and appear heterogeneous or it may appear mobile when the stalk is elongated (Fig. 6). The search for polyps requires rigorous review through each segment of the colon using focused magnified axial views. When a potential lesion is identified a bookmark is placed and reviews of the multiplanar reformats and 3D images are performed to help distinguish a true polyp. Advantages of the primary 2D-interpretation method includes the inherent ability to discriminate density of lesions and the relatively shorter interpretation times compared with primary 3D interpretation.[6]

Primary 3D interpretation consists of endoluminal navigation through the colon along an automatically generated centerline. Typically four complete navigations are needed, once in antero-grade and retrograde directions in both supine and prone positions. When a possible polyp is identified, it is bookmarked and the reader can review 2D axial or multiplanar reformatted views to help evaluate density and mobility of the lesion. Computer software for CTC is available that offers a translucency view or color map overlay based on lesion density that can be used for the 3D view. The translucency view is typically used to help differentiate tagged stool from the soft tissue density of polyps on 3D views. Software is also available that tracks the portions of the colonic wall that have been visualized and then paints these surfaces a different color so that the reader can

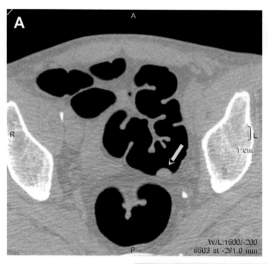
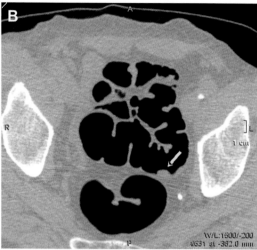
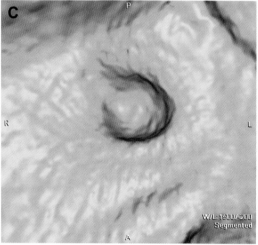

Fig. 4. (*A*) Supine axial view shows the typical homogeneous soft tissue density and ovoid morphology of a polyp (*arrow*). (*B*) The polyp appears fixed in a similar location (*arrow*) on the opposing prone view. (*C*) The 3D endoluminal image shows the typical appearance of a polyp.

review the "missing patches." This method helps to assure that all of the colonic surfaces have been reviewed by the reader. The advantages of using the primary 3D-interpretation method include the ease of use by novice readers. Additionally, polyps located on or near folds may be easier to detect on 3D views. However, interpretation times for primary 3D reads is often longer than for primary 2D reads.

The American College of Radiology Practice Guidelines recommend that physicians should have reviewed at least 50 cases in a variety of formats to be a qualified reader for CTC.[11] These formats include formal hands-on interactive training, supervision by a CTC-trained physician acting as a double reader, and/or correlation of findings in patients undergoing both CTC and colonoscopy. Adequate reader training is essential for CTC because search patterns and appearances of true lesions and pitfalls are different than for routine CT scan of the abdomen and pelvis. An additional number of cases will be needed if the physician does not have recent experience in the interpretation of CT scan of the abdomen and pelvis.

Novel displays have been developed and are increasingly available such as the virtual dissection view, which allows visualization of larger regions of the colon wall for evaluation. The colon is opened along its long axis and then flattened for display. The dissection view has the potential to decrease interpretation times while maintaining the ability to accurately detect polyps. Computer-aided detection (CAD) or computer-assisted readers (CAR) for CTC are now available. Strategies are being developed regarding whether

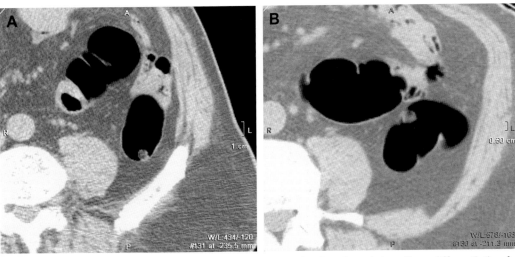

Fig. 5. (A) Supine axial image demonstrates the heterogeneous density of stool that allows differentiation from a true polyp. (B) Another typical feature of stool is mobility to the dependent wall in this prone view.

optimum use is as a primary versus secondary reader. Improvements in sensitivity for polyp detection using CAD or CAR must be balanced with adequate specificity so that interpretation times are acceptable.

There is increasing experience with stool and fluid tagging using oral barium and/or iodinated contrast material to help to decrease false positives encountered from residue in the colon. Electronic or digital subtraction of the tagged material may then be performed to allow visualization of a greater portion of the colonic surface and to allow easier identification of true polyps. Non-cathartic CTC was performed in 114 patients who had known or suspected colorectal neoplasms.[51] Tagging was performed using 21.6 g of barium in nine divided doses. The per-patient sensitivity for detecting adenomas ≥ 10 mm or 6–9 mm ranged from 84%–93% and 53%–88% without stool subtraction. When stool subtraction was included the per-patient sensitivity for detecting adenomas ≥ 10 mm or 6–9 mm improved and ranged from 93%–94% and 68%–92%.

A consensus proposal of a CTC Reporting and Data System (C-RADS) has been developed by the Working Group on Virtual Colonoscopy and published to help facilitate clear and consistent communication of CTC results.[52] In this report, the descriptive features of polyps and masses are suggested and include lesion morphology, size, location and attenuation. Classification and suggested follow-up of colonic findings are presented using a C0 (inadequate study) to C4 (likely malignant mass) system. There is also a classification scheme for extracolonic findings using E0 (limited examination) to E4 (potentially important finding) grading.

CT COLONOGRAPHY APPLICATIONS

The American College of Radiology Practice Guidelines include indications for CTC. CTC may be performed as a screening or surveillance examination, as well as a diagnostic test in symptomatic patients.[11] The 2008 Guidelines for Screening and Surveillance for the Early Detection of Colorectal Cancer and Adenomatous Polyps from the American Cancer Society, the U. S. Multi-Society Task Force, and the American College of Radiology endorses CTC as a screening option every five years.[53]

Patients who have incomplete colonoscopy due to various etiologies including redundant segment, patient intolerance, and distally stenosing benign or malignant lesion may undergo CTC. Other patients who are at increased risk for complications during fiberoptic colonoscopy, such as elderly patients who have comorbid conditions, patients who are a sedation risk, patients who are on anticoagulation therapy, and patients who have a history of failed colonoscopy, may elect to undergo CTC. Patients who are at high risk for the development of colorectal carcinoma, such as individuals who have ulcerative colitis or Crohn's disease as well as those patients who have hereditary colorectal polyposis or cancer syndromes should undergo fiberoptic colonoscopy because of the increased likelihood of need for biopsy or polypectomy.

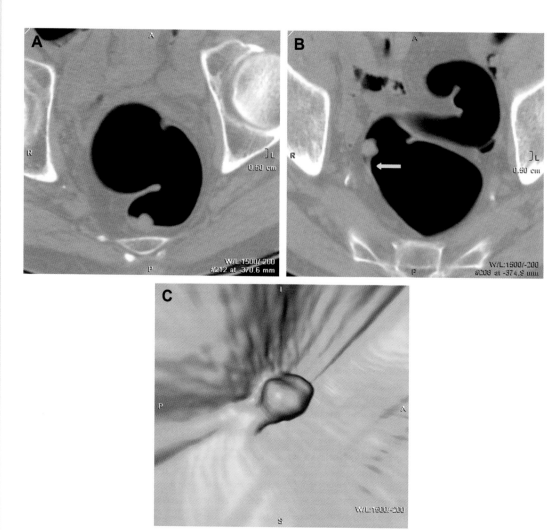

Fig. 6. (*A*) A mildly lobulated soft tissue density lesion is identified along the posterior wall of the rectosigmoid in the supine view. (*B*) In the prone view the stalk of this pedunculated polyp has elongated (*arrow*) and the head of the polyp appears to have shifted in location from the wall. (*C*) The stalk and the head of this pedunculated polyp are visualized on the 3D endoluminal view.

COMPLICATIONS

Perforation of the colon associated with CTC is very uncommon. A survey by the Working Group for Virtual Colonoscopy of 16 medical centers from five countries was evaluated the perforation rate and the overall significant complication rate of CTC.[54] A total of 21,923 CTC studies were evaluated. There were about an equal number of screening and diagnostic examinations. Two patients undergoing diagnostic CTC had perforations. Manual room air insufflation was employed in the two patients. One patient was asymptomatic and did not require treatment. The second patient was symptomatic and required treatment. Therefore, the symptomatic perforation rate was

determined to be 0.0046% (1/21,923) and the overall perforation rate was 0.0091%. Two other patients developed renal failure related to the bowel preparation and one patient had chest pain. This resulted in a significant complication rate of 0.018% (4/21,923). The overall conclusion was that CTC is very safe.

Other reports of colonic perforation have been documented in patients undergoing CTC. Some of these patients had an abnormal colon with inflammatory and/or obstructive lesions (ulcerative colitis, Crohn's disease, or obstructive carcinoma).[55–57] However, there are reports of patients without known colonic disease who have had colonic perforation during CTC. These results have occurred with both manual room air and electronic CO_2 insufflation of the colon. Typically, these patients have no significant symptoms and do not require surgical treatment.[58,59]

REFERENCES

1. Ferruci JT. Colon cancer screening with virtual colonoscopy: promise, polyps, politics. Am J Roentgenol 2001;177:975–88.

2. Fenlon HM, Nunes DP, Schroy PC III, et al. A comparison of virtual and conventional colonoscopy for the detection of colorectal polyps. N Engl J Med 1999;341:1540–2.

3. Yee J, Akerkar GA, Hung RK, et al. Colorectal neoplasia: performance characteristics of CT colonography for detection in 300 patients. Radiology 2001; 219:685–92.

4. Macari M, Bini EJ, Jacobs SL, et al. Colorectal polyps and cancers in asymptomatic average-risk patients: evaluation with CT colonography. Radiology 2004;230:629–36.

5. Pickhardt PJ, Choi JR, Hwang I, et al. CT virtual colonoscopy to screen for colorectal neoplasia in asymptomatic adults. N Engl J Med 2003;349: 2191–200.

6. Johnson CD, Chen MH, Toledano AY, et al. Accuracy of CT colonography for detection of large adenomas and cancers. N Engl J Med 2008;359:1207–17.

7. Sosna J, Morrin MM, Kruskal JB, et al. CT colonography of colorectal polyps: a metaanalysis. AJR Am J Roentgenol 2003;181:1593–8.

8. Halligan S, Altman DG, Taylor SA, et al. CT colonography in the detection of colorectal polyps and cancer: systematic review, meta-analysis, and proposed minimum data set for study level reporting. Radiology 2005;237:893–904.

9. Mulhall BP, Veerappan GR, Jackson JL. Meta-analysis: computed tomographic colonography. Ann Intern Med 2005;142:635–50.

10. Yee J, Kumar NN, Hung RK, et al. Comparison of supine, prone and both supine and prone scans in CT colonography. Radiology 2003;226:653–61.

11. American College of Radiology. ACR practice guideline for the performance of computed tomography (CT) colonography in adults. In: Practice guidelines and technical standards 2005. Reston, VA: American College of Radiology; 2005. p. 295–9.

12. Bartram CI. Bowel preparation- principles and practice. Clin Radiol 1994;49:365–7.

13. Gelfand DW, Chen MYM, Ott DJ. Preparing the colon for the barium enema examination. Radiology 1991;178:609–13.

14. DeLegge M, Kaplan R. Efficacy of bowel preparation with the use of a prepackaged, low fiber diet with a low sodium, magnesium citrate cathartic vs. a clear liquid diet with a standard sodium phosphate cathartic. Aliment Pharmacol Ther 2005;15:1491–5.

15. Sharma VK, Chockalingham SK, Ugheoke EA, et al. Prospective, randomized, controlled comparison of the use of polyethylene glycol electrolyte lavage solution in four-liter versus two-liter volumes and pretreatment with either magnesium citrate or bisacodyl for colonoscopy preparation. Gastrointest Endosc 1998;47:167–71.

16. Golub RW, Kerner BA, Wise WE, et al. Colonoscopic bowel preparations- which one? A blinded, prospective, randomized trial. Dis Colon Rectum 1995;38: 594–9.

17. Afridi SA, Barthel JS, King PD, et al. Prospective, randomized trial comparing a new sodium phosophate-bisacodyl regimen with conventional PEG-ES lavage for outpatient colonoscopy preparation. Gastrointest Endosc 1995;41:485–9.

18. Marshall JB, Pineda JJ, Barthel JS, et al. Prospective, randomized trial comparing sodium phosphate solution with polyethylene glycol-electrolyte lavage for colonoscopy preparation. Gastrointest Endosc 1993;39:631–4.

19. Cohen SM, Wexner SD, Binderow SR, et al. Prospective, randomized, endoscopic-blinded trial comparing precolonoscopy bowel cleansing methods. Dis Colon Rectum 1994;37:689–96.

20. Kolts BE, Lyles WE, Achem SR, et al. A comparison of the effectiveness and patient tolerance of oral sodium phosphate, castor oil, and standard electrolyte lavage for colonoscopy or sigmoidoscoopy preparation. Am J Gastroenterol 1993;88:1218–23.

21. Vanner SJ, MacDonald PH, Paterson WG, et al. A randomized prospective trial comparing oral sodium phosphate with standard polyethylene glycol-based lavage solution (golytely) in the preparation of patients for colonoscopy. Am J Gastroenterol 1990;4: 422–7.

22. Hsu CW, Imperiale TF. Meta-analysis and cost comparison of polyethylene glycol lavage versus sodium phosphate for colonoscopy preparation. Gastrointest Endosc 1998;48:276–82.

23. Ehrenpreis ED, Nogueras JJ, Botoman VA, et al. Serum electrolyte abnormalities secondary to Fleet's phospho-soda colonscopy prep. Surg Endosc 1996;10:1022–4.

24. Vukasin P, Weston LA, Beart RW. Oral fleet phosphosoda laxative-induced hyperphosphatemia and hypocalcemic tetany in an adult. Dis Colon Rectum 1997;40:497–9.

25. Markowitz GS, Stokes MB, Radhakrishnan J, et al. Acute phosphate nephropathy following oral sodium phosphate bowel purgative: an under-recognized cause of chronic renal failure. J Am Soc Nephrol 2005;16:3389–96.

26. Khurana A, McLean L, Atkinson S, et al. The effect of oral sodium phosphate drug products on renal

function in adults undergoing bowel endoscopy. Arch Intern Med 2008;168:593–7.

27. Fass R, Do S, Hixson LJ. Fatal hyperphosphatemia following Fleet phospho-soda in a patient with colonic ileus. Am J Gastroenterol 1993;88:929–32.

28. Food and Drug Administration. Science background: safety of sodium phosphates oral solution, Center for drug evaluation and research. Washington, DC: Food and Drug Administration; 2002.

29. Gryspeerdt S, Lefere P, Herman M, et al. CT colonography with fecal tagging after incomplete colonoscopy. Eur Radiol 2005;15:1192–202.

30. Lefere PA, Gryspeerdt SS, Dewyspelaere J, et al. Dietary fecal tagging as a cleansing method before CT colonography: initial results polyp detection and patient acceptance. Radiology 2002;224:393–403.

31. Taylor SA, Slater A, Burling DN, et al. CT colonography: optimization, diagnostic performance and patient acceptability of reduced-laxative regimens using barium-based fecal tagging. Eur Radiol 2008;18:32–42.

32. Zalis ME, Perumpillichira JJ, Magee C, et al. Tagging-based, electronically cleansed CT colonography: evaluation of patient comfort and image readability. Radiology 2006;239:149–59.

33. Bielen D, Thomeer M, Vanbeckevoort D, et al. Dry preparation for virtual CT colonography with fecal tagging using water-soluble contrast medium: initial results. Eur Radiol 2003;3:453–8.

34. Iannaccone R, Laghi A, Catalano C, et al. Computed tomographic colonography without cathartic preparation for the detection of colorectal polyps. Gastroenterology 2004;127:1300–11.

35. Pickhardt PJ, Taylor AJ, Kim DH, et al. Screening for colorectal neoplasia with CT colonography: initial experience from the first year of coverage by third-party payers. Radiology 2006;241:417–25.

36. Callstrom MR, Johnson CD, Fletcher JG, et al. CT colonography without cathartic preparation: feasibility study. Radiology 2001;219:693–8.

37. Lefere P, Gryspeerdt S, Marrannes J, et al. CT colonography after fecal tagging with a reduced cathartic cleansing and a reduced volume of barium. AJR Am J Roentgenol 2005;184:1836–42.

38. Jensch S, deVries AH, Peringa J, et al. CT Colonography with limited bowel preparation: performance characteristics in an increased-risk population. Radiology 2008;247:122–32.

39. Burling D, Taylor SA, Halligan S, et al. Automated insufflation of carbon dioxide for MDCT colonography: distention and patient experience compared with manual insufflation. Am J Roentgenol 2006;186:96–103.

40. Kim SY, Park SH, Choi EK, et al. Automated carbon dioxide insufflation for CT colonography:effectiveness of colonic distention in cancer patients with severe luminal narrowing. Am J Roentgenol 2008;190:698–706.

41. Morrin MM, Farrell RJ, Keogan MT, et al. CT colonography: colonic distention improved by dual positioning but not intravenous glucagon. Eur Radiol 2002;12:525–30.

42. Rogalla P, Lembcke A, Ruckert JC, et al. Spasmolysis at CT colonography: butyl scopolamine versus glucagon. Radiology 2005;236:184–8.

43. Yee J, Hung RK, Akerkar GA, et al. The usefulness of glucagon hydrochloride for colonic distention in CT colonography. Am J Roentgenol 1999;173:1–4.

44. Yee J, Hung RK, Steinauer-Gebauer AM, et al. Colonic distention and prospective evaluation of colorectal polyp detection with and without glucagon during CT colonography. Radiology 1999;213:256.

45. Lui YW, Macari M, Israel G, et al. CT colonography data interpretation: effect of different section thicknesses-preliminary observations. Radiology 2003;229:791–7.

46. Macari M, Bini EJ, Xue X, et al. Colorectal neoplasms: prospective comparison of thin-section low-dose multi-detector row CT colonography and conventional colonoscopy for detection. Radiology 2002;224:383–92.

47. Luz O, Buchgeister M, Klabunde M, et al. Evaluation of dose exposure in 64-slice CT colonography. Eur Radiol 2007;17:2616–21.

48. Liedenbaum MH, Venema HW, Stoker J. Radiation dose in CT colonography-trends in time and differences between daily practice and screening protocols. Eur Radiol 2008;18:2222–30.

49. van Gelder RE, Venema HW, Florie J, et al. CT colonography: feasibility of substantial dose reduction-comparison of medium to very low doses in identical patients. Radiology 2004;232:611–20.

50. Hara AK, Johnson CD, MacCarty RL, et al. CT colonography: single- versus multi-detector row imaging. Radiology 2001;219:461–5.

51. Johnson CD, Manduca A, Fletcher JG, et al. Noncathartic CT colonography with stool tagging: performance with and without electronic stool subtraction. Am J Roentgenol 2008;190:361–6.

52. Zalis ME, Barish MA, Choi JR, et al. For the Working Group on Virtual Colonoscopy. CT colonography reporting and data system: a consensus proposal. Radiology 2005;236:3–9.

53. Levin B, Lieberman DA, McFarland B, et al. Screening and surveillance for the early detection of colorectal cancer and adenomatous polyps, 2008: a joint guideline from the American cancer society, the US multi-society task force on colorectal cancer, and the American college of radiology. CA Cancer J Clin 2008;58:130–60.

54. Pickhardt PJ. Incidence of colonic perforation at CT colonography: review of existing data and implications for screening of asymptomatic adults. Radiology 2006;239:313–6.

55. Kamar M, Portnoy O, Bar-Dayan A, et al. Actual colonic perforation in virtual colonoscopy: report of a case. Dis Colon Rectum 2004;47:1242–6.

56. Coady-Fariborzian L, Angel LP, Procaccino JA. Perforated colon secondary to virtual colonoscopy: report of a case. Dis Colon Rectum 2004;47:1247–9.

57. Triester SL, Hara AK, Young-Fadok TM, et al. Colonic perforation after computed tomographic colonography in a patient with fibrostenosing crohn's disease. Am J Gastroenterol 2006;101:189–92.

58. Young BM, Fletcher JG, Earnest F, et al. Colonic perforation at CT colonography in a patient without known colonic disease. AJR Am J Roentgenol 2006;186:119–21.

59. Bassett JT, Liotta RA, Barlow D, et al. Colonic perforation during screening CT colonography using automated CO_2 insufflation in an asymptomatic adult. Abdom Imaging 2008;33:598–600.

Positron Emission Tomography/Computed Tomography: The Current Technology and Applications

Erik Mittra, MD, PhD*, Andrew Quon, MD

KEYWORDS

- Positron emission tomography
- Fluorodeoxyglucose
- Novel radiopharmaceuticals
- Physics • Oncology • Neurology • Cardiology
- Infection and inflammation

The first positron emission tomography (PET) scanners were developed in the 1950s and produced relatively low-quality images. Although of limited clinical usefulness, these images showed the potential for functional imaging. The quality of PET imaging evolved steadily through the decades with vast improvements in resolution and scanning speed. Additionally, modern PET scanners are now hybrid devices in which PET and CT scanners are fused together. These integrated units greatly improved the usefulness of PET imaging because they allowed for far more accurate anatomic localization. In addition to the evolution of scanner design, the success of clinical PET imaging can also be attributed to the usefulness of the radiotracer [F-18]-fluoro-2'-deoxy-D-glucose (FDG). PET/CT is now commonly used for a multitude of clinical indications in oncology, cardiology, and neurology using this single radiotracer.

This article reviews the fundamentals and state of the art in PET/CT instrumentation, and the current clinical applications of this technology. Future directions with regard to PET technology are also discussed.

POSITRON EMISSION TOMOGRAPHY TECHNOLOGY: THE FUNDAMENTALS AND THE FUTURE
Positron Emission Tomography Radiopharmaceuticals

At its core, PET imaging depends on detection of pairs of photons (511 KeV each) resulting from the annihilation of a positron with an electron. Any isotope that decays by releasing positrons can be used for PET imaging. The common isotopes include ^{11}C, ^{13}N, ^{15}O, and ^{18}F. By far, the leading radiopharmaceutical (an isotope bound to a ligand) for PET imaging is FDG. The cyclotron-produced ^{18}F isotope has a half-life of 109.7 minutes and returns with a beta positive decay scheme to ^{18}O water.

Novel Radiopharmaceuticals

A multitude of new PET radiopharmaceuticals are currently being developed—primarily for use in cancer imaging—to complement FDG for use in cancer imaging. These can be categorized as nonspecific tracers that take advantage of the

Division of Nuclear Medicine, Stanford Hospital and Clinics, 300 Pasteur Drive, Room H0101, Stanford, CA 94305, USA
* Corresponding author.
E-mail address: erik.mittra@stanford.edu (E. Mittra).

Radiol Clin N Am 47 (2009) 147–160
doi:10.1016/j.rcl.2008.10.005
0033-8389/08/$ – see front matter © 2009 Published by Elsevier Inc.

increased metabolic activity and vascularity of malignant tumors, and specific agents that bind to tumor-specific antigens or receptors. Metabolic agents, such as FDG, typically trace the enzymatic turnover of a parent compound. A promising tracer compound is the thymidine analog 3′-deoxy-3′-[18F]fluorothymidine (FLT), which provides a measure of DNA replication. Potential advantages of FLT over FDG include fewer false-positive lesions due to inflammation, increased sensitivity of detecting brain lesions because of decreased neuronal uptake, and theoretically greater reliability in monitoring response to selective (cytostatic) chemotherapies. PET radiopharmaceuticals that exploit the high vascularity of many tumors include pure perfusion tracers, such as ^{15}O-labeled water or $^{13}NH_3$, or measures of angiogenesis, such as the ^{18}F-labeled glycosylated tripeptide ^{18}F-galacto-RGD, which targets $\alpha_v\beta_3$-integrin, a protein selectively expressed on activated endothelial cells. Related to these in principle are tracers that clear slowly from hypoxic tissues, leading to relatively increased activity on delayed images in areas at risk for poor response to chemotherapeutics requiring adequate tumor oxygenation. Hypoxia-sensitive agents include [18F]fluoromisonidazole, an analog of 2-nitroimidazole, and Cu(II)-diacetyl-bis (N4-methylthiosemicarabaone), a copper bis (thiosemicarbazone). Although nonspecific tracers provide useful imaging of aggressive neoplasms, they typically exhibit decreased sensitivity in detecting tumors with low growth rates. It is therefore essential that PET agents be developed that bind selectively and with high tumor-to-background ratio to intracellular and cell-surface receptors up-regulated in cancer cells. Radiolabeled steroid

analogs of estrogen and androgen derivatives are expected to be useful for evaluating response to hormonal therapy of breast and prostate cancer. Examples of cell-surface receptor radioligands are ^{18}F-labelled spiperone, which binds dopamine receptors on pituitary adenomas, and ^{64}Cu-labeled octreotide and 68-Ga-labelled octreotide analogs for targeting somatostatin-receptor–positive tumors. A potentially useful class of tumor imaging agents uses radio-chelated monoclonal antibodies labeled with relatively long half-life positron emitters ^{64}Cu and ^{124}I, which target tumor-specific antigens, such as carcinoembryonic antigen (CEA). From an imaging standpoint, plasma clearance of the bulky antibody molecule must be optimized to improve tumor-to-background activity, and so smaller engineered antibody fragments with rapid renal clearance are being developed.

Photon Detection, Conversion to light, and Signal Amplification: Present and Future

Detection of the coincident annihilation photons begins with scintillation crystals. When a photon strikes a crystal, the photon is absorbed and visible light is emitted—an intrinsic feature of the crystal. This light is then detected and converted to photoelectrons by a photocathode. The photoelectrons in turn are greatly amplified by a photomultiplier tube (PMT) coupled to the photocathode (**Fig. 1**). The electronic signal generated by the PMT is then further increased by preamplifiers and amplifiers before being passed onto the computer circuitry for further analysis.

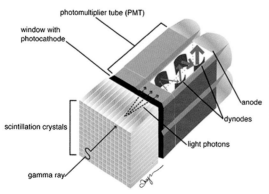
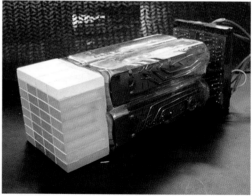

Fig. 1. (*Left*) Scintillation crystals coupled to photomultiplier tubes show the basic process of photon detection. When a photon interacts with a crystal, the photon is absorbed and visible light is emitted. This light is received and transformed into photoelectrons by the photocathode. The photomultiplier tube then greatly amplifies the photoelectron signal through the use of successive dynodes of greater charge. An actual system is shown on the right. (*Courtesy of* C. Levin and H. Peng, Stanford University, Stanford, CA.)

The crystals are made of various composite materials with different attributes (**Table 1**). The principal design considerations for PET scintillation crystals include having a high density to interact with the high-energy 511 KeV photons, a high light output per megaelectron volt, and a short scintillation decay time to improve coincident detection. The first scintillation crystals used in PET imaging were the same sodium iodide (Nal-Tl) crystals used in planar and single photon emission computed tomography (SPECT) imaging, but understandably had poor stopping power for the higher-energy photons. The next generation crystal, bismuth germinate (BGO), had much better attributes, whereas the newest crystals, including lutetium oxyorthosilicate (LSO) and its derivate lutetium yttrium orthosilicate (LYSO), continue to improve the sensitivity of PET.

Determining the optimal size of a scintillation crystal requires a tradeoff between sensitivity and spatial resolution. In general, the smaller the cross-sectional size of the crystal, the greater the spatial resolution. If the size becomes too small, the increased amount of data may create convergence issues during reconstruction. Additionally, the inherent physical limitations of positron range and photon non-colinearity limit the theoretic size to 0.4 mm in the reconstructed image. Positron range refers to the small distance a positron travels before interacting with an electron (usually 1.2 mm for ^{18}F in water). Photon non-colinearity refers to the slight deviation away from a true 180° path that annihilation photons sometimes take. Developing very small crystals is also a manufacturing challenge and increases cost. As such, the crystals used in clinical scanners will likely remain comparatively larger (roughly 4 × 4 mm), whereas small animal scanners will gain the most benefit from smaller crystal size (roughly 1 × 1 mm) (**Fig. 2**).[1]

The length of the scintillation crystal is also important. A longer crystal provides a greater chance of interaction and, therefore, increased sensitivity. Because a longer crystal also accepts a greater number of tangential photons striking along its entire vertical dimension, the spatial resolution is diminished. This problem can theoretically be overcome by detecting the depth of interaction (DOI) within the crystal, either by having two layers of crystals stacked on each other or by mathematically resolving the DOI continuously in one long crystal.[2] This process is especially important in those systems in which the resolution must be maintained at all costs, such as small animal PET scanners.

The purpose of the PMT is to receive the light output from a scintillation crystal/photocathode, and further amplify this signal before transferring it to the computer electronics of the PET system. A PMT is a large vacuum tube that accelerates electrons against dynodes of increasing electric charge to amplify their signal. Although a relatively old design, PMTs are still in widespread use because they provide good performance with respect to noise and timing properties. The next generation of light detectors, however, may be avalanche photodiodes (APDs; **Fig. 3**).[3,4] APDs are compact, solid-state, semiconductor devices. The primary advantages of APDs over PMTs lies in their small size, potential for inexpensive production, and insensitivity to magnetic fields. The latter is especially important with the development

Table 1
Attributes of common scintillation crystals for positron emission tomography

Property	Nal(Tl)	BGO	LSO	YSO	BaF	LaBr$_3$	LYSO
Density (g/cm^3)	3.67	7.13	7.4	4.53	4.89	5.3	5.31
Effective Z	50.6	74.2	65.5	34.2	52.2	—	54
Attenuation length	2.88	1.05	1.16	2.58	2.2	2.1	2.0
Decay constant	230	300	40	70	0.6	15	53
Relative light output (%)	100	15	75	118	5	160	76
Wavelength (λ [nm])	410	480	420	420	220	360	420
Index of refraction	1.85	2.15	1.82	1.8	1.56	1.9	1.81
Hygroscopic?	Yes	No	No	No	No	Yes	No

Abbreviations: BaF, barium fluoride; BGO, bismuth germinate; LaBr$_3$, lanthanum tribromide; LSO, lutetium oxyorthosilicate; Nal(Tl), sodium iodide (thallium); YSO, yttrium oxyorthosilicate.
Data from Pichler BJ, Wehrl HF, Judenhofer MS. Latest advances in molecular imaging instrumentation. J Nucl Med 2008;49 Suppl 2:5S–23S.

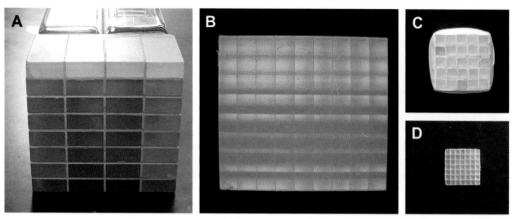

Fig. 2. Scintillation crystals can be manufactured of various sizes for use in clinical and preclinical work. All images are shown at the same magnification for ease of comparison. (*A*) Crystal from an extant scanner. (*B–D*) Crystals destined for various types of preclinical work. (*Courtesy of* C. Levin and H. Peng, Stanford University, Stanford, CA.)

of integrated PET/MR imaging systems.[5] PMTs are not optimal for PET/MR imaging systems given their relatively large size and loss of gain due to the magnetic field of the MR imaging causing deflection of the electrons. The primary disadvantage of APDs is a limited electronic gain of approximately 1000 to 10,000 less than PMTs, thus requiring additional dedicated, integrated preamplifiers. The latter problem is solved with the advent of silicon photomultipliers (siPM) which are a type of APD running in Geiger-mode. siPMs have gains on the order of 10^6 and so require only basic preamplifiers.[1] With further development, siPMs will likely become the light detector of choice for future PET/CT and PET/MR imaging systems.

Line of Response and Time of Flight

Because the photons are emitted in all directions, a ring of crystals is placed around the patient. When the two paired annihilation photons strike opposing crystals, a line of response (LOR) is created within which the original source of the positron is known to be located (**Fig. 4**). An LOR is created only if two photons of the appropriate energy strike opposing detectors within a preset time window (usually 10 nanoseconds). The latter is required because the opposing photons (traveling at the speed of light) strike their respective crystals at slightly different times. Not all true coincident photons are captured, however, and not all random events are excluded. Both these factors lead to degradation in image quality. Coincident photons may not be captured if one photon is scattered (and thus of lower energy) or is out plane. Conversely, false LORs may be created if a scattered photon is not appropriately excluded, or two

independent events strike opposing detectors within the allowed time window.

Standard reconstruction algorithms based on the LOR result in a somewhat noisy image; this is because it is unknown from where the original photon originated within the LOR. Narrowing the location of the source photon to a smaller range (or ideally a point) within the LOR would improve the signal-to-noise (SNR) ratio, which is the goal of time of flight (TOF) (**Fig. 4**).[6,7] Unless the original photon originated in exactly the center of the detector ring (ie, patient), there will be slight time delay between the arrival of the two photons. Based on the simple formula shown in **Fig. 4**, this time delay can be used to calculate the location of the source photon within the original LOR. The primary limitation to TOF is in the intrinsic scintillator decay time and the net time resolution of the detectors and electronics. At the time of writing, the fastest systems have a time resolution of approximately

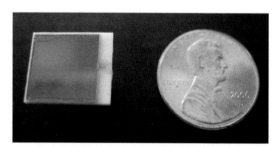

Fig. 3. Compared with standard photomultiplier tubes, the newest generation silicone photodiodes (avalanche photodiodes) are considerably smaller, potentially less expensive, and insensitive to magnetic fields. As with standard PMTs, APDs can be arranged in arrays of various dimensions depending on the specific manufacturing requirements. (*Courtesy of* C. Levin and H. Peng, Stanford University, Stanford, CA.)

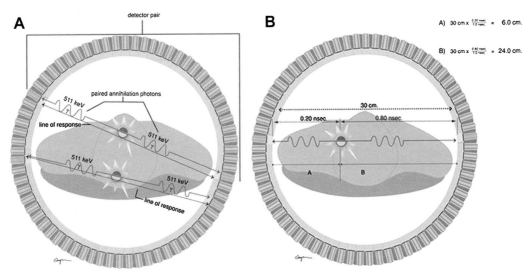

Fig. 4. Coincident annihilation photon detection (*A*), and time of flight (*B*). In time of flight, the time delay between detection of the coincident annihilation photons allows more precise localization of the source using the simple calculation shown.

500 picoseconds. This resolution can narrow the location of the annihilation event to a few centimeters. Practically, this is most helpful in reducing noise for larger patients in whom the SNR is inherently low. It is theoretically interesting to note that if the time resolution could be reduced to 15 picoseconds, the position of the original photon could be reduced to a few millimeters, and image reconstruction would be obviated.[1]

Multiple detector rings are placed together to form a cylindric detector, which has a usual length

in the range of 15 to 25 cm. Moveable tungsten septa are located between the adjacent rings. When these septa are present between the rings, the imaging is termed two-dimensional (2D); when the septa are retracted, the imaging is termed three-dimensional (3D) (**Fig. 5**). All PET scanners are capable of imaging in 3D. The presence of septa limits the number of counts detected by the scanner, but also improves the contrast by reducing the number of scattered and unrelated photons leading to increased background and degrading contrast.

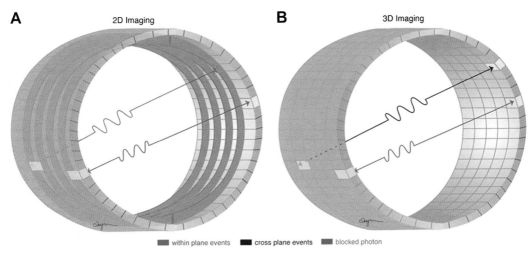

Fig. 5. 2D versus 3D imaging. With the septa in (*A*), 2D imaging blocks cross-plane events, but leads to decreased counts. With the septa out (*B*), 3D imaging allows more photons to be counted, but inevitably includes cross-plane or random events leading to increased background and decreased contrast. Ultimately, the choice of 2D or 3D imaging depends on the clinical or research question.

Image Reconstruction

The raw data, once collected, must be reconstructed to form a diagnostic image. The standard reconstruction algorithms include either filtered back projection or iterative reconstruction. Iterative methods, including maximum likelihood expectation maximization (MLEM) and ordered subsets expectation maximization (OSEM), have largely become the standard method in PET reconstruction, secondary to less star artifact and because corrections for attenuation, scatter, and resolution can be directly incorporated. Although computationally demanding, certain mathematical techniques—such as in OSEM—and faster computers have made this clinically viable. The details of these standard reconstruction algorithms are covered in other sources.[8,9]

One new technique in image reconstruction involves use of a point spread function (PSF). The PSF is a reflection of the widened LOR that occurs especially near the edge of the field of view (FOV) and especially with longer scintillation crystals. This new technique uses spatially variant PSFs in the reconstruction technique to improve the resolution over the entire FOV.[10] Ultimately, this can lower noise and improve contrast (**Fig. 6**). Similar to TOF, this process may be of greatest benefit in larger patients with more information near the edge of the FOV and an inherently lower SNR.[1]

Attenuation Correction and Concurrent Positron Emission Tomography/CT

The reconstructed emission scan provides diagnostic quality images that are successfully used in clinical practice. These images suffer from photon attenuation (photons emanating from deeper structures are attenuated while photons from near the surface are attenuated less). This attenuation can be mathematically corrected using a transmission attenuation map. Traditionally, this attenuation map came from a rotating positron source, usually [68]Ge. The transmission scan is acquired first with and without the patient in the scanner. The difference between these two scans forms the attenuation map, which can be used as a template to correct the emission scan.

All modern PET scanners are now manufactured as combined PET/CT systems (**Fig. 7**). The CT provides two primary advantages over PET alone. First, the CT images provide a faster and equally reliable transmission map for use in attenuation correction. Second, they provide a detailed anatomic map for correlation of the PET findings. Furthermore, diagnostic quality CT scans (with contrast, breath-hold, and so forth) can also be performed during the same examination—either concurrently or in series. **Fig. 8** demonstrates two commonly used PET/CT image acquisition protocols.

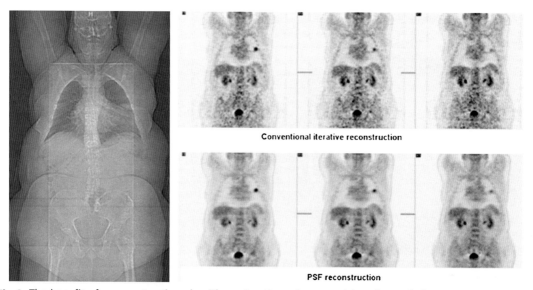

Conventional iterative reconstruction

PSF reconstruction

Fig. 6. The benefit of a reconstruction algorithm using the point spread function technique over conventional reconstruction algorithms is particularly evident in a larger patient. (*Courtesy and copyright* Siemens Medical Solutions USA, Inc.; with permission).

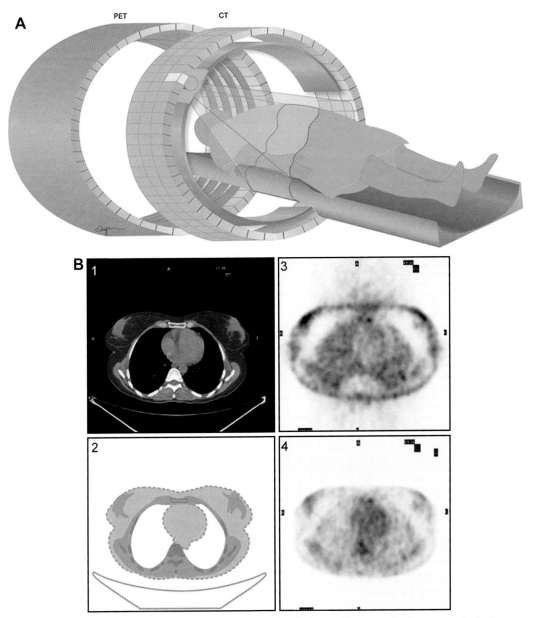

Fig. 7. Modern PET scanners are coupled to CT scanners (*A*), which provides several advantages. Aside from anatomic location of radiotracer activity, the CT scan (*B1*) provides an attenuation map (*B2*) that can be used to correct the raw PET data (*B3*) into an attenuation-corrected image (*B4*).

CLINICAL APPLICATIONS OF POSITRON EMISSION TOMOGRAPHY/CT

FDG PET is an effective diagnostic tool in several clinical scenarios that fall under the general categories of oncology, cardiology, neurology, and infection/inflammation imaging. In the United States, FDG PET has been approved for reimbursement by the Centers for Medicare Services (CMS) for several clinical conditions (**Table 2**). This approval has hastened the acceptance of PET as a standard imaging examination. By far, FDG PET has found its leading role in oncologic imaging, primarily for lung, esophageal, colorectal, head and neck, and breast cancer, and melanoma and lymphoma. For these malignancies, FDG PET has proved to be effective and, in many cases, superior to conventional anatomic imaging for the diagnosis, staging, and restaging of tumors and for monitoring therapy. The following reviews the clinical applications of FDG PET.

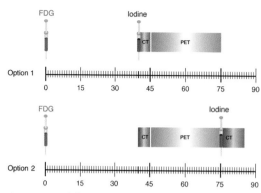

Fig. 8. Two different scanning protocols for concurrent PET/CT are shown. The use of iodinated intravenous or oral contrast is optional. If they are to be used, the intravenous contrast should be given just before the CT, whereas the oral contrast should be ingested between the FDG administration and the start of scanning.

Oncologic Applications

Lung cancer

FDG PET is helpful for the evaluation of solitary pulmonary nodules and for the staging and restaging of established non–small cell lung cancer. As demonstrated by a meta-analysis by Gould in 2001,[11] PET has a sensitivity of greater than 96%

for detecting and characterizing malignant lung nodules greater than 1 cm while maintaining an overall specificity of 77%. Sources of false-positive results include granulomatous diseases, such as histoplasmosis, coccidiomycosis, and sarcoidosis. Active tuberculosis can also be a frequent source of false positives. False-negative PET scans occur predominantly because of lesions that are too small to be evaluated by PET. Also, bronchioloalveolar carcinoma seems to have poor FDG avidity and can be a source of false negative.

The detection of metastatic lymph nodes in the pulmonary hila and mediastinum and the detection of distant metastatic disease is of paramount importance because malignant disease in these areas largely determines the clinical management of patients who have non–small cell lung cancer. Although CT scanning remains the mainstay diagnostic examination for initial staging, FDG PET is rapidly becoming equally routine. Because the main criteria by CT for the determining the presence of nodal metastases is size (generally lymph nodes greater than 1 cm are considered malignant), smaller lymph nodes that harbor cancer can be potentially overlooked and larger nodes can be a source of false positives. FDG PET is an excellent modality for staging mediastinal and

---

Table 2
Medicare coverage indications for [F-18]-fluoro-2′-deoxy-ᴅ-glucose positron emission tomography

Clinical Condition	Coverage Specifics
Oncology	
Breast cancer	Staging, restaging, and evaluating response to therapy
Colorectal cancer	Diagnosis, staging, and restaging
Esophageal cancer	Diagnosis, staging, and restaging
Head and neck cancers[a]	Diagnosis, staging, and restaging
Non–small cell lung cancer	Diagnosis, staging, and restaging
Solitary pulmonary nodules	Characterization of nodules indeterminate on CT
Lymphoma	Diagnosis, staging, and restaging
Melanoma[b]	Diagnosis, staging, and restaging
Thyroid cancer	Restaging
Cervical cancer	Staging as an adjunct to conventional imaging
Cardiology	
Myocardial viability	Primary or initial diagnosis, or following an inconclusive SPECT before revascularization
Neurology	
Refractory seizures	Covered for presurgical evaluation only
Dementia	Differentiating frontotemporal and Alzheimer types

[a] Excludes primary CNS and thyroid cancers.
[b] Excludes evaluation of regional lymph nodes.
   Data from PET Imaging Institute of South Florida. Available at: http://www.petimagingflorida.com/hp/pet_indications.html.

hilar lymph nodes with an overall sensitivity range of 85% and specificity of 80%. A meta-analysis that directly compared patients staged by both FDG PET and CT showed that PET is superior with a sensitivity range of 85% to 95% and specificity range of 81% to 100% on PET versus a sensitivity of 64% and specificity of 62% on CT.[12] Additionally, PET is well suited for detecting distant metastases because it is routinely performed as a whole body examination (from the base of the skull to the mid-thigh). PET is particularly useful for evaluating metastatic disease within the adrenal glands that may pose a diagnostic challenge on CT.

For patients undergoing treatment, FDG PET can be used for monitoring response to chemotherapy and radiation therapy. Again, CT relies on evaluating changes in size and morphology to determine response to therapy, which may at times prove to be inaccurate. Although the data for using PET in this clinical scenario are not as strong as for staging, there is nevertheless reasonable validation in patients who have non-resectable disease that reduction of FDG activity after chemotherapy correlates with intermediate-term survival.

Esophageal cancer

In esophageal cancer, the initial diagnostic workup of cancer includes evaluation by a combination of endoscopy, endoscopic ultrasound (EUS), and CT. FDG PET plays an adjunctive role and is used primarily for initial staging and evaluating response to neoadjuvant treatment of adenocarcinoma and squamous cell carcinoma. Direct comparisons of the staging sensitivity and specificity of PET, CT, and combination CT plus EUS have yielded mixed results. Locoregional lymph node staging seems to be most accurate with EUS, whereas PET seems to have greater sensitivity than CT in upstaging patients who have distant nodal and organ metastases. Ultimately, the optimal strategy for staging may be the combination of FDG PET with EUS and fine needle aspiration biopsy.[13]

In patients who have locally advanced disease undergoing initial neoadjuvant therapy before possible surgical resection, PET seems to be effective in selecting those who have had a sufficient response to therapy to merit surgery. In this clinical setting, FDG PET is typically performed at initial staging and after completion of chemotherapy. Several reports have demonstrated that a diminishment in FDG uptake at tumor sites correlates well with pathologic results of successfully treated disease. This pattern seems to hold true for evaluating response to radiation therapy also. One study specifically demonstrated that using a decrease in FDG activity of greater than 50%, PET scanning has a positive predictive value of 72% for residual disease and a negative predictive value of 100% for good response.[14]

Colorectal cancer

Because of the presence of nonspecific normal variant bowel activity and its relatively high cost, FDG PET is generally not recommended for colorectal cancer screening despite some reports suggesting that premalignant and malignant lesions can be detected by this modality. Further, PET is not effective in evaluating tumor depth or locoregional nodal disease (T and N staging, respectively). FDG PET does have a high sensitivity for detecting distant metastatic disease, particularly in the liver, and may alter surgical management (from curative to palliative measures). The role of PET in the initial management is therefore limited, because surgery is generally performed regardless of PET results at initial diagnosis. FDG PET is useful for detecting and restaging recurrent disease after initial therapy has been completed, however. Several recent reports have demonstrated that PET has a sensitivity of greater than 90% and specificity of greater than 75% in detecting recurrent colorectal cancer with significant impact on subsequent patient management.[15–17] PET is particularly helpful for detecting liver metastases and for ruling out distant disease for those patients who have proven liver metastases in which curative local resection is being contemplated.[18] Moreover, PET is helpful in confirming and localizing sites of disease in patients who have increasing CEA levels after treatment. Using FDG PET for monitoring therapy, including neoadjuvant chemotherapy, has had mixed results in the literature with several studies showing that PET is more accurate than CT and others showing relatively poor accuracy due to nonspecific inflammation, particularly after irradiation.[19]

Melanoma

FDG PET has been shown to be useful in detecting metastatic melanoma, particularly in sites that are not always imaged using conventional imaging modalities. A retrospective analysis of 104 patients who had melanoma demonstrated the superiority of stand-alone FDG PET compared with CT in sensitivity (84% versus 58%) and specificity (97% versus 70%) of detecting metastatic disease,[20] with general agreement in other similar studies. Further prospective analysis of a subgroup of 53 patients in the same study demonstrated a continued advantage of PET over CT in detecting metastasis (81% versus 57% detection rate). Despite the strong FDG avidity of melanoma, PET has difficulty in detecting early-stage disease (stage I–II). A study of 144 early-stage patients detected only 21% of regional lymph node metastases, with no confirmed true positive findings in distal sites.[21] There is no role for FDG PET in detecting sentinel nodes because of the inability to detect micrometastases. Several studies have shown a sensitivity of less than 15% of detecting biopsy-proven sentinel node metastases found with conventional sentinel node mapping.[22,23] Sensitivity is also reduced in small lesions and brain metastases.[24]

Lymphoma

FDG PET has several advantages in the management of patients who have lymphoma. PET shows a functional metabolic status and gives quantitative information—especially important for differentiating indolent versus aggressive lymphomas and assessing early treatment response. In addition, PET provides whole-body images that give a comprehensive assessment of disease extent during the staging and follow-up period. Based on the present literature, FDG PET is at least equivalent to CT for the initial staging of lymphomas.[25] The impact of new technologies of combined PET/CT and fast-scanning CT with contrast has yet to be evaluated in the management of lymphoma patients, however. At this point, FDG PET and CT provide complementary staging information. FDG PET also has high diagnostic accuracy for restaging lymphoma after initial treatment. FDG PET has shown high accuracy in the early prediction of response to chemotherapy and in the evaluation of residual masses after chemotherapy or radiation therapy.[26] PET is therefore likely to play a major role in tailoring the intensity of the treatment to the individual patient. A pretreatment PET study is essential for accurate assessment of residual masses and early monitoring of response to the treatment. In addition, a baseline PET scan helps detect relapse or residual disease, because relapse occurs most often in the region of previous disease.

Head and neck cancer

The use of FDG PET for the identification and characterization of head and neck tumors has been described primarily for squamous cell carcinoma and, less commonly, for salivary gland tumors. Generally, PET does not play a significant role in the characterization of a primary head and neck tumor, largely because FDG PET, even when performed as an integrated PET/CT, does not provide greater information than MR imaging or CT regarding the locoregional anatomy of the primary tumor.

The primary usefulness of FDG PET in head and neck cancer is for the detection of locoregional nodal disease and distant metastases. Numerous studies that directly compare FDG PET to CT or clinical examination show that PET has a higher sensitivity and specificity than either CT or physical examination for the initial pretreatment evaluation of metastatic lymph nodes of the head and neck.[27–29] Further, FDG PET and MR imaging have comparable sensitivities but PET has superior specificity in evaluating metastatic lymph nodes.[30,31] PET is most commonly used for those patients who have suspected local lymph node metastases in whom the identification of additional contralateral or distant malignant lymph nodes needs to be elucidated. In those patients who have negative nodal disease by clinical examination and CT or MR imaging, however, the role of PET is uncertain, likely because of the limited spatial resolution of PET. In current practice, such patients undergo minimally invasive sentinel lymph node biopsy to determine the presence of locoregional nodal metastases and subsequent need for an elective neck dissection. In patients who have more advanced disease, however, PET is superior to CT for detecting distant sites of disease and synchronous tumors.[32]

PET also has usefulness in following response to chemotherapy and radiation. Several authors have described reduced specificity with PET scanning in postradiation cases, however, particularly when performed within 3 months of therapy.[33] Long-term surveillance may also be accomplished by FDG PET, for which it is more sensitive than CT alone.

Other cancers

Although the above malignancies form the cornerstone of oncologic imaging with FDG PET, several other tumor types also show promise, but have yet to be fully approved for reimbursement by CMS. The top three on this list include breast, thyroid, and cervical cancer. FDG PET has a limited role in the diagnosis of breast cancer,[34] but it is important in detecting locoregional (including nodal) and distant disease, in helping to plan surgical and medical treatment, in monitoring response to treatment, and in finding recurrence.[35–41] PET also has the potential to evaluate novel treatment agents rapidly by detecting their effects on specific receptors[37,42] and has been shown to improve prediction of the clinical outcome in patients who have previously treated breast cancer.[43,44]

For thyroid cancer, FDG PET is approved for restaging patients who have thyroglobulin-positive, iodine-negative disease. For these patients, FDG PET provides a viable alternative for assessing extent of disease and response to therapy when iodine scans cannot be used. For cervical cancer, FDG PET is approved for staging as an adjunct to conventional imaging. Studies show good results for restaging and monitoring therapy in cervical cancer also.

Cancers that show reliable FDG uptake but are not approved by CMS include gastrointestinal stromal tumors, endometrial carcinoma, testicular and bladder cancer, and glioblastoma multiforme. FDG is helpful in the evaluation of the latter especially after initial treatment and with equivocal MR imaging findings. Malignancies that are still being evaluated or show variable uptake include renal cell carcinoma, neuroendocrine tumors, and sarcomas. The latter is particularly difficult because the group includes a heterogenous collection of soft tissue and skeletal malignancies, some of which show intense and reliable FDG uptake, whereas others do not. Primary renal cell carcinoma (RCC) is difficult to interpret given the high physiologic background activity in urine, although this can be lessened with the administration of furosemide between radiopharmaceutical administration and imaging. It is also interesting that metastatic RCC often has more intense FDG uptake compared with the primary, possibly secondary to the more aggressive nature of the metastases.

Equally, certain tumor types show poor FDG uptake such that PET is likely of limited value. These malignancies include ovarian, prostate, pancreatic, primary central nervous system (except for glioblastoma multiforme), hepatoma, and bronchoalveolar carcinoma. This is not to say that these carcinomas are never FDG avid. The sensitivity remains low enough, however, that reliable evaluation of these malignancies cannot be performed with FDG PET.

Cardiac Applications

Myocardial SPECT imaging uses various tracers to assess the relative perfusion of the myocardium at stress and in rest (sestamibi and tetrofosmin) and to evaluate the degree of viability (thallium). Although this forms a cornerstone of general nuclear medicine, cardiac PET and PET/CT imaging can take this further. Primarily, PET provides improved resolution compared with SPECT (approximately 8 mm for PET versus 15 mm for SPECT) and allows gated analysis of wall motion and ejection fraction. PET can evaluate myocardial perfusion using several positron-emitting perfusion agents, including ^{13}N-ammonia and ^{82}Rb. Standard stress protocols can be performed before the perfusion agents are administered to obtain both stress and rest studies. The short half-life of these agents (^{13}N = 9.97 minutes; ^{82}Rb = 76 seconds) requires an efficient technical set-up, however. PET viability studies can be performed with ^{18}F-FDG and currently provide the main indication for PET cardiac studies. Indeed, PET viability studies are often coupled with SPECT perfusion studies.[45] The basis of FDG uptake in viable myocardium differs, however, from thallium. For the latter, assessment of viability depends on redistribution over time. For FDG, assessment of viability depends on the theorized preferential uptake of glucose over fatty acids in poorly perfused but living myocardial cells. Several early reports showed favorable and concordant results between thallium SPECT and FDG PET for assessment of viability.[46,47] More recently, however, the improved resolution of PET and ability to perform gated studies somewhat favors its use over thallium SPECT.

Additionally, with the use of PET/CT, and particularly those coupled to faster multislice CT scanners, it is possible to combine coronary CT angiograms with the functional data from PET. As such, there is the potential for a comprehensive examination of the heart, including coronary anatomy and function perfusion and viability information, all displayed on a 3D volume rendering of the myocardium.[48–50]

Neurologic Applications

There are three primary applications of PET and PET/CT in the brain. These include assessment and differentiation of dementias, evaluation of seizure foci, and evaluation of primary brain tumors. FDG PET can be used to evaluate several types of dementias including Alzheimer dementia (AD), frontotemporal dementia (FTD), Lewy-body dementia (LBD), and multi-infarct dementia, based on the pattern of FDG uptake/glucose metabolism. AD is characterized by parietotemporal hypometabolism, with involvement of the frontal lobe in advanced cases but relative sparing of the motor cortices. LBD has a similar pattern to AD but also involves the visual cortices. FTD, as the name implies, primarily affects the frontotemporal regions. Multi-infarct dementia has scattered regions of hypometabolism corresponding to the areas of prior infarct. Several studies have shown good sensitivity and specificity with FDG PET for the differentiation of these different types of dementias. Early evaluation of AD can also be done with alternative compounds. These include ^{11}C bound to a selective ligand for peripheral benzodiazepine binding sites, or Pittsburgh Compound B, which binds to the amyloid protein. In these cases, there is increased uptake of tracer in the appropriate regions on PET rather than regional hypometabolism.[51]

Seizure foci are primarily evaluated with electroencephalogram (EEG) or video-EEG. When additional corroboration is required, however, FDG PET can be used. The greatest benefit of PET seems to be in the evaluation of patients who have temporal lobe epilepsy,[48–50] although PET can and has been done to evaluate for unknown seizure foci.

Infection and Inflammation Imaging

One of the reasons for the decreased specificity of FDG PET in oncologic imaging is that the tracer also shows uptake in infection and inflammation. This feature can be used to the advantage of the clinician if FDG PET is specifically used to query for infection or inflammation. General nuclear medicine studies are often used to answer these questions with radiolabeled leukocyte studies or gallium scans. The primary advantages of PET over these studies lie in its superior resolution, faster time to results, high sensitivity, and inherent quantitation to allow treatment monitoring.[52] The physiology behind FDG activity in infection and inflammation lies in its uptake in activated granulocytes and macrophages with increased rates of glucose metabolism. As such, FDG PET can be used to evaluate infections of soft tissue and the musculoskeletal system. A normal FDG PET study essentially rules out infection, and unlike radiolabeled leukocytes, FDG also differentiates between hematopoietic bone marrow and activated white cells. PET/CT can also be used for the evaluation of fever of unknown origin. A recent review on this application found that PET can be helpful in this regard, but primarily as a second-line test for those patients who have normal or equivocal anatomic imaging.[53] FDG PET is positive in sterile inflammatory disease, including autoimmune vasculitis, subacute thyroiditis, sarcoidosis, inflammatory bowel disease, pancreatitis, rheumatoid arthritis, osteoarthritis, and pigmented villonodular sinovitis.[52]

SUMMARY

The fundamental strength of PET over conventional imaging is the ability to convey functional information that even the most exquisitely detailed anatomic image cannot provide. Although the basic physics behind the technology has remained unchanged—detection of coincident annihilation photons—advances in crystal structure, photomultiplier tube construction, electronics, and reconstruction algorithms have greatly improved image quality, cost, and availability of this modality. The newest technologic advances have been reviewed, including improved crystal design, depth of interaction analysis, TOF, and PSF integration in iterative reconstruction algorithms. These advancements will continue to improve contrast, decrease noise, and increase resolution. Furthermore, combined PET/CT systems provide faster attenuation correction and useful anatomic correlation all in one study. Multiple studies show that the sum of the two modalities is better than either used separately and also may be an extremely useful tool in pre–radiation therapy planning. PET/MR imaging is just now becoming clinically available and may provide similar gains. Other new scanning devices are also being developed, including small gantry PET scanners designed specifically for breast imaging and handheld PET probes for direct intraoperative localization of FDG foci.

The current clinical applications of PET and PET/CT are widespread, and include oncology, cardiology, and neurology. As the standard PET radiotracer in current clinical use, FDG is a glucose analog that is taken up by cells in proportion to their rate of glucose metabolism. A multitude of new PET tracers are under development, many of which are aimed at targeting cellular processes that are more specific than glucose metabolism.

ACKNOWLEDGEMENTS

The authors would like to thank Amy Morris for the illustrations found in this article.

REFERENCES

1. Pichler BJ, Wehrl HF, Judenhofer MS, et al. Latest advances in molecular imaging instrumentation. J Nucl Med 2008;49(Suppl 2):5S–23S.
2. Yang Y, Wu Y, Qi J, et al. A prototype PET scanner with DOI-encoding detectors. J Nucl Med 2008; 49(7):1132–40.
3. McCallum S, Clowes P, Welch A, et al. A four-layer attenuation compensated PET detector based on APD arrays without discrete crystal elements. Phys Med Biol 2005;50(17):4187–207.
4. Pichler BJ, Swann BK, Rochelle J, et al. Lutetium oxyorthosilicate block detector readout by avalanche photodiode arrays for high resolution animal PET. Phys Med Biol 2004;49(18):4305–19.
5. Pichler BJ, Judenhofer MS, Catana C, et al. Performance test of an LSO-APD detector in a 7-T MRI scanner for simultaneous PET/MRI. J Nucl Med 2006;47(4):639–47.

6. Karp JS, Surti S, Daube-Witherspoon ME, et al. Benefit of time-of-flight in PET: experimental and clinical results. J Nucl Med 2008;49(3):462–70.

7. Surti S, Karp JS, Popescu LM, et al. Investigation of time-of-flight benefit for fully 3-D PET. IEEE Trans Med Imaging 2006;25(5):529–38.

8. Defrise M, Gullberg GT. Image reconstruction. Phys Med Biol 2006;51(13):R139–54.

9. Tarantola G, Zito F, Gerundini P, et al. PET instrumentation and reconstruction algorithms in whole-body applications. J Nucl Med 2003;44(5):756–69.

10. De Bernardi E, Zito F, Baselli G, et al. Assessment of PSF modeling in PET AWOSEM reconstruction. Conf Proc IEEE Eng Med Biol Soc 2007;2007:6548–51.

11. Gould MK, Maclean CC, Kuschner WG, et al. Accuracy of positron emission tomography for diagnosis of pulmonary nodules and mass lesions: a meta-analysis. J Am Med Assoc 2001;285(7):914–24.

12. Gould MK, Kuschner WG, Rydzak CE, et al. Test performance of positron emission tomography and computed tomography for mediastinal staging in patients with non-small-cell lung cancer: a meta-analysis. Ann Intern Med 2003;139(11):879–92.

13. Wallace MB, Nietert PJ, Earle C, et al. An analysis of multiple staging management strategies for carcinoma of the esophagus: computed tomography, endoscopic ultrasound, positron emission tomography, and thoracoscopy/laparoscopy. Ann Thorac Surg 2002;74(4):1026–32.

14. Brucher BL, Weber W, Bauer M, et al. Neoadjuvant therapy of esophageal squamous cell carcinoma: response evaluation by positron emission tomography. Ann Surg 2001;233(3):300–9.

15. Esteves FP, Schuster DM, Halkar RK, et al. Gastrointestinal tract malignancies and positron emission tomography: an overview. Semin Nucl Med 2006; 36(2):169–81.

16. Pelosi E, Deandreis D. The role of 18F-fluoro-deoxy-glucose positron emission tomography (FDG-PET) in the management of patients with colorectal cancer. Eur J Surg Oncol 2007;33(1):1–6.

17. Soyka JD, Veit-Haibach P, Strobel K, et al. Staging pathways in recurrent colorectal carcinoma: is contrast-enhanced 18F-FDG PET/CT the diagnostic tool of choice? J Nucl Med 2008;49(3):354–61.

18. Wiering B, Ruers TJ, Oyen WJ, et al. Role of FDG-PET in the diagnosis and treatment of colorectal liver metastases. Expert Rev Anticancer Ther 2004;4(4): 607–13.

19. Lubezky N, Metser U, Geva R, et al. The role and limitations of 18-fluoro-2-deoxy-D-glucose positron emission tomography (FDG-PET) scan and computerized tomography (CT) in restaging patients with hepatic colorectal metastases following neoadjuvant chemotherapy: comparison with operative and pathological findings. J Gastrointest Surg 2007;11(4): 472–8.

20. Swetter SM, Carroll LA, Johnson DL, et al. Positron emission tomography is superior to computed tomography for metastatic detection in melanoma patients. Ann Surg Oncol 2002;9(7):646–53.

21. Wagner JD, Schauwecker D, Davidson D, et al. Inefficacy of F-18 fluorodeoxy-D-glucose-positron emission tomography scans for initial evaluation in early-stage cutaneous melanoma. Cancer 2005; 104(3):570–9.

22. Belhocine T, Pierard G, De Labrassinne M, et al. Staging of regional nodes in AJCC stage I and II melanoma: 18FDG PET imaging versus sentinel node detection. Oncologist 2002;7(4):271–8.

23. Fink AM, Holle-Robatsch S, Herzog N, et al. Positron emission tomography is not useful in detecting metastasis in the sentinel lymph node in patients with primary malignant melanoma stage I and II. Melanoma Res 2004;14(2):141–5.

24. Stas M, Stroobants S, Dupont P, et al. 18-FDG PET scan in the staging of recurrent melanoma: additional value and therapeutic impact. Melanoma Res 2002;12(5):479–90.

25. Pelosi E, Pregno P, Penna D, et al. Role of whole-body [18F] fluorodeoxyglucose positron emission tomography/computed tomography (FDG-PET/CT) and conventional techniques in the staging of patients with Hodgkin and aggressive non Hodgkin lymphoma. Radiol Med 2008;113(4):578–90.

26. Altamirano J, Esparza JR, de la Garza Salazar J, et al. Staging, response to therapy, and restaging of lymphomas with 18F-FDG PET. Arch Med Res 2008;39(1):69–77.

27. Yamazaki Y, Saitoh M, Notani K, et al. Assessment of cervical lymph node metastases using FDG-PET in patients with head and neck cancer. Ann Nucl Med 2008;22(3):177–84.

28. Murakami R, Uozumi H, Hirai T, et al. Impact of FDG-PET/CT imaging on nodal staging for head-and-neck squamous cell carcinoma. Int J Radiat Oncol Biol Phys 2007;68(2):377–82.

29. Jeong HS, Baek CH, Son YI, et al. Use of integrated 18F-FDG PET/CT to improve the accuracy of initial cervical nodal evaluation in patients with head and neck squamous cell carcinoma. Head Neck 2007; 29(3):203–10.

30. Schoder H, Carlson DL, Kraus DH, et al. 18F-FDG PET/CT for detecting nodal metastases in patients with oral cancer staged N0 by clinical examination and CT/MRI. J Nucl Med 2006;47(5):755–62.

31. Yen TC, Chang JT, Ng SH, et al. Staging of untreated squamous cell carcinoma of buccal mucosa with 18F-FDG PET: comparison with head and neck CT/ MRI and histopathology. J Nucl Med 2005;46(5): 775–81.

32. Krabbe CA, Pruim J, van der Laan BF, et al. FDG-PET and detection of distant metastases and simultaneous tumors in head and neck squamous cell

carcinoma: a comparison with chest radiography and chest CT. Oral Oncol 2008; [epub ahead of print].

33. Tan A, Adelstein DJ, Rybicki LA, et al. Ability of positron emission tomography to detect residual neck node disease in patients with head and neck squamous cell carcinoma after definitive chemoradiotherapy. Arch Otolaryngol Head Neck Surg 2007;133(5): 435–40.

34. Raylman RR, Majewski S, Smith MF, et al. The positron emission mammography/tomography breast imaging and biopsy system (PEM/PET): design, construction and phantom-based measurements. Phys Med Biol 2008;53(3):637–53.

35. Buscombe JR, Holloway B, Roche N, et al. Position of nuclear medicine modalities in the diagnostic work-up of breast cancer. Q J Nucl Med Mol Imaging 2004;48(2):109–18.

36. Byrne AM, Hill AD, Skehan SJ, et al. Positron emission tomography in the staging and management of breast cancer. Br J Surg 2004;91(11):1398–409.

37. Esserman L. Integration of imaging in the management of breast cancer. J Clin Oncol 2005;23(8):1601–2.

38. Isasi CR, Moadel RM, Blaufox MD, et al. A meta-analysis of FDG-PET for the evaluation of breast cancer recurrence and metastases. Breast Cancer Res Treat 2005;90(2):105–12.

39. Quon A, Gambhir SS. FDG-PET and beyond: molecular breast cancer imaging. J Clin Oncol 2005;23(8): 1664–73.

40. Rieber A, Schirrmeister H, Gabelmann A, et al. Preoperative staging of invasive breast cancer with MR mammography and/or PET: boon or bunk? Br J Radiol 2002;75(898):789–98.

41. Zangheri B, Messa C, Picchio M, et al. PET/CT and breast cancer. Eur J Nucl Med Mol Imaging 2004; 31(Suppl 1):S135–42.

42. Flanagan FL, Dehdashti F, Siegel BA, et al. PET in breast cancer. Semin Nucl Med 1998;28(4): 290–302.

43. Bombardieri E, Crippa F. PET imaging in breast cancer. Q J Nucl Med 2001;45(3):245–56.

44. Vranjesevic D, Filmont JE, Meta J, et al. Whole-body (18)F-FDG PET and conventional imaging for predicting outcome in previously treated breast cancer patients. J Nucl Med 2002;43(3):325–9.

45. Sawada SG, Allman KC, Muzik O, et al. Positron emission tomography detects evidence of viability in rest technetium-99m sestamibi defects. J Am Coll Cardiol 1994;23(1):92–8.

46. Marin-Neto JA, Dilsizian V, Arrighi JA, et al. Thallium scintigraphy compared with 18F-fluorodeoxyglucose positron emission tomography for assessing myocardial viability in patients with moderate versus severe left ventricular dysfunction. Am J Cardiol 1998;82(9):1001–7.

47. Bonow RO, Dilsizian V. Thallium 201 for assessment of myocardial viability. Semin Nucl Med 1991;21(3): 230–41.

48. Namdar M, Hany TF, Koepfli P, et al. Integrated PET/CT for the assessment of coronary artery disease: a feasibility study. J Nucl Med 2005;46(6):930–5.

49. Berman DS, Hachamovitch R, Shaw LJ, et al. Roles of nuclear cardiology, cardiac computed tomography, and cardiac magnetic resonance: assessment of patients with suspected coronary artery disease. J Nucl Med 2006;47(1):74–82.

50. Di Carli MF, Dorbala S, Curillova Z, et al. Relationship between CT coronary angiography and stress perfusion imaging in patients with suspected ischemic heart disease assessed by integrated PET-CT imaging. J Nucl Cardiol 2007;14(6):799–809.

51. Koeppe RA, Gilman S, Junck L, et al. Differentiating Alzheimer's disease from dementia with Lewy bodies and Parkinson's disease with (+)-[11C]dihydrotetrabenazine positron emission tomography. Alzheimers Dement 2008;4(1 Suppl 1):S67–76.

52. Kaim A. Sterile inflammatory disease. In: Schulthess GKV, editor. Clinical molecular anatomic imaging. 2 edition. Philadelphia: Lippincott Williams & Wilkins; 2003. p. 429–37.

53. Meller J, Sahlmann CO, Scheel AK, et al. 18F-FDG PET and PET/CT in fever of unknown origin. J Nucl Med 2007;48(1):35–45.

Body Perfusion CT: Technique, Clinical Applications, and Advances

Avinash R. Kambadakone, MD, FRCR, Dushyant V. Sahani, MD*

KEYWORDS
- Functional imaging • Perfusion CT • Contrast media
- Tumor angiogenesis • Surrogate bio-marker

Perfusion CT is an exciting CT technology that allows functional evaluation of tissue vascularity. Perfusion CT measures the temporal changes in tissue density after intravenous injection of a contrast medium (CM) bolus using a series of dynamically acquired CT images. Because of rapid technologic advancements in multidetector CT (MDCT) systems and the availability of commercial software, perfusion CT offers a wide array of clinical and research applications. The greatest impact of perfusion CT has been on the assessment of patients who have had strokes, wherein the rapid scan timing and faster image processing have cemented its role as the modality of choice for evaluation of the structural and functional status of cerebral vasculature.[1] In the field of oncology, perfusion CT has found applications in diagnosis, staging, prognostic evaluation, and monitoring of response to therapies.[2–9] Although still primarily considered a research tool, perfusion CT has the potential to become the preferred technique for the assessment of tumor response to antiangiogenic drugs.[10,11] In this article, the authors review the basic principles and technique of perfusion CT and discuss its various oncologic and nononcologic clinical applications in body imaging.

WHY PERFUSION CT?

Although an array of other imaging techniques allow tissue perfusion assessment, CT is particularly ideal for this purpose in day-to-day clinical practice for several reasons, primarily due to its widespread availability and prevalence of better experience.[1,12] This is particularly true in acute settings, such as in the evaluation of patients who have had a stroke, wherein round-the-clock accessibility and easy image acquisition permit early therapeutic intervention.[1] Another key advantage of perfusion CT is the linear relation between iodine concentration and tissue density changes, which makes mathematic modeling straightforward and relatively simpler compared with MR imaging, in which the contrast-signal relation and quantification are complex.[1] Moreover, routine availability of commercial software for perfusion CT makes quantification of tissue relatively easier. Because MDCT is already established as a modality of choice for tumor diagnosis and response assessment, protocol modifications to include perfusion analysis seem attractive and are fairly convenient.[12]

PERFUSION CT TECHNIQUE: BASIC PRINCIPLES

The fundamental principle of perfusion CT is based on the temporal changes in tissue attenuation after intravenous administration of iodinated CM. This enhancement of tissues depends on the tissue iodine concentration and is an indirect reflection of tissue vascularity and vascular physiology.[13,14] After intravenous injection of the iodinated CM, the ensuing tissue enhancement can be divided into two phases based on its distribution in the intravascular or extravascular compartment.[13]

Division of Abdominal Imaging and Intervention, Department of Radiology, Massachusetts General Hospital, 55 Fruit Street, White 270, Boston, MA 02114, USA
* Corresponding author.
E-mail address: dsahani@partners.org (D.V. Sahani).

Radiol Clin N Am 47 (2009) 161–178
doi:10.1016/j.rcl.2008.11.003
0033-8389/08/$ – see front matter © 2009 Elsevier Inc. All rights reserved.

In the initial phase, the enhancement is mainly attributable to the distribution of contrast within the intravascular space, and this phase usually lasts approximately 40 to 60 seconds from the time of contrast arrival.[13–16] Later, in the second phase, as contrast passes from the intravascular to the extravascular compartment across the capillary basement membrane, tissue enhancement results from contrast distribution between the two compartments.[13] Thus, in the initial phase, the enhancement is determined to a great extent by the tissue blood flow (BF) and blood volume (BV), whereas in the second phase, it is influenced by the vascular permeability to the CM.[13] By obtaining a series of CT images in quick succession in the region of interest during these two phases, the temporal changes in tissue attenuation after CM injection can be recorded, and by applying appropriate mathematic modeling, tissue perfusion can be quantitated.[13] The two most commonly used analytic methods to estimate tissue perfusion from the dynamic CT data are compartmental analysis and deconvolution analysis.[15,16]

Compartmental Analysis

In this kinetic modeling technique, analysis can be undertaken using the single compartment or double-compartment method.[15–17] The single-compartmental method assumes that the intravascular and extravascular spaces are a single compartment and calculates tissue perfusion based on the conservation of mass within the system (ie, using Fick's principle).[16,17] It estimates perfusion using the maximal slope or the peak height of the tissue concentration curve normalized to the arterial input function.[14,16,17] Conversely, the double-compartmental method assumes that the intravascular and extravascular spaces are separate compartments and estimates capillary permeability and BV using a technique called Patlak analysis, which quantifies the passage of contrast from the intravascular space into the extravascular space.[13,14,16,17]

Deconvolution Analysis

This CM kinetic modeling is based on the use of arterial and tissue time-concentration curves to calculate the impulse residue function (IRF) for the tissue. The IRF is a theoretic tissue curve that is obtained from the direct arterial input, assuming that the concentration of contrast material in the tissue is linearly dependent on the input arterial concentration when the BF is constant.[15–17] After accounting for the flow correction, the height of this curve reflects the tissue perfusion and the

area under the curve provides the relative BV estimation.[16] For the estimation of capillary permeability, a distributed parameter model is used, which is essentially an extended deconvolution model.[17]

Compartmental and deconvolution modeling methods have been found to be generally comparable, with differences in their theoretic assumptions and their susceptibility to noise and motion.[16,18] Compartmental analysis is based on the assumption that the bolus of CM has to be retained within the organ of interest at the time of measurement, which may result in underestimation of perfusion values in organs with rapid vascular transit or with a large bolus injection.[16] Deconvolution analysis, however, assumes that the shape of the IRF is a plateau with a single exponential washout.[16] Although this assumption is believed to work for most organs, it might not be suitable for assessing perfusion in such organs as the spleen and kidney, which have complex microcirculations.[16] Hence, it is preferable to use compartmental analysis for organs with complex circulatory pathways. Deconvolution methods are appropriate for measuring lower levels of perfusion (<20 mL/min per 100 mL) because they are able to tolerate greater image noise attributable to the inclusion of the complete time series of images for calculation.[16] This is particularly beneficial for the accurate measurement of lower perfusion values typically seen in tumors after treatment response.[16] A potential drawback of including all the acquired images for calculation is the possibility of image misregistration secondary to motion of the patient.[16] Conversely, compartmental analysis effectively uses three images for perfusion measurement: the baseline image and the images immediately before and after the moment the maximal rate of contrast tissue enhancement is reached.[16] Hence, patient motion has relatively less impact on the compartmental analysis. The mathematic modeling technique employed also has implications on the CT protocol used. The deconvolution method, being less sensitive to noise, allows the use of a lower tube current and permits scanning with higher temporal resolution for the dynamic cine acquisition.[16,17] For the compartmental model, the presence of image noise results in miscalculation of perfusion values; hence, a higher tube current with lower image frequency is preferred for the dynamic study.[16]

The analytic methods used and the acquisition protocols vary from scanner to scanner and among commercial vendors. General Electric works on the deconvolution approach and allows calculation of parametric maps of BF, BV, mean transit time (MTT), and permeability measurements (**Tables 1, 2**).[8,9,14] The Philips CT perfusion software uses the slope method to calculate the perfusion maps, and it estimates the tissue peak enhancement, time to peak enhancement, and MTT.[5,14] Siemens perfusion software similarly exploits the slope method to calculate perfusion and also estimates the BV and time to peak enhancement.[16,19]

PERFUSION CT PROTOCOLS

A variety of perfusion CT protocols have been proposed, and they typically depend on the target organ, mathematic modeling technique, CT scan configuration, and clinical objective. Nevertheless, a typical perfusion CT protocol consists of a baseline acquisition without contrast enhancement, followed by a dynamic acquisition performed sequentially after intravenous injection of CM (**Fig. 1**).[16] The dynamic image acquisition includes a first-pass study, a delayed study, or both, depending on the pertinent physiologic parameter that needs to be analyzed.[16]

Unenhanced CT Acquisition

The baseline unenhanced CT acquisition should provide wide coverage to include the organ of interest. This study basically serves as a localizer to select the appropriate tissue area to be included in the contrast-enhanced dynamic imaging range.

Depending on the scanner configuration, a 2-cm coverage area (for a 4- or 16-row CT scanner) or a 4-cm coverage area (for a 64-row CT scanner) can be selected for dynamic scanning. Larger coverage (8–16 cm) is now feasible with the availability of newer scanners with 128 to 320 rows of detectors.

Dynamic CT Acquisition

The first-pass study for perfusion measurements comprises images acquired in the initial cine phase for a total of approximately 40 to 60 seconds. For the typical first-pass study based on the deconvolution method, image acquisition is done every 1 second, whereas for the compartmental method, image acquisition is done every 3 to 5 seconds.[9,16,17]

For obtaining permeability measurements, a second phase ranging from 2 to 10 minutes is supplemented after the first-pass study.[16,17] The second phase images are acquired every 10 seconds for 2 minutes after the first-pass study for a deconvolution method–based study.[16,17] For permeability measurements with the compartmental model, images are acquired every 10 to 20 seconds.[16,17]

Contrast Medium

One of the important considerations for adequate assessment of tissue perfusion is the CM bolus

---

Table 1
Glossary of terms commonly used in CT perfusion

Perfusion Parameter	Definition	Marker (In Oncology)	Units
BF or Perfusion	Flow rate through vasculature in tissue region	Tumor vascularity Tumor grade	mL per 100 g/min
BV	Volume of flowing blood within a vasculature in tissue region	Tumor vascularity	mL per 100 g
MTT	Average time taken to travel from artery to vein	Perfusion pressure	Seconds
PS	Total flux from plasma to interstitial space	Immature leaky vessels	mL per 100 g/min
TTP	Time from arrival of the contrast in major arterial vessels to the peak enhancement	Perfusion pressure	Seconds
PEI	Maximum increase in tissue density after contrast injection	Tissue blood volume	HU

Abbreviations: BF, blood flow; BV, blood volume; MTT, mean transit time; PEI, peak enhancement intensity; PS, permeability surface area product; TTP, time to peak.
Data from[1,3,5–9,13–16]

Table 2
CT perfusion analytic methods and parameters evaluated with different vendors

	CT Perfusion (GE Healthcare, Milwaukee, Wisconsin)	Functional CT (Siemens, Erlangen, Germany)	Brilliance Perfusion (Philips Medical Systems, Best, The Netherlands)
Mathematic model	Deconvolution method	Two-compartment model	Slope method
Principle of the model	IRF, which is the time enhancement curve of tissue attributable to idealized instantaneous injection of contrast	One-way transfer of CM from IVS to EVS, proportional to blood clearance constant	Perfusion is ratio of maximum slope of tissue enhancement curve to maximum arterial enhancement
Parameters measured	BF, BV, MTT, PS	Perfusion, BV, PE, TTP and permeability	Perfusion, BV, PEI, TTP
Advantages	BF, BV, MTT, and PS can be calculated using a single CT study	Simple analysis. Efficient in calculation of rate-constant K value	Short scan duration. "No venous outflow" is true. No recirculation
Limitations	Partial volume-averaging correction required	Assumes that backflux of CM from EVS to IVS is negligible for first 1 to 2 minutes	Sensitive to image noise

Abbreviations: BF, blood flow; BV, blood volume; CM, contrast material; EVS, extravascular space; IRF, impulse residue function; IVS, intravascular space; MTT, mean transit time; PE, peak enhancement; PEI, peak enhancement intensity; PS, permeability surface area product; TTP, time to peak.
Data from[5,8,9,14,16,19,49,50]

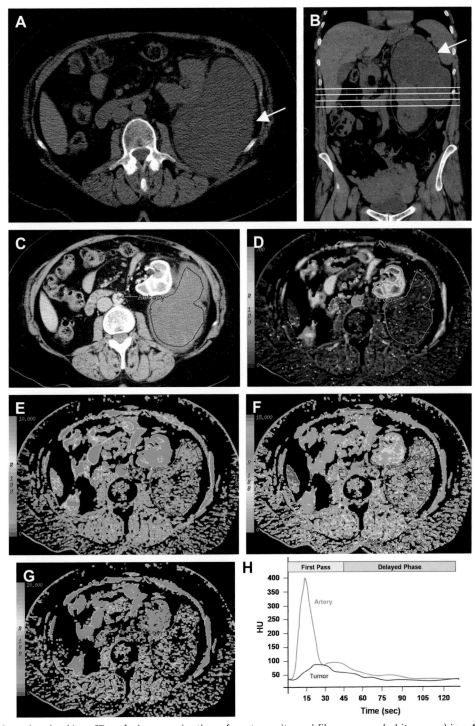

Fig. 1. Steps involved in a CT perfusion examination of a retroperitoneal fibrosarcoma (*white arrow*) in a 46-year-old man. (*A*) Step I involves the acquisition of unenhanced CT images to cover the entire region of interest. (*B*) Step II involves the selection of slices for dynamic imaging. The selected slices should be chosen to cover the maximum tumor area. The total tumor coverage area is 2 cm for 16-MDCT and 4 cm for 64-MDCT. (*C*) Step III involves contrast-enhanced dynamic image acquisition. The tumor ROI drawn for estimation of perfusion measurements is shown demarcated with a pink curved line. Step IV is postprocessing of CT data to generate colored perfusion maps of blood flow (*D*), blood volume (*E*), mean transit time (*F*), and permeability surface area product (*G*). (*H*) Time attenuation curves showing the enhancement characteristics of the artery and the tumor during the first pass and the delayed phase of the perfusion CT acquisition.

used for the intravenous injection.[15–17] A contrast bolus of 40 to 70 mL and an injection rate ranging from 3.5 to 10 mL/s are typically adequate for optimal perfusion analysis.[15–17] Because of the linear relation between iodine concentration and tissue enhancement, a higher concentration of CM is preferred (iodine, 370 mg/mL).[15,16] For the compartment method, a short sharp bolus with an injection rate of 5 to 10 mL/s is preferred for adequate perfusion assessment. Although the deconvolution method can tolerate lower injection rates, such as less than 5 mL/s, higher injection rates, such as 7 to 10 mL/s, are considered beneficial to maximize the tissue enhancement and to improve the signal-to-noise ratio.[15–17] The scan delay for cine acquisition from the start of CM injection is determined by the CM circulation time to the region of interest. Typically, for most body applications, a scan delay of 5 to 10 seconds is considered suitable (5–8 seconds for neck/chest/abdomen studies and 10–15 seconds for studies of the pelvis and extremities).

Acquisition Parameters

The selection of acquisition parameters for perfusion CT needs to be done judiciously in keeping with the body part scanned, modeling technique used, and radiation exposure. Use of lower tube voltage (kilovolt peak, kVp) and tube current (milliampere-second, mAs) is recommended to reduce the radiation exposure. In the authors' experience, a tube potential of 80 to 100 kVp is typically appropriate for most body applications. For a deconvolution method–based protocol, a tube current of 50 to 100 mAs is considered optimal, whereas for a compartment method–based protocol, a tube current of 100 to 250 mAs is suitable.[16,17]

Other Important Considerations

Motion during data acquisition can lead to image misregistration and can cause errors in the estimation of perfusion values. Hence, efforts should be made to minimize motion by appropriate approaches, such as breath-holding instructions to the patient for chest and upper abdominal applications. Likewise, anterior abdominal wall motion can be restricted by the use of abdominal straps.[20–23] Use of motility-inhibiting agents, such as hyoscine butylbromide or glucagon, is recommended to curtail bowel peristalsis during the perfusion examination of bowel.[20–23] In addition, luminal distention with water or saline is encouraged for studies of hollow viscera to enable optimal tumor delineation.[9] This is particularly relevant in follow-up examinations after therapy, in which tumor conspicuity is often in question

after successful treatment. Metallic stents, prostheses, and surgical implants cause beam-hardening artifacts and can negatively influence the perfusion measurements.[14] Finally, selecting the region of interest is crucial, and areas with excessive tumor necrosis or those located along organs with motion (in chest examinations) and areas near metallic prostheses or stents should be avoided.

VALIDATION AND REPRODUCIBILITY

CT perfusion methods have been validated against various techniques, including microsphere methods in animal studies and stable xenon washout methods in human studies.[14,24–29] In addition, few studies have attempted to correlate histologic markers of tissue vascularity with CT perfusion.[9,10,30] Reproducibility studies show good correlation for perfusion CT measurements with a variability of 13% to 30% in studies involving normal brain tissue, colorectal carcinoma (CRC), lung cancer, and hepatocellular carcinoma (HCC).[8,22,31–34] Sahani and colleagues[8] reported excellent correlation ($r = 0.9$, $P<0.01$) for perfusion CT values in HCC, with a mean variability of 4% when repeat studies were performed within 24 hours of each other. In their study, BF showed the least variability (1%).[8] Similarly, Goh and colleagues[34] compared the perfusion CT reproducibility in CRC and skeletal muscle; they found that perfusion CT values were reproducible and also noted that variability was less for tumor than for skeletal muscle. Baseline reproducibility studies may be desirable to ensure the accuracy of perfusion measurements in clinical trials relying on functional techniques.[22] Unlike MR imaging, however, wherein reproducibility studies are more often performed, CT heightens radiation concerns and occasional concerns of contrast-induced nephropathy; hence, reproducibility is not routinely tested in clinical studies. In situations in which the expected change in perfusion after treatment is small, it is also preferable that the same reviewer perform the follow-up measurements to avoid interobserver variability.[22]

CLINICAL APPLICATIONS
In Oncology

There has been a gradual increase in the utility of perfusion CT in oncology, with a wide spectrum of clinical applications, including (1) lesion characterization (differentiation between benign and malignant lesions); (2) identification of occult malignancies; (3) provision of prognostic information based on tumor vascularity; and (4) monitoring therapeutic effects of the various treatment regimens, including chemoradiation and antiangiogenic drugs.[17]

An emerging aspect of cancer care is the individualized approach, in which the treatment strategies are targeted according to the tumor biology.[15] One of the key elements of tumor physiology that influences the aggressiveness of cancer and its response to treatment is tumor microvasculature (neoangiogenesis), and the presence of high vascularity usually suggests aggressive behavior and is associated with a poor outcome.[35] Tumor angiogenesis is defined as the process of developing new capillary blood vessels, resulting in vascularization of the tumor.[36] This process, which is integral to the growth and spread of tumors, consists of several dynamic processes mediated by a host of growth factors, such as vascular endothelial growth factor, fibroblast growth factor, and platelet-derived endothelial cell growth factor.[36,37] Perfusion CT displays and permits quantification of the abnormal vasculature within tumors, thus allowing assessment of tumor aggressiveness.

Development of newer antiangiogenic drugs has necessitated the use of functional imaging techniques, such as perfusion CT or dynamic contrast-enhanced MR, to monitor their therapeutic effects, because conventional methods of monitoring response are not effective for these drugs.[15,36,38,39] Moreover, given that functional changes precede morphologic changes after treatment, techniques like perfusion CT allow earlier assessment of treatment effect than conventional methods, which rely on tumor size.[36] Perfusion CT can measure vascular physiologic changes by virtue of changes in the CM enhancement characteristics of tissues. Accordingly, perfusion CT can be considered a surrogate (indirect) imaging biomarker for the in-vivo

evaluation of response to antiangiogenic drugs.[40] This is in contrast to microvessel density (MVD), which represents the actual tumor blood vessels (ie, direct biomarker) that form the target of antiangiogenic drugs, and hence is considered the "gold standard" for quantifying and monitoring angiogenesis.[40] MVD has also been established as a prognostic indicator for many cancers. The most direct strategy for the measurement of MVD, and hence for monitoring antiangiogenic therapy, would require periodic biopsies.[40,41] There are several limitations in its routine use as a biomarker, however, including (1) the requirement of invasive tissue sampling, such as biopsy; (2) the need for standardization; (3) the presence of random sampling errors; and (4) the fact that such studies do not explore the entire tumor volume, which can hamper evaluation because of the heterogeneity of malignant tumors.[36] Surrogate biomarkers like perfusion CT are hence used because of their observed benefits like noninvasiveness, they can be repeated frequently, and they dynamically reflect the microcirculatory function in a living individual.[40] Several investigators have validated the utility of CT perfusion as a biomarker for measuring angiogenesis and monitoring response to treatment (**Figs. 2, 3**).[10,11]

Head and neck tumors
Perfusion CT is increasingly being used as an alternative to direct laryngoscopy for evaluating tumor response to neoadjuvant treatment.[42–44] Evaluation of head and neck tumors using deconvolution-based techniques has demonstrated that squamous cell carcinoma shows substantially increased BF, BV, PS and reduced MTT in comparison to adjacent normal tissues.[3] Rumboldt and

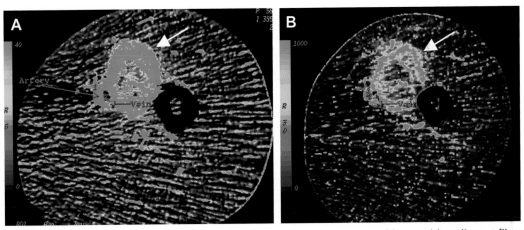

Fig. 2. Pre- and post-antiangiogenic treatment CT perfusion images in a 65-year-old man with malignant fibrous histiocytoma (*arrow*) of the thigh. (*A*) Colored perfusion map of BF at baseline before antiangiogenic treatment shows a high tumor BF (110 mL per 100 g/min). (*B*) Colored perfusion map after treatment shows a significant reduction in tumor BF (60 mL per 100 g/min).

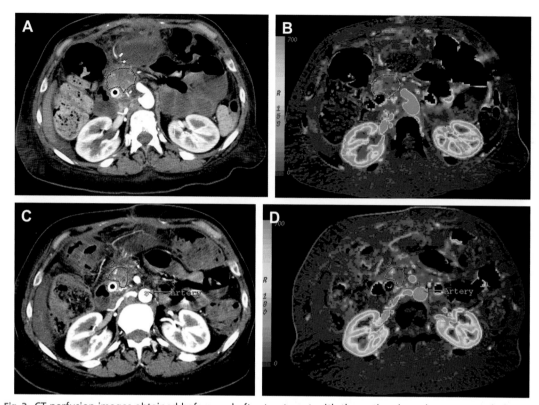

Fig. 3. CT perfusion images obtained before and after treatment with the antiangiogenic agent avastin in a 50-year-old woman with pancreatic adenocarcinoma. An axial contrast-enhanced CT image (A) shows the enhancing mass (ROI, region of interest, marked around the tumor) in the pancreatic head, with the corresponding functional colored map of BF (B) showing increased perfusion (76 mL per 100 g/min). After treatment with avastin, the contrast-enhanced CT image shows reduced enhancement (C), with the corresponding colored perfusion map of BF (D) demonstrating a reduction in perfusion (50 mL per 100 g/min).

colleagues[44] were able to differentiate between benign and malignant processes in the neck based on CT perfusion differences. Benign tissues show lower BF and longer MTTs compared with malignant tissue.[44]

Hermans and colleagues[43] studied the role of perfusion CT in predicting local and regional failure in patients who had head and neck cancer and were receiving radiotherapy. It was found that tumors with lower perfusion values showed a poor response to radiotherapy with high local failure, which was independent of tumor volume.[43] Similarly, Gandhi and colleagues[3,45] found that the presence of high tumor perfusion parameters predicted a favorable response to induction chemotherapy. The poor treatment response of tumors with low perfusion values could be attributed to the presence of tissue hypoxia within the tumor, which hinders the treatment delivery and, thereby, the therapeutic effect of chemoradiation.[3,43,45] Perfusion CT thus performed before treatment initiation can predict treatment response and help to dictate management strategies.

Lung cancer

Dynamic CT has been used for characterization of solitary pulmonary nodules as benign or malignant based on the enhancement characteristics, and nodules demonstrating higher perfusion are more likely to harbor malignancy.[46–48] Several investigators have attempted to study the utility of perfusion CT in lung cancer.[5,49–51] Kiessling and colleagues[50] did not find any correlation between the various histologic types of lung cancer and CT perfusion characteristics, whereas Li and colleagues[5,49] reported that the perfusion values of small cell carcinoma are the highest, followed by adenocarcinoma, squamous cell carcinoma, and large cell carcinoma. Several authors have observed that increasing tumor size resulted in lower CT perfusion values and this has been attributed to several factors, including infection, hypoxia, and necrosis.[5,49,50,52] For obvious reasons, necrotic tumors also exhibit significantly lower perfusion than nonnecrotic tumors (Fig. 4).[5,49] In keeping with biology of tumor angiogenesis, lung cancers with distant metastases

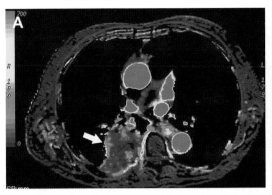
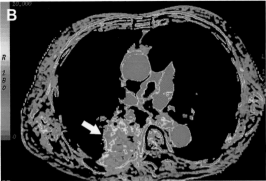

Fig. 4. Colored perfusion maps obtained in a 76-year-old man with adenocarcinoma of lung in the right lower lobe (*white arrow*) with no areas of necrosis. Functional CT maps of the blood flow (*A*) and blood volume (*B*) demonstrate increased blood flow (mean = 52 mL per 100g/min) and increased blood volume (mean = 3.7 mL per 100g) within the non-necrotic tumor.

have been reported to have higher perfusion values.[5]

Liver tumors

Earlier identification of hepatic metastatic disease has far-reaching implications in the management of patients by dictating treatment strategies with regard to surgical resection or targeted chemo-therapeutic regimens.[53] Perfusion CT has been shown to have potential applications in the enhanced detection and characterization of hepatic metastases.[53–57] Patients who have known metastatic disease of the liver have been found to have increased arterial perfusion compared with those without metastases.[54–57] This concept has relevance in the characterization of focal hepatic lesions and in the early detection of liver metastases that are too small to be detected by conventional CT.[53–55] Meijerink and colleagues[58] reported that total liver volume perfusion improves the detection of colorectal liver metastases. The presence of higher perfusion in the metastatic lesions on CT is considered to be a good prognostic indicator, suggesting optimal response to treatment.[55–58] This is in contrast to tumors with lower perfusion, which present with progressive disease.

Perfusion CT used for in-vivo assessment of HCC has benefits in making the differential diagnosis, evaluating tumor aggressiveness, monitoring therapeutic effects, and determining the final patient outcome.[59] Indeed, Ippolito and colleagues[60] confirmed that the perfusion parameters of HCC are considerably different compared with the background liver parenchyma. HCC demonstrates higher BF, BV, and PS and lower MTT measurements compared with background liver.[8,60] Sahani and colleagues,[8] in their study of 22 patients who had locally advanced HCC,

demonstrated gross differences between CT perfusion values of well-differentiated tumors and those of moderately and poorly differentiated tumors. Well-differentiated HCC demonstrated relatively higher tumor BF, BV, and PS and lower MTT measurements than did moderately and poorly differentiated HCC.[8] Because HCCs are preferentially supplied by hepatic arteries, no significant difference in the perfusion parameters is seen in the presence or absence of tumor thrombus in the portal vein.[8] The presence of background changes of cirrhosis in the liver also did not significantly alter the perfusion values in HCC.[8] Interestingly, the perfusion parameters of metastases from HCC to other tissues show similar values as compared with the primary lesion in the liver.[8] Earlier identification of tumor recurrence after various intervention procedures is also potentially possible with perfusion CT.[53]

Perfusion CT allows accurate quantification of changes in liver tumor perfusion during and after an embolization procedure, thus helping to optimize the therapeutic outcomes.[61] Kan and colleagues[4] also reported that perfusion CT was able to assess changes in liver tumor perfusion in response to anti-angiogenic treatment. Zhu and colleagues[11] demonstrated that after bevacizumab treatment, HCCs demonstrate reduction in the perfusion values, and the changes seen in MTT after therapy correlated with the clinical outcome (**Fig. 5**).

Pancreatic neoplasms

The perfusion values of normal human pancreas show an age-dependent physiologic decline.[62,63] Miles and colleagues[62] reported that pancreatic perfusion values were higher in patients who had Wilson's disease and reduced in patients who had diabetes and in failing pancreatic transplants.

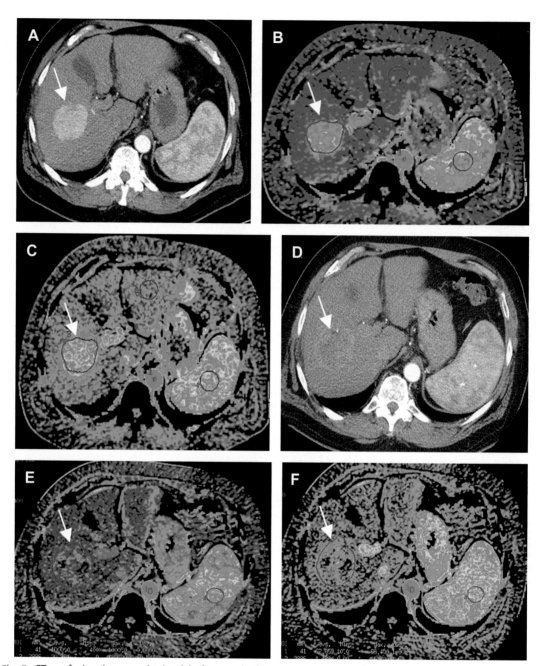

Fig. 5. CT perfusion images obtained before and after treatment with the antiangiogenic agent avastin in a 64-year-old man with HCC. An axial contrast-enhanced CT image in the dynamic phase shows the avidly enhancing rounded HCC (*arrow*) in the right lobe (*A*), with the corresponding colored perfusion maps demonstrating increased BF (82 mL per 100 g/min) (*B*) and increased BV (5.4 mL per 100 g) (*C*). After treatment with avastin, an axial contrast-enhanced CT image shows reduced enhancement (*D*), with corresponding colored perfusion maps demonstrating a reduction in the BF (20 mL per 100 g/min) (*E*) and reduced BV (1.41 mL per 100 g). (*F*) Tissue ROIs were drawn on the normal liver parenchyma in the left lobe and spleen for comparison. ROI, region of interest.

Substantially high blood perfusion was observed in hypervascular tumors, such as insulinomas, compared with background pancreatic parenchyma.[62] Moreover, Abe and colleagues[29] found that the pancreatic tumor perfusion measurements performed with CT were comparable to those performed with xenon CT, a more validated technique of tissue perfusion.

Colorectal carcinoma
CRC is the fourth most commonly diagnosed cancer in the United States, and the 5-year survival rate depends on the tumor stage at presentation.[9] Tumors of an advanced stage are usually given preoperative chemotherapy to decrease the tumor stage, facilitating curative resection and minimizing recurrence.[9] The predominant application of

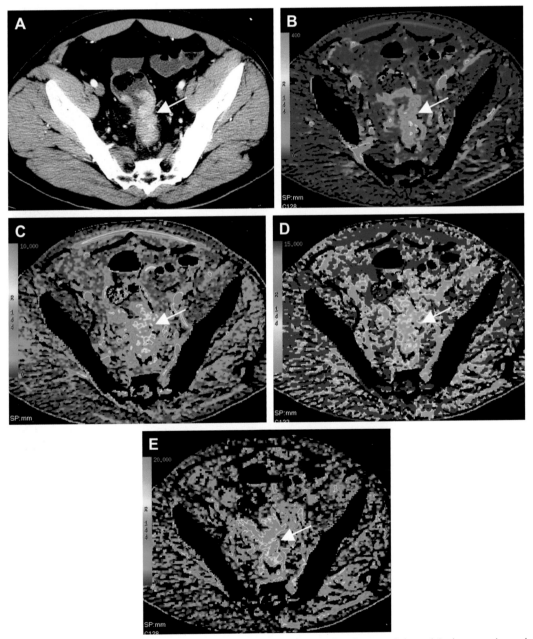

Fig. 6. Perfusion CT scans of rectal cancer. (*A*) Axial contrast-enhanced CT image of the pelvis shows an irregular enhancing mass (*arrow*) in the rectum causing wall thickening. Functional CT perfusion color maps of BF (mean = 96.7 mL per 100 g/min) (*B*), BV (mean = 6.9 mL per 100 g) (*C*), MTT (mean = 9.2 seconds) (*D*), and PS (mean = 15 mL per 100 g/min) (*E*) show the perfusion changes in rectal cancer.

Table 3
Literature review on the Oncological applications of Perfusion CT

Clinical Application	Author (Journal/Year)	Observations
Diagnosis		
Head and neck	Rumboldt et al[44] (AJNR 2005), Gandhi et al[3] (JCAT 2003)	Head and neck cancers have high BF and low MTT values compared to normal and benign tissues
Lung	Ma et al[7] (BMC Cancer, 2008)	Lung cancers have high BF, BV and PS values compared to benign nodules
Liver	Meijerink et al[58] (Eur Radiol 2008)	Total liver volume perfusion improves the detection of colorectal liver metastases
	Ippolito et al[60] (Acad Radiol 2008)	HCCs have high BF and BV values compared to surrounding cirrhotic liver tissue
Colon and rectum	Goh et al[64] (Radiology 2007)	Colorectal cancer have high BF, BV, PS and low MTT values as compared to diverticular disease
	Sahani et al[9] (Radiology 2005), Bellomi et al[79] (Radiology 2007)	Rectal cancer have high BF and low MTT values as compared to normal rectal wall
Prostate	Henderson et al[35] (Phys Med Biol 2003)	Prostate cancer foci have high BF, BV and PS values
Staging, Grading, and Prognosis		
Head and neck	Zima et al[42] (AJNR 2007)	Upper aerodigestive tract cancers with high BF and BV values respond well to induction chemotherapy
	Hermans et al[43] (Int J Radiat Oncol Biol Phy 2003)	Head and neck cancers with lower perfusion rate (BF) show poor response to radiotherapy (high local failure)
Lung	Li et al[5] (Clinical Radiology 2008)	Lung cancers with distant metastases have high BF, BV and PEI and different histological types of lung cancer show no difference in perfusion characteristics
Breast	Hirasawa et al[80] (Acad Radiol 2007)	Nonscirrhous carcinomas have high BF values compared to scirrhous carcinomas
Liver	Zhu et al[11] (The Oncologist 2008)	Patients with progressive disease (HCC) had lower baseline MTT values
	Sahani et al[8] (Radiology 2007)	Well differentiated HCCs show high BF, BV, PS and low MTT values than poorly differentiated HCCs

Pancreas	d'Assignies et al[78] (Radiology 2008)	Benign endocrine tumors have high BF values. Malignant tumors with liver & lymphnodal metastases have long MTT
	Park et al[81] (Radiology 2009)	Pancreatic cancers with high baseline K^{Trans} values responded better to concurrent chemoradiation
Colon and rectum	Sahani et al[9] (Radiology 2005),	Rectal cancers with high baseline BF and low MTT responded poorly to chemoradiation
	Bellomi et al[79] (Radiology 2007)	Rectal cancers with high baseline BF and BV showed good response to chemoradiation
Monitoring Treatment Response		
Liver	Zhu et al[11] (The Oncologist 2008)	Fall in BF, BV, PS and rise in MTT after antiangiogenic treatment in HCC
Colon and rectum	Sahani et al[9] (Radiology 2005)	Fall in BF and rise in MTT after chemoradiation in rectal cancer
	Bellomi et al[79] (Radiology 2007)	Fall in BF, BV and PS after chemoradiation in rectal cancer
	Willett et al[10] (Nature Medicine 2004)	Fall in BF and BV after antiangiogenic treatment in rectal cancer
Validation, Reproducibility, and Correlation with MVD		
Lung	Ma et al[7] (BMC Cancer, 2008)	BF, BV and PS values of peripheral lung cancer correlated positively with MVD
Liver	Sahani et al[8] (Radiology 2007)	Reproducibility of BF, BV, PS and MTT values with high correlation and variability of 4% in HCC
Pancreas	d'Assignies et al[78] (Radiology 2008)	BF values of pancreatic endocrine tumors correlated well with MVD
	Abe et al[29] (Radiat Med 2005)	Good linear correlation of BF measured by Xenon CT and CTp in pancreatic tumors
Colon and rectum	Goh et al[34] (AJR 2006)	Quantitative perfusion measurements are reproducible in colorectal cancer
	Li et al[6] (World J Gastroenterol 2005)	BF values of colorectal carcinomas did not correlate with MVD

Abbreviations: BF, blood flow/perfusion; BV, blood volume; HCC, hepatocellular carcinoma; MTT, mean transit time; PS, permeability surface area product; MVD, microvessel density; PEI, peak enhancement intensity.

perfusion CT in CRC is in the diagnosis and in assessing the response to treatment.

The MVD in CRC is significantly increased as compared with adenomas and normal colonic mucosa.[6] Li and colleagues[6] found that superficially invasive carcinomas are capable of eliciting neovascularization similar to those with distant metastases. Rectal cancer shows high BF and a shorter MTT compared with normal rectum (**Fig. 6**).[9] Similarly, CT was able to distinguish colonic wall thickening attributable to diverticulitis from CRC based on the high perfusion values in the latter.[64]

CT perfusion has been used to evaluate tumor vascularity in rectal cancer and to determine whether CT perfusion can predict tumor response to chemoradiotherapy and antiangiogenic treatment.[9,10] In their initial observations in patients who had rectal cancer, Sahani and colleagues[9] found that tumors with high BF and a low MTT tended to have a poor prognosis, which was attributed to the presence of a high rate of angiogenesis. High perfusion values in association with a poor response to chemotherapy and radiation therapy can be explained by large numbers of intratumoral arteriovenous shunts with a high perfusion rate and low exchange of oxygen.[9] It was observed in their study that after completion of chemoradiotherapy, rectal cancers showed a consistent decrease in BF and an increase in MTT.[9] In a clinical trial of patients who had rectal cancer treated with antiangiogenic therapy (bevacizumab), Willett and colleagues[10] not only found that CT perfusion characteristics correlated with the tumor MVD but monitored antiangiogenic changes within 2 weeks after treatment.

Prostate carcinoma

In a small series of nine patients who had prostate cancer, Henderson and colleagues[35] studied the CT perfusion characteristics and found that malignant foci within the prostate showed considerably increased perfusion values. A potential application of this is in the identification of tumor foci within the prostate, thus enabling targeted radiotherapy for the tumor foci with minimal radiation to the surrounding tissues.[35,65]

Lymphoma

CT is currently the imaging modality of choice for the diagnosis, staging, and follow-up of lymphoma. The data on the utility of perfusion CT in patients who have lymphoma are limited, however.[66] The chief reason for this is that angiogenesis is not a predominant feature of lymphoma. Dugdale and colleagues[66] performed perfusion CT on 26 patients who had lymphoma and observed that intermediate- and high-grade lymphoma had a higher perfusion compared with low-grade tumors. Active lymphoma also showed an increase in perfusion compared with inactive lymphoma, and progression from inactive to active disease showed an increase in perfusion on serial evaluation.[66]

Nononcologic Applications

Perfusion CT facilitates assessment of tissue perfusion and has several nononcologic applications.[67] Blomley and colleagues[68] reported that perfusion CT could quantify perfusion in the liver, kidney, and spleen. In nephrology, dynamic CT has been used to study the relative glomerular filtration rate and to determine the relative function of each kidney.[68–70] Paul and colleagues[71] reported that in patients who had renovascular hypertension attributable to unilateral renal artery stenosis, perfusion CT was capable of distinguishing between renal stenosis with and without preserved perfusion. A future application in this regard would be in the differentiation of rejection from other causes of dysfunction in transplant kidneys.[67] Studies have also explored the utility of perfusion CT in evaluating the perfusion changes in hepatic cirrhosis.[72,73] The hemodynamic changes observed in cirrhosis, characterized by reduced portal perfusion and elevated arterial perfusion, can be demonstrated on perfusion CT.[73] The perfusion changes as estimated by perfusion CT also correlate well with the severity of chronic liver disease, and this has implications in the follow-up of patients who have chronic liver disease and in the prognostication of their outcome.[73]

In acute pancreatitis, perfusion CT has been found to have a sensitivity and specificity of 100% and 95.3%, respectively, in detection of pancreatic ischemia.[74] Areas with pancreatic ischemia show a reduction in perfusion values compared with normal pancreas, and identification of these areas can help to predict the later development of pancreatic necrosis.[74] Because pancreatic necrosis substantially increases patient morbidity and mortality, its early detection and identification allow induction of intensive care for these patients at the earliest possible time so as to prevent infective complications and improve their prognosis.[74] Although further studies are needed before its routine use, it has enormous clinical implications, particularly in improving the prognosis of patients who have severe acute pancreatitis.

OTHER CONSIDERATIONS

A major concern of perfusion CT is the risk for exposure to ionizing radiation, especially in patients who require serial perfusion studies for monitoring treatment effects. Several techniques, including the use of reduced tube current and tube potential, can be employed to reduce radiation dose. Likewise, protocol modifications involving the use of higher temporal sampling rates, such as scanning every 2 to 3 seconds instead of 1 second during the first-pass and limiting the scan duration of cine acquisition to 40 to 50 seconds, can substantially minimize the radiation exposure from each examination without compromising the data.[75,76] Likewise, tailoring the perfusion CT protocol to the clinical objective or the relevant parameter can also diminish the radiation dose to the patient. For example, in clinical situations requiring tissue perfusion parameters like BF or MTT, it would be prudent to perform only the first-pass study.

Limited coverage of the organ or site for cine acquisition is another limitation of the technique, because a maximum of 4 cm of tissue can be interrogated with the present 64-slice CT scanners. The recent introduction of CT scanners with 128, 256, and 320 detector rows in addition to concurrent advancements in scanner technology enabling shuttle mode scanning could potentially facilitate whole-organ perfusion.[76,77] In patients with compromised renal function, contrast-induced nephropathy is a valid concern and should be dealt with cautiously

One of the impediments in accurate quantification of tissue perfusion is the degradation of CT data that occurs as a result of motion, particularly that secondary to respiratory misregistration. Respiratory gating could minimize misregistration artifacts, and sophisticated software programs, such as "motion-tracking algorithms," may allow more precise functional estimation.[14] Integrated positron emission tomography (PET)–CT systems with prospects of combining perfusion measurements with PET data represent an exciting new innovation that has wide-ranging implications in the investigation of ischemic tissue and tumors.[14]

SUMMARY

Perfusion CT has achieved great strides as a functional technique since its inception, and its scope in the clinical and research settings is rising (**Table 3**). Development of newer MDCT scanners with increased detector arrays and advanced features may soon allow perfusion analysis of greater volumes of tissue. Greater anatomic coverage would not only permit a comprehensive evaluation of tumor vascularity but enable perfusion evaluation of multiple organs concurrently. This would facilitate simultaneous functional evaluation of primary tumors and their metastases. Low-dose MDCT techniques with improved reconstruction algorithms generating high-resolution images may allow reduction in radiation exposure, which would benefit patients undergoing multiple perfusion examinations.

To conclude, perfusion CT, which has turned out to be the modality of choice in the evaluation of patients who have a stroke, is strengthening its role as a preferred functional imaging tool in the field of oncology. Despite its shortcomings, perfusion CT has the potential to play a crucial role in the management of patients who have cancer, particularly as a biomarker for monitoring the response to antiangiogenic drugs. More collaborative research and robust validation are imperative before this innovative technique can find utility in routine clinical practice, however.

REFERENCES

1. Miles KA. Perfusion imaging with computed tomography: brain and beyond. Eur Radiol 2006;16(Suppl 7):M37–43.
2. Ellika SK, Jain R, Patel SC, et al. Role of perfusion CT in glioma grading and comparison with conventional MR imaging features. AJNR Am J Neuroradiol 2007; 28(10):1981–7.
3. Gandhi D, Hoeffner EG, Carlos RC. Computed tomography perfusion of squamous cell carcinoma of the upper aerodigestive tract. Initial results. J Comput Assist Tomogr 2003;27(5):687–93.
4. Kan Z, Phongkitkarun S, Kobayashi S, et al. Functional CT for quantifying tumor perfusion in antiangiogenic therapy in a rat model. Radiology 2005;237(1):151–8.
5. Li Y, Yang ZG, Chen TW, et al. Whole tumour perfusion of peripheral lung carcinoma: evaluation with first-pass CT perfusion imaging at 64-detector row CT. Clin Radiol 2008;63(6):629–35.
6. Li ZP, Meng QF, Sun CH, et al. Tumor angiogenesis and dynamic CT in colorectal carcinoma: radiologic-pathologic correlation. World J Gastroenterol 2005; 11(9):1287–91.
7. Ma SH, Le HB, Jia BH, et al. Peripheral pulmonary nodules: relationship between multi-slice spiral CT perfusion imaging and tumor angiogenesis and VEGF expression. BMC Cancer 2008;8:186.
8. Sahani DV, Holalkere NS, Mueller PR, et al. Advanced hepatocellular carcinoma: CT perfusion of liver and tumor tissue—initial experience. Radiology 2007;243(3):736–43.
9. Sahani DV, Kalva SP, Hamberg LM, et al. Assessing tumor perfusion and treatment response in rectal

cancer with multisection CT: initial observations. Radiology 2005;234(3):785–92.

10. Willett CG, Boucher Y, di Tomaso E, et al. Direct evidence that the VEGF-specific antibody bevacizumab has antivascular effects in human rectal cancer. Nat Med 2004;10(2):145–7.

11. Zhu AX, Holalkere NS, Muzikansky A, et al. Early antiangiogenic activity of bevacizumab evaluated by computed tomography perfusion scan in patients with advanced hepatocellular carcinoma. Oncologist 2008;13(2):120–5.

12. Goh V, Padhani AR. Imaging tumor angiogenesis: functional assessment using MDCT or MRI? Abdom Imaging 2006;31(2):194–9.

13. Miles KA. Tumour angiogenesis and its relation to contrast enhancement on computed tomography: a review. Eur J Radiol 1999;30(3):198–205.

14. Miles KA, Griffiths MR. Perfusion CT: a worthwhile enhancement? Br J Radiol 2003;76(904):220–31.

15. Miles KA. Functional computed tomography in oncology. Eur J Cancer 2002;38(16):2079–84.

16. Miles KA. Perfusion CT for the assessment of tumour vascularity: which protocol? Br J Radiol 2003; 76(Spec No 1):S36–42.

17. Miles KA, Charnsangavej C, Lee FT, et al. Application of CT in the investigation of angiogenesis in oncology. Acad Radiol 2000;7(10):840–50.

18. Cao J, Yang A, Long XY, et al [CT hepatic volume measurement combined with CT perfusion imaging in evaluating the hepatic functional reserve]. Zhong Nan Da Xue Xue Bao Yi Xue Ban 2007;32(3):422–6 [in Chinese].

19. Koenig M, Klotz E, Luka B, et al. Perfusion CT of the brain: diagnostic approach for early detection of ischemic stroke. Radiology 1998;209(1):85–93.

20. Goh V, Halligan S, Gartner L, et al. Quantitative colorectal cancer perfusion measurement by multidetector-row CT: does greater tumour coverage improve measurement reproducibility? Br J Radiol 2006;79(943):578–83.

21. Goh V, Halligan S, Gharpuray A, et al. Quantitative assessment of colorectal cancer tumor vascular parameters by using perfusion CT: influence of tumor region of interest. Radiology 2008;247(3):726–32.

22. Goh V, Halligan S, Hugill JA, et al. Quantitative assessment of colorectal cancer perfusion using MDCT: inter- and intraobserver agreement. AJR Am J Roentgenol 2005;185(1):225–31.

23. Goh V, Halligan S, Hugill JA, et al. Quantitative colorectal cancer perfusion measurement using dynamic contrast-enhanced multidetector-row computed tomography: effect of acquisition time and implications for protocols. J Comput Assist Tomogr 2005;29(1): 59–63.

24. Cenic A, Nabavi DG, Craen RA, et al. Dynamic CT measurement of cerebral blood flow: a validation study. AJNR Am J Neuroradiol 1999;20(1):63–73.

25. Gobbel GT, Cann CE, Fike JR. Comparison of xenon-enhanced CT with ultrafast CT for measurement of regional cerebral blood flow. AJNR Am J Neuroradiol 1993;14(3):543–50.

26. Gobbel GT, Cann CE, Iwamoto HS, et al. Measurement of regional cerebral blood flow in the dog using ultrafast computed tomography. Experimental validation. Stroke 1991;22(6):772–9.

27. Purdie TG, Henderson E, Lee TY. Functional CT imaging of angiogenesis in rabbit VX2 soft-tissue tumour. Phys Med Biol 2001;46(12):3161–75.

28. Wintermark M, Thiran JP, Maeder P, et al. Simultaneous measurement of regional cerebral blood flow by perfusion CT and stable xenon CT: a validation study. AJNR Am J Neuroradiol 2001;22(5):905–14.

29. Abe H, Murakami T, Kubota M, et al. Quantitative tissue blood flow evaluation of pancreatic tumor: comparison between xenon CT technique and perfusion CT technique based on deconvolution analysis. Radiat Med 2005;23(5):364–70.

30. Yi CA, Lee KS, Kim EA, et al. Solitary pulmonary nodules: dynamic enhanced multi-detector row CT study and comparison with vascular endothelial growth factor and microvessel density. Radiology 2004;233(1):191–9.

31. Cenic A, Nabavi DG, Craen RA, et al. A CT method to measure hemodynamics in brain tumors: validation and application of cerebral blood flow maps. AJNR Am J Neuroradiol 2000;21(3):462–70.

32. Gillard JH, Antoun NM, Burnet NG, et al. Reproducibility of quantitative CT perfusion imaging. Br J Radiol 2001;74(882):552–5.

33. Nabavi DG, Cenic A, Dool J, et al. Quantitative assessment of cerebral hemodynamics using CT: stability, accuracy, and precision studies in dogs. J Comput Assist Tomogr 1999;23(4):506–15.

34. Goh V, Halligan S, Hugill JA, et al. Quantitative assessment of tissue perfusion using MDCT: comparison of colorectal cancer and skeletal muscle measurement reproducibility. AJR Am J Roentgenol 2006;187(1):164–9.

35. Henderson E, Milosevic MF, Haider MA, et al. Functional CT imaging of prostate cancer. Phys Med Biol 2003;48(18):3085–100.

36. Cuenod CA, Fournier L, Balvay D, et al. Tumor angiogenesis: pathophysiology and implications for contrast-enhanced MRI and CT assessment. Abdom Imaging 2006;31(2):188–93.

37. Phongkitkarun S, Kobayashi S, Kan Z, et al. Quantification of angiogenesis by functional computed tomography in a Matrigel model in rats. Acad Radiol 2004;11(5):573–82.

38. Miles KA. Functional CT imaging in oncology. Eur Radiol 2003;13(Suppl 5):M134–8.

39. Li WW. Tumor angiogenesis: molecular pathology, therapeutic targeting, and imaging. Acad Radiol 2000;7(10):800–11.

40. Provenzale JM. Imaging of angiogenesis: clinical techniques and novel imaging methods. AJR Am J Roentgenol 2007;188(1):11–23.

41. Tae K, El-Naggar AK, Yoo E, et al. Expression of vascular endothelial growth factor and microvessel density in head and neck tumorigenesis. Clin Cancer Res 2000;6(7):2821–8.

42. Zima A, Carlos R, Gandhi D, et al. Can pretreatment CT perfusion predict response of advanced squamous cell carcinoma of the upper aerodigestive tract treated with induction chemotherapy? AJNR Am J Neuroradiol 2007;28(2):328–34.

43. Hermans R, Meijerink M, Van den Bogaert W, et al. Tumor perfusion rate determined noninvasively by dynamic computed tomography predicts outcome in head-and-neck cancer after radiotherapy. Int J Radiat Oncol Biol Phys 2003;57(5):1351–6.

44. Rumboldt Z, Al-Okaili R, Deveikis JP. Perfusion CT for head and neck tumors: pilot study. AJNR Am J Neuroradiol 2005;26(5):1178–85.

45. Gandhi D, Chepeha DB, Miller T, et al. Correlation between initial and early follow-up CT perfusion parameters with endoscopic tumor response in patients with advanced squamous cell carcinomas of the oropharynx treated with organ-preservation therapy. AJNR Am J Neuroradiol 2006;27(1):101–6.

46. Swensen SJ, Viggiano RW, Midthun DE, et al. Lung nodule enhancement at CT: multicenter study. Radiology 2000;214(1):73–80.

47. Yamashita K, Matsunobe S, Tsuda T, et al. Solitary pulmonary nodule: preliminary study of evaluation with incremental dynamic CT. Radiology 1995; 194(2):399–405.

48. Zhang M, Kono M. Solitary pulmonary nodules: evaluation of blood flow patterns with dynamic CT. Radiology 1997;205(2):471–8.

49. Li Y, Yang ZG, Chen TW, et al. Peripheral lung carcinoma: correlation of angiogenesis and first-pass perfusion parameters of 64-detector row CT. Lung Cancer 2008;61(1):44–53.

50. Kiessling F, Boese J, Corvinus C, et al. Perfusion CT in patients with advanced bronchial carcinomas: a novel chance for characterization and treatment monitoring? Eur Radiol 2004;14(7):1226–33.

51. Ma SH, Xu K, Xiao ZW, et al. Peripheral lung cancer: relationship between multi-slice spiral CT perfusion imaging and tumor angiogenesis and cyclin D1 expression. Clin Imaging 2007;31(3):165–77.

52. Costouros NG, Diehn FE, Libutti SK. Molecular imaging of tumor angiogenesis. J Cell Biochem Suppl 2002;39:72–8.

53. Pandharipande PV, Krinsky GA, Rusinek H, et al. Perfusion imaging of the liver: current challenges and future goals. Radiology 2005;234(3):661–73.

54. Blomley MJ, Coulden R, Dawson P, et al. Liver perfusion studied with ultrafast CT. J Comput Assist Tomogr 1995;19(3):424–33.

55. Miles KA, Hayball MP, Dixon AK. Functional images of hepatic perfusion obtained with dynamic CT. Radiology 1993;188(2):405–11.

56. Leggett DA, Kelley BB, Bunce IH, et al. Colorectal cancer: diagnostic potential of CT measurements of hepatic perfusion and implications for contrast enhancement protocols. Radiology 1997;205(3):716–20.

57. Perkins AC, Whalley DR, Ballantyne KC, et al. Reliability of the hepatic perfusion index for the detection of liver metastases. Nucl Med Commun 1987; 8(12):982–9.

58. Meijerink MR, van Waesberghe JH, van der Weide L, et al. Total-liver-volume perfusion CT using 3-D image fusion to improve detection and characterization of liver metastases. Eur Radiol 2008;18(10):2345–54.

59. Chen WX, Min PQ, Song B, et al. Single-level dynamic spiral CT of hepatocellular carcinoma: correlation between imaging features and density of tumor microvessels. World J Gastroenterol 2004; 10(1):67–72.

60. Ippolito D, Sironi S, Pozzi M, et al. Hepatocellular carcinoma in cirrhotic liver disease: functional computed tomography with perfusion imaging in the assessment of tumor vascularization. Acad Radiol 2008;15(7):919–27.

61. Kan Z, Kobayashi S, Phongkitkarun S, et al. Functional CT quantification of tumor perfusion after transhepatic arterial embolization in a rat model. Radiology 2005;237(1):144–50.

62. Miles KA, Hayball MP, Dixon AK. Measurement of human pancreatic perfusion using dynamic computed tomography with perfusion imaging. Br J Radiol 1995;68(809):471–5.

63. Tsushima Y, Kusano S. Age-dependent decline in parenchymal perfusion in the normal human pancreas: measurement by dynamic computed tomography. Pancreas 1998;17(2):148–52.

64. Goh V, Halligan S, Taylor SA, et al. Differentiation between diverticulitis and colorectal cancer: quantitative CT perfusion measurements versus morphologic criteria—initial experience. Radiology 2007;242(2):456–62.

65. Jeukens CR, van den Berg CA, Donker R, et al. Feasibility and measurement precision of 3D quantitative blood flow mapping of the prostate using dynamic contrast-enhanced multi-slice CT. Phys Med Biol 2006;51(17):4329–43.

66. Dugdale PE, Miles KA, Bunce I, et al. CT measurement of perfusion and permeability within lymphoma masses and its ability to assess grade, activity, and chemotherapeutic response. J Comput Assist Tomogr 1999;23(4):540–7.

67. Dawson P. Functional imaging in CT. Eur J Radiol 2006;60(3):331–40.

68. Blomley MJ, Coulden R, Bufkin C, et al. Contrast bolus dynamic computed tomography for the measurement of solid organ perfusion. Invest Radiol 1993;28(Suppl 5):S72–7 [discussion S78].

69. Frennby B, Almen T. Use of spiral CT and the contrast medium iohexol to determine in one session aortorenal morphology and the relative glomerular filtration rate of each kidney. Eur Radiol 2001;11(11):2270–7.

70. Tsushima Y. Functional CT of the kidney. Eur J Radiol 1999;30(3):191–7.

71. Paul JF, Ugolini P, Sapoval M, et al. Unilateral renal artery stenosis: perfusion patterns with electron-beam dynamic CT—preliminary experience. Radiology 2001;221(1):261–5.

72. Tsushima Y, Blomley JK, Kusano S, et al. The portal component of hepatic perfusion measured by dynamic CT: an indicator of hepatic parenchymal damage. Dig Dis Sci 1999;44(8):1632–8.

73. Van Beers BE, Leconte I, Materne R, et al. Hepatic perfusion parameters in chronic liver disease: dynamic CT measurements correlated with disease severity. AJR Am J Roentgenol 2001;176(3):667–73.

74. Tsuji Y, Yamamoto H, Yazumi S, et al. Perfusion computerized tomography can predict pancreatic necrosis in early stages of severe acute pancreatitis. Clin Gastroenterol Hepatol 2007;5(12):1484–92.

75. Kambadakone AR, Sharma A, Catalano OA, et al. Protocol modifications for the CT perfusion of abdominal tumors: impact on radiation dose and data processing [abstract 6015424]. In: Programs and abstracts of the 94th scientific assembly and annual meeting of RSNA 2008. Chicago: RSNA; 2008. p. 590.

76. Goh V, Liaw J, Bartram CI, et al. Effect of temporal interval between scan acquisitions on quantitative vascular parameters in colorectal cancer: implications for helical volumetric perfusion CT techniques. AJR 2008;191:W288–92.

77. Mori S, Obata T, Nakajima N, et al. Volumetric perfusion CT using prototype 256-Detector row CT scanner: Preliminary study with healthy porcine model. Am J Neuroradiol 2005;26:2536–41.

78. d'Assignies G, Couvelard A, Bahrami S, et al. Pancreatic Endocrine Tumors: Tumor blood flow assessed with perfusion CT reflects angiogenesis and correlates with prognostic factors. Radiology 2008;18 [in press].

79. Bellomi M, Petralia G, Sonzogni A, et al. CT perfusion for the monitoring of neoadjuvant chemotherapy and radiation therapy in rectal carcinoma: initial experience. Radiology 2007;244(2):486–93.

80. Hirasawa H, Tsushima Y, Hirasawa S, et al. Perfusion CT of breast carcinoma: arterial perfusion of nonscirrhous carcinoma was higher than that of scirrhous carcinoma. Acad Radiol 2007;14(5):547–52.

81. Park MS, Klotz E, Kim MJ, et al. Perfusion CT: noninvasive surrogate marker for stratification of pancreatic cancer response to concurrent chemo- and radiation therapy. Radiology 2009;250(1):110–7.

Index

Note: Page numbers of article titles are in **boldface** type.

A

Abdomen
    and computer-aided detection, 70–73
Advanced postprocessing and the emerging role of
    computer-aided detection, **59–77**
Arterial enhancement
    and contrast medium dynamics, 15–16
    effect of injection duration on, 16
    effect of injection flow rate on, 16
    pharmacokinetics and physiology of, 14–16
    physiologic parameters affecting, 16
Atherosclerotic plaque
    and coronary CT angiography, 92, 100–103
Automatic exposure control
    and image quality selection, 32

B

Body perfusion CT: Technique, clinical applications,
    and advances, **161–178**
Bowel cleansing
    and CT colonography, 134–135
    and magnesium citrate, 134
    and sodium phosphate, 134–135
Bowel distention
    and CT colonography, 136–138
    and glucagon, 138
Breast cancer
    and positron emission tomography, 156
Bypass grafts
    and coronary CT angiography, 99–100

C

CAD. See *Computer-aided detection.*
CAD. See *Coronary artery disease.*
Calcium
    in dual-energy CT, 41–42, 50, 52–53, 55
Cancer screening
    and CT colonography, 133–143
Cardiac CT, 79–90
    and cardiac coverage per gantry resolution, 86
    and cardiac dosimetry, 88–89
    and electrocardiographic gating, 80, 84–85, 88–89
    and electrocardiography-based tube current
        modulation, 35–36
    and reduction of radiation, 34–36
    and signal to noise ratio, 82

    and spatial resolution, 81–83
    and temporal resolution, 83–86
Cardiac imaging
    and CT with contrast medium enhancement,
        14, 16, 19–20, 22
Children
    and radiation from CT, 34
CM. See *Contrast medium.*
Collateral blood flow
    and multimodal CT, 109, 111–112
Colon
    and computer-aided detection, 70–71
    and virtual endoscopy, 63–64
Colonoscopy
    virtual, 63–64, 133–143
Colorectal cancer
    and positron emission tomography, 155
Colorectal carcinoma
    and CT colonography, 133–142
    and perfusion CT, 171–174
Colorectal polyps
    and CT colonography, 133–142
Compartmental analysis
    and perfusion CT, 162
Computed tomography
    abdominal, 41–57
    and advantages and disadvantages of fast
        acquisitions, 20–22
    and automated bolus triggering, 20
    and automated tube current modulation, 20
    cardiac, 34–36
    cardiovascular, 22–23
    colonography, 134–143
    contrast media for, 14
    and contrast medium injection strategies, 22–23
    and double-layer detectors, 8
    dual-source, 5–7
    dynamic volume, 8–10
    enterography, 177–128
    injection time equals scan time, 22
    multidetector, 59–74, 79–90
    multimodal, 109–114
    and new detector materials, 7–8
    noncontrast, 109–111
    pelvic, 41–57
    perfusion, 112–114, 161–175
    radiation output of, 27–37
    and scanning and injection protocol design, 20–25
    and scanning delay, 22

radiologic.theclinics.com

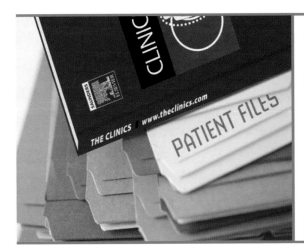
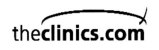

Moving?

Make sure your subscription moves with you!

To notify us of your new address, find your **Clinics Account Number** (located on your mailing label above your name), and contact customer service at:

E-mail: elspcs@elsevier.com

800-654-2452 (subscribers in the U.S. & Canada)
314-453-7041 (subscribers outside of the U.S. & Canada)

Fax number: 314-523-5170

Elsevier Periodicals Customer Service
11830 Westline Industrial Drive
St. Louis, MO 63146

*To ensure uninterrupted delivery of your subscription, please notify us at least 4 weeks in advance of move.